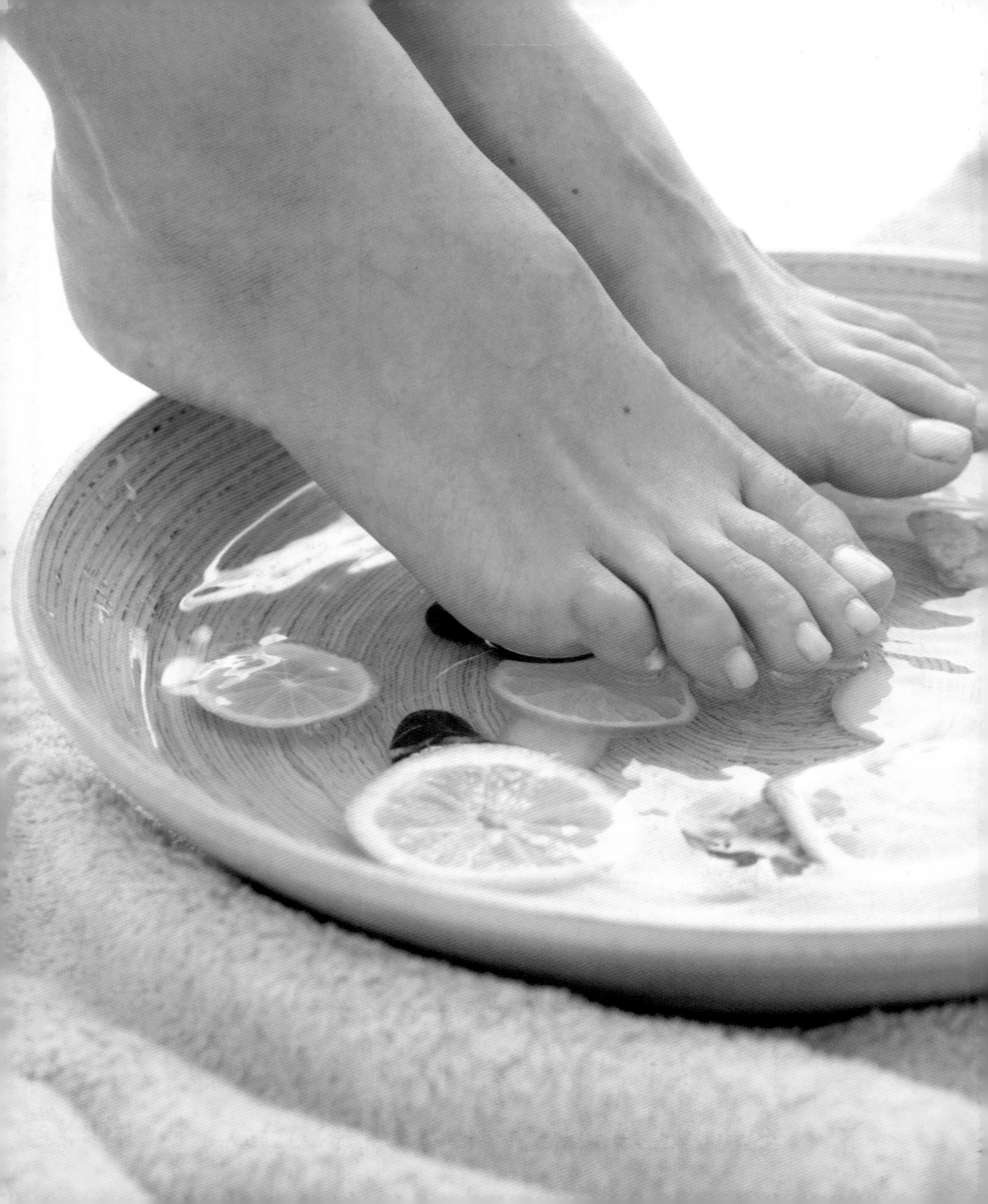

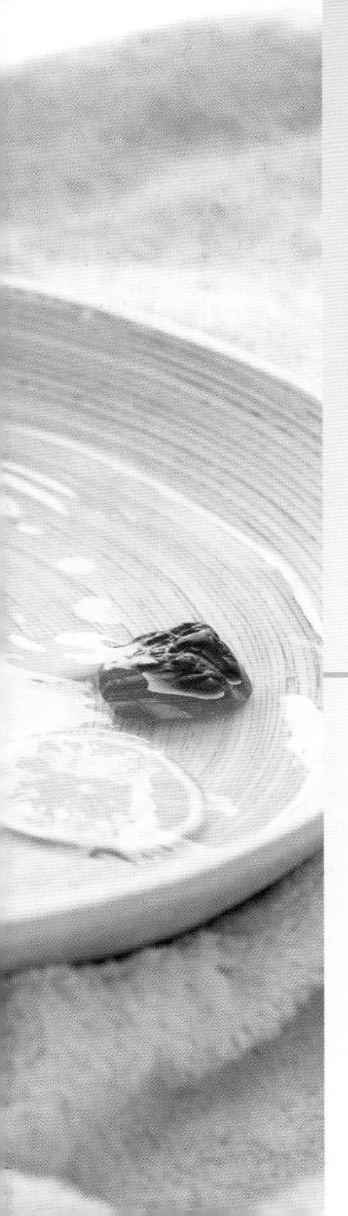

THE Reflexology Bible

LOUISE KEET

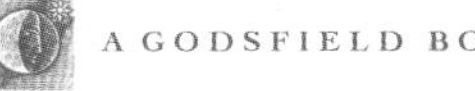

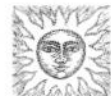

An Hachette Livre UK Company
www.hachettelivre.co.uk
First published in Great Britain in 2008 by
Godsfield, a division of Octopus Publishing Group Ltd
2–4 Heron Quays, London E14 4JP
www.octopusbooks.co.uk

ISBN: 978-1-841-81341-7

A CIP catalogue record of this book is available from the British Library.

Printed and bound in China

10 9 8 7 6 5 4 3

CAUTION
This book is not intended as a substitute for medical advice. The reader should consult a physician in all matters relating to health and particularly in respect of any symptoms that may require diagnosis or medical attention. While the advice and information are believed to be accurate and true at the time of going to press, neither the author nor the publisher can accept legal responsibility or liability for any errors or omissions that may have been made.

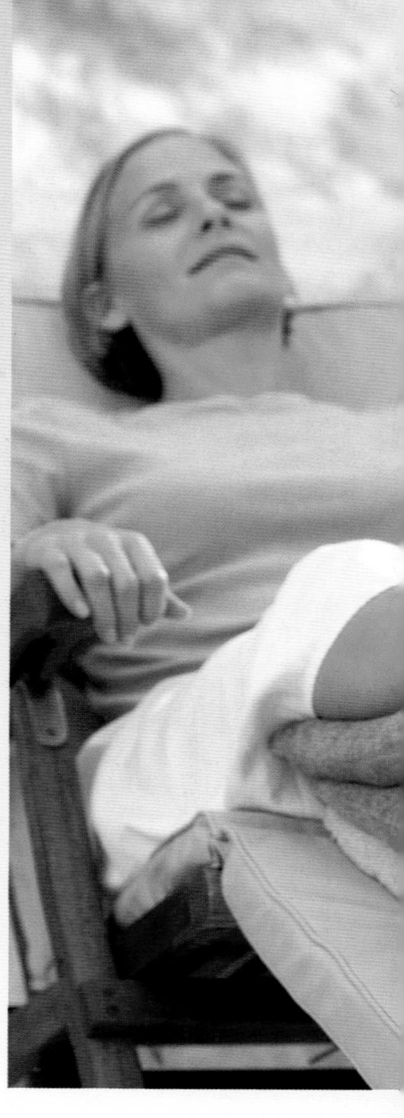

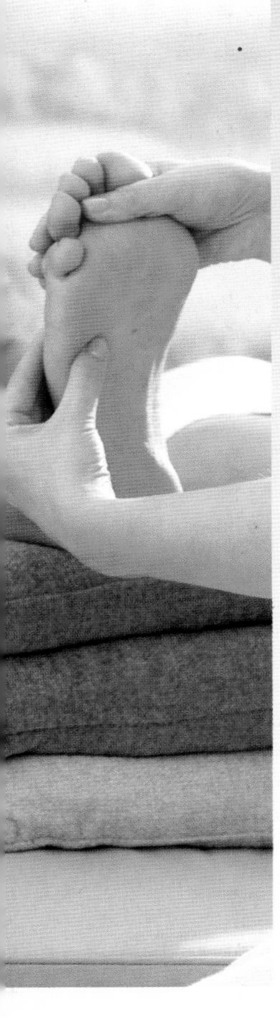

Contents

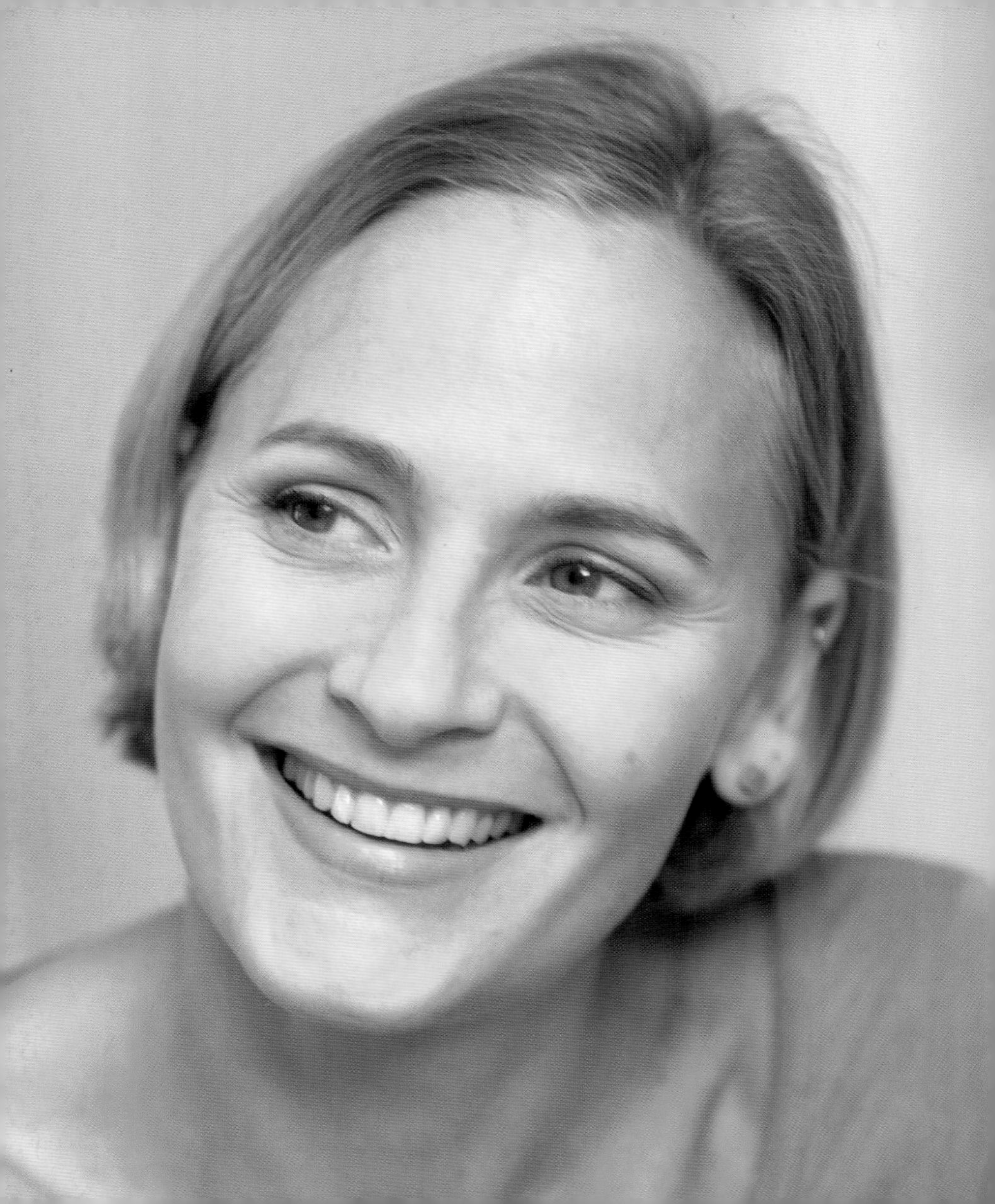

PART 1

Introduction

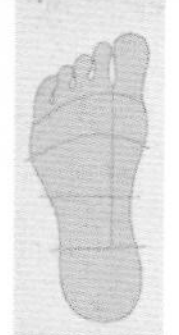

What is reflexology?

Reflexology is the technique of applying gentle pressure to reflex areas on the feet or hands to bring about a state of deep relaxation and to stimulate the body's own healing processes. It is a natural therapy that can also facilitate more vital energy, help boost the immune system and create a stronger body and calmer mind.

Reflexology is a safe, natural therapy that helps to give your body what it needs – that might be conceiving or carrying a baby to full term, a reduction in the symptoms of irritable bowel syndrome, assistance in losing weight or in feeling younger and looking healthier. In this book you will discover how reflexology and a holistic approach to health can help you achieve and fulfil both emotional and physical goals.

The theory of reflexology

The theory underlying reflexology is that the organs, nerves, glands and other parts of the body are connected to reflex areas or reflex points on the feet and hands. These areas are found on the soles of the

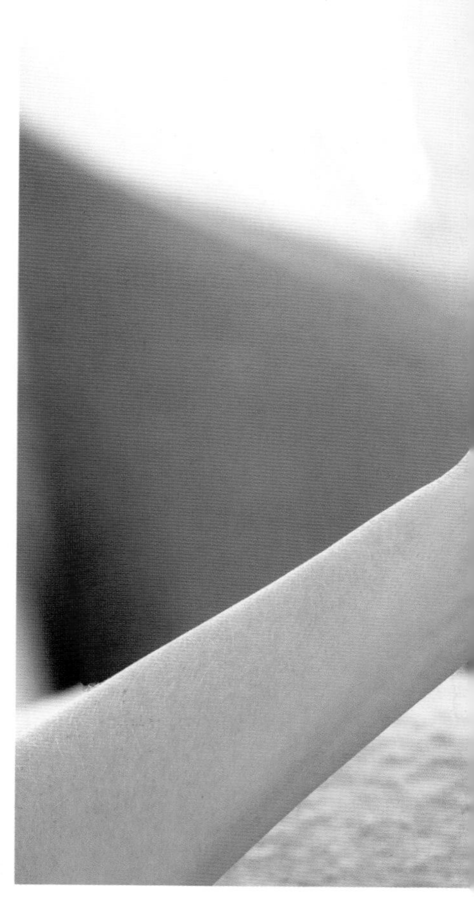

Better emotional and physical health can be promoted through the help of healing hands and reflexology.

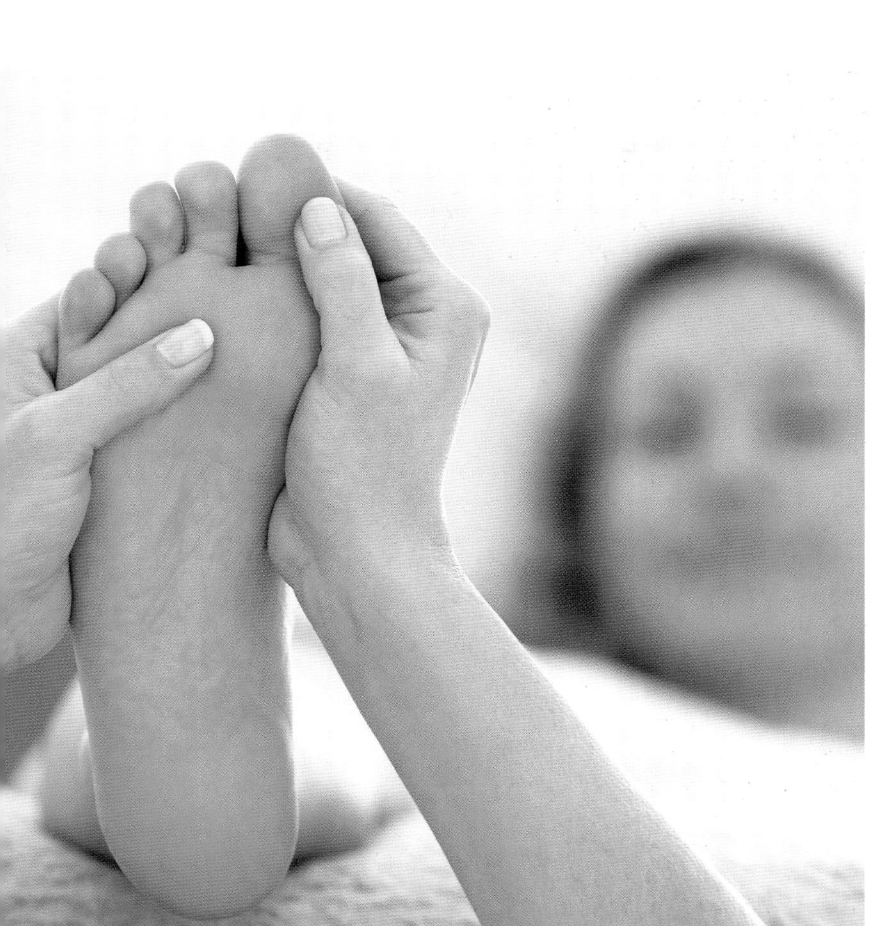

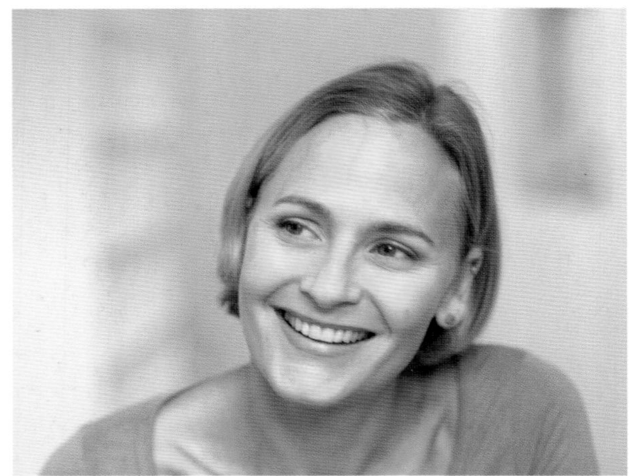

Reflexology can create a healthier and happier you.

feet and palms of the hands, as well as on the top and sides of the feet and hands. By stimulating these areas using a compression technique and a form of massage with your thumbs, fingers and hands, you can create a direct response in a related body area. For example, by working on the head reflex (which is found on the big toe), you can activate the body's own healing processes to help alleviate headaches.

The right foot and hand represent the right side of the body, while the left foot and hand represent the left side; and according to 'zone therapy' (see page 16), there are ten different zones in the body. The feet are most commonly worked on in reflexology, because practitioners feel they are normally more responsive to treatment than the hands, since they contain a larger treatment area and so the reflex points are easier to identify; and, because the feet are usually protected by shoes and socks, they are more sensitive to treatment. However, the hands can be used for treatments just as effectively and are great to work on, especially when giving yourself reflexology.

Creating a state of balance

Reflexology is all about bringing balance, harmony and a sense of well-being to the body. At times, we find ourselves feeling 'out of sorts or ungrounded', and our body needs equilibrium in order to keep working healthily. Even a very light reflexology treatment can help create this sense of balance.

Reflexology is not a therapy used to diagnose illness; it is not a medical treatment. It does not cure – only the body can do that. Instead it facilitates healing within the body. It is virtually impossible to determine how long it will take an individual to feel and enjoy the benefits of reflexology. Everything starts with one small step, but it is the commitment to reflexology that can drive forward a positive outcome.

How to use this book

This book is designed to give you a comprehensive approach to reflexology and a holistic approach to health, including diet and lifestyle changes. It incorporates a variety of treatment sequences that aim to suit the needs of you, your friends and your family, and which are suitable for all ages. After an introduction to the way reflexology works and essential preparation steps, Parts 4, 5 and 6 offer numerous foot-reflexology and power-treatment sequences, while Part 7 presents some hand-reflexology sequences. All the treatment sequences are simple to follow and are the same sequences that you could expect from a professional treatment.

You can apply the foot-reflexology treatments and any of the specialized treatment sequences daily, every other day, weekly, or as you wish. The general foot treatment in Part 4 (see pages 136–167) covers all the systems and parts of the body and can help with most conditions, as well as reducing the effects of stress on the body. In Part 5 the focus is on specific ailments, and here you will find power-reflexology treatment sequences that will help you treat common conditions in the body, ranging from acne and asthma to psoriasis and a sore throat. Part 6 contains specialized treatment sequences and focuses separately on moods and emotions, women, men, pregnancy, young children, the golden years and couples. These sequences will help you adjust your treatments to treat certain medical problems and ailments.

Hand reflexology is perfect for self-treatment, treating the elderly, giving a treatment in a few minutes or while on the move, and for deep relaxation. The general treatment sequence in Part 7 (see page 374–389) should suit everyone's needs and is a great experience to give as well as to receive. Working on your own hands is self-empowering.

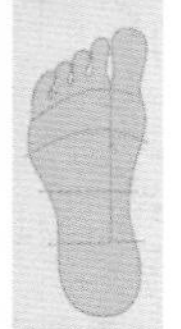

The roots of reflexology

The very roots of reflexology and its relationship with healthcare and astrology are believed to date back to ancient Egypt, where astrologer/physicians looked towards the stars to provide a theoretical basis on which to treat patients.

Ancient Egypt

The oldest documentation depicting the practice of reflexology was discovered in the tomb of an Egyptian physician called Ankmahor, dated around 2500 BCE. Ankmahor was considered one of the most influential people at that time, second only to the king. Within his tomb were found many medically related paintings, and the one shown here is believed to be the earliest example of reflexology. Two patients are receiving reflexology on their hands and feet. 'Don't hurt me', one patient says in the inscription; and the practitioner's reply is, 'I shall act so you praise me'.

Reflexology was obviously being practised either as a preventative to ill health or to help ease patients' medical conditions; either way, it is clear that the practitioners wished to meet their patients' needs. Working with a reflexologist, the physician would have devised individual treatment plans for his patients that focused on the prevention of illness or on treating a current condition – so that practitioners were acting 'so you praise me'.

Over the years, various forms of reflexology have been practised and developed in America, Africa and the Far East. These often developed in different ways, with different lengths of treatment, heavier or lighter pressure, and even the use of implements such as small sticks or the end of a pipe.

Modern reflexology: the pioneers

Dr William Fitzgerald was one of the pioneers of modern reflexology. An American laryngologist who carried out his most significant work in the early 1900s, he had been aware that Native Americans were using techniques of pressure-point therapy to relieve pain. He also found that there was a lot of research developing in Europe on the functioning of the nervous system and the effects of stimulation of the sensory pathways on the

This early painting of reflexology was found in the tomb of the ancient Egyptian physician Ankmahor.

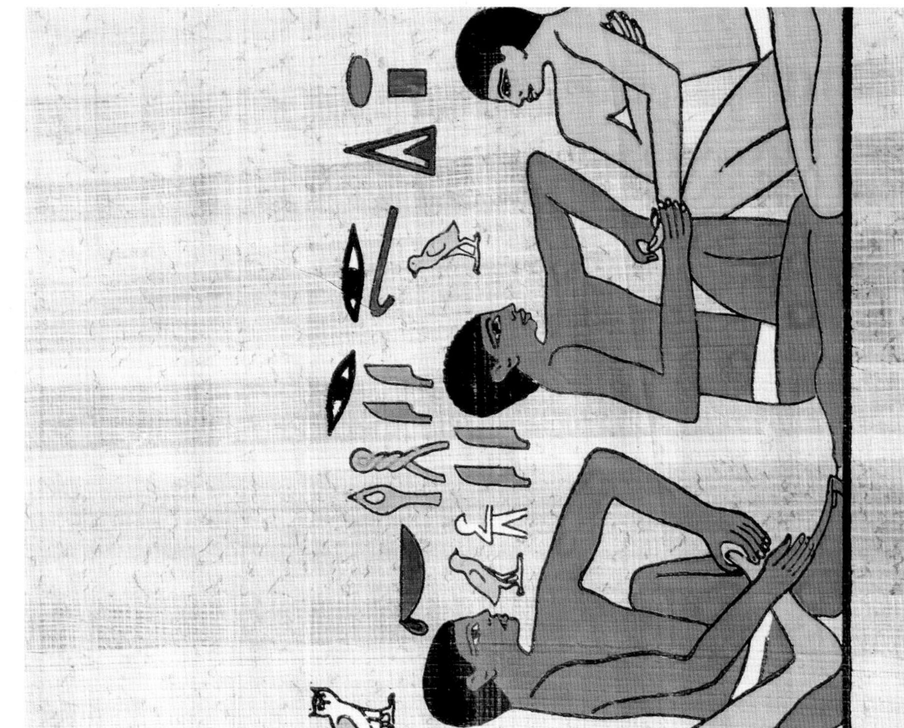

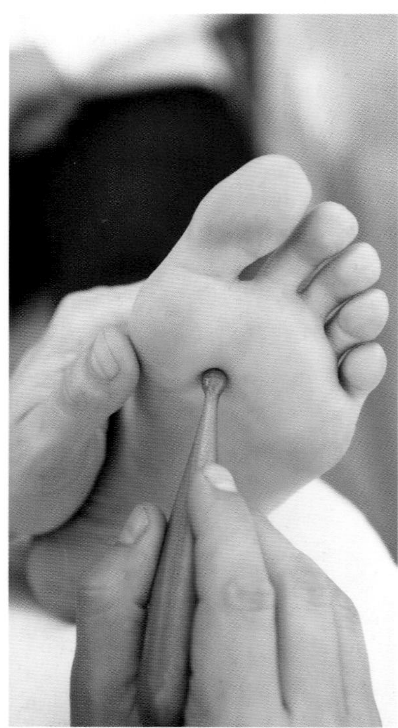

The Asian Rwo Shur method, which focuses on revitalization rather than than relaxation, using a small stick.

rest of the body. Inspired by his research, Dr Fitzgerald decided to experiment on his patients with pain relief for minor surgery, and the result was the discovery of 'zone therapy', with energy lines running through the body (see page 16), on which the modern form of reflexology was subsequently based.

The Rwo Shur method

In many parts of Asia, including Taiwan, China and Singapore, the Rwo Shur method of reflexology is practised. This can be quite painful to receive because it involves a combination of thumb-sliding and pressure techniques, incorporating the knuckles and sometimes small wooden sticks. The pressure is very firm and the therapist uses a cream rather than a powder; this allows for a fast, efficient and flowing motion. You can normally expect a session to last for about 30 minutes, with the focus being on revitalization rather than relaxation.

The Rwo Shur method was developed in Taiwan by Father Joseph Eugster, a Swiss missionary. Having experienced the benefits of reflexology himself, he saw the potential to help thousands of needy people and began to treat and then train others in reflexology.

The Ingham method

This technique forms the basis for the way in which most reflexology is practised around the world today. It was pioneered and developed in America in the early

1930s by the late Eunice Ingham, who is considered by most to be the 'mother of reflexology'. She made the feet specific targets for reflexology because they are particularly sensitive, and developed maps of the entire body on the feet (see pages 40–49), based on her research in the practice of reflexology.

She also developed a method of using the thumbs and fingers known as the Ingham compression technique. In this method, pressure is applied by 'thumb-walking', in which the thumb or finger bends and straightens while maintaining constant pressure across the area of the foot that is being worked.

Eunice Ingham introduced her work to the non-medical community because she realized how reflexology could help the general public. Her techniques were simple to apply, and people could learn how to use reflexology to help themselves, their family and friends. She wrote two books on reflexology, *Stories the Feet Can Tell* (1938) and *Stories the Feet Have Told* (1963).

A reflexologist practising the Ingham method uses powder rather than cream, and a session generally lasts for about 60 minutes, although this depends on the health of the client. The focus is on relaxation and balancing the body systems, and the therapist works with a pressure that is constantly adjusted in order to avoid discomfort. The session is holistic, with the reflexologist considering the impact that the client's lifestyle has on their health. He or she will adjust the treatment sequence to suit each person, and although all the reflexes are worked, some are emphasized a little more than others.

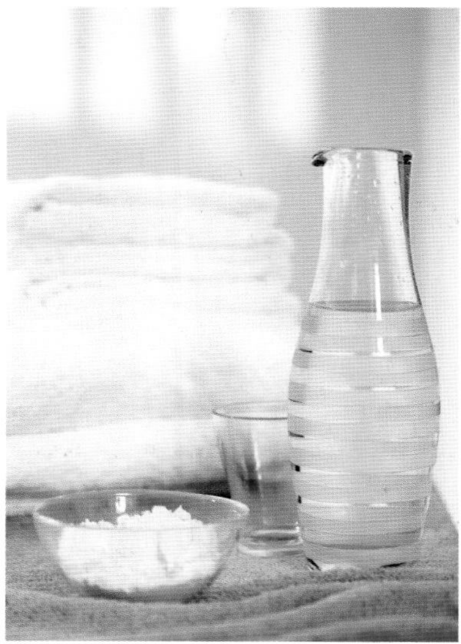

Powder, towels and water should be laid out in readiness before the client arrives and treatment begins.

Zone therapy

Zone therapy is the foundation of modern reflexology, whereby reflexologists apply pressure to (or massage) specific areas of the feet or hands, stimulating the circulation and nerve impulses to promote health throughout 'zones' of the body.

The principle of energy zones, and the disease and rejuvenation of energy pathways, has been known for centuries. Harry Bond Bressler, who investigated the possibility of treating organs in the body through pressure points, stated in his book *Zone Therapy* (1955) that 'Pressure therapy was well known in the middle countries in Europe and was practised by the working classes of those countries as well as by those who catered to the diseases of royalty and the upper classes.' This form of reflexology seems to have been practised as far back as the 14th century.

Dr William Fitzgerald

The American Dr William Fitzgerald is considered to be the founder of zone therapy. During his research into pain relief he established that pressure applied to one part of the body could have an anaesthetic effect on another part, away from the pressure site. For example, applying wooden clothes pegs to the fingers created an anaesthetic affect on the ear, nose, face, jaw, shoulder, arm and hand, and in this way he was able to perform minor surgery using just zone therapy, without anaesthetics.

Dr Fitzgerald finally published a book on zone therapy in 1917, which divided the body into ten longitudinal sections, and then charted the longitudinal zones of the body, with five on each side (see page 18). Modern reflexology is based on this idea of zone therapy. Using pressure on the toes, for instance, reflexologists can help with the pain associated with sinusitis, can drain the sinuses and strengthen them, in order to avoid future bouts of sinusitis. This pressure, applied to any of the ten zones, creates a signal throughout the nervous system to the brain, which in turn stimulates the internal organs to regulate and improve the way they function.

Applying pressure to an area can help with pain relief. The roots of this form of treatment date back to the Middle Ages.

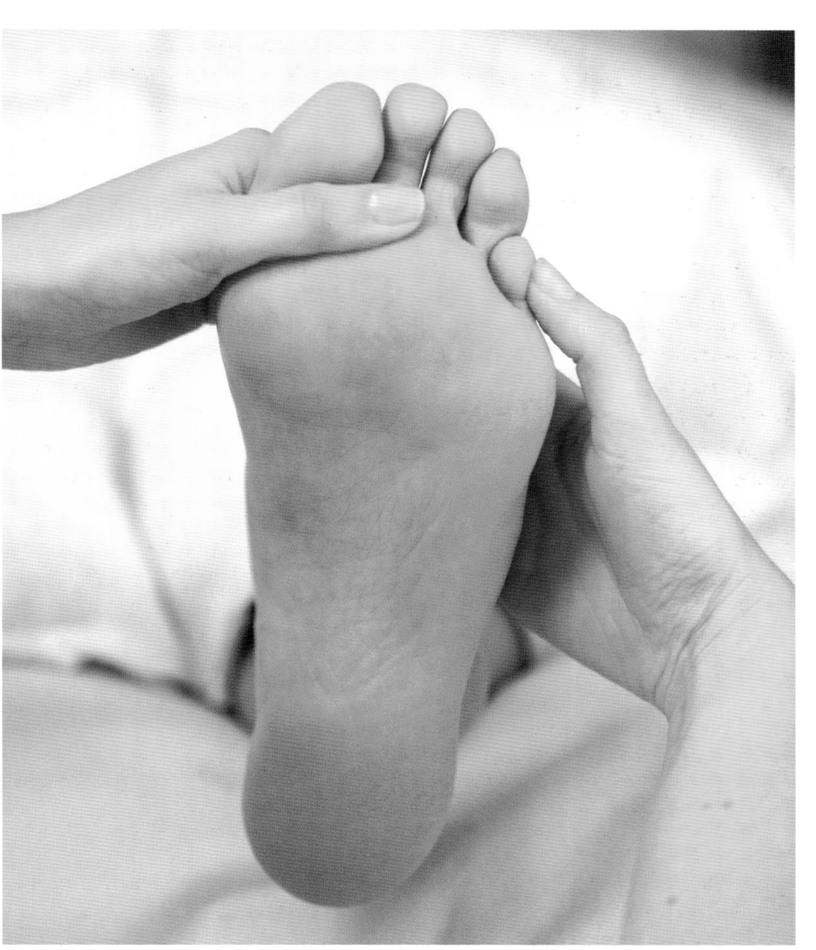

The zone therapy chart

The body is divided into ten longitudinal zones, which provide a simple numbering sequence. Each toe falls into one zone, and there are five zones in each foot, with the big toe as zone one, through to the little toe, which is zone five; the fingers link up to the zones in the same way. Zones are distributed up the body like slices, and when you work on the feet, you are automatically working through the whole of the human body.

The principle is that, within these zones, energy runs up and down between all the parts of the body. This energy connection should be free-flowing, in order that all the parts of the body – organs, muscles, nerves, glands and blood supply – work in harmony and at the optimum level for good health. If there is a block of the body's natural energy, it will have an effect on any organ or part of the body that lies within that particular zone.

Balancing the zones

If a reflexologist finds sensitivity in one spot of the feet or hands, this indicates that there is an imbalance in the entire length of that zone. For example, if someone is suffering from conjunctivitis in the right eye, zone therapy would suggest that this creates an energy imbalance in the right kidney and in any other bodily structure lying in that zone, causing it not to function as effectively as it should.

Each organ or part of the body is represented on the hands and feet. Massaging or pressing each area can stimulate the flow of energy, blood, nutrients and nerve impulses to the corresponding body zone, and thereby relieve ailments in that zone. The reflexes on the feet and hands are effective because they are situated at the ends of the zones and are therefore more sensitive than other parts of the body.

ENERGY ZONES

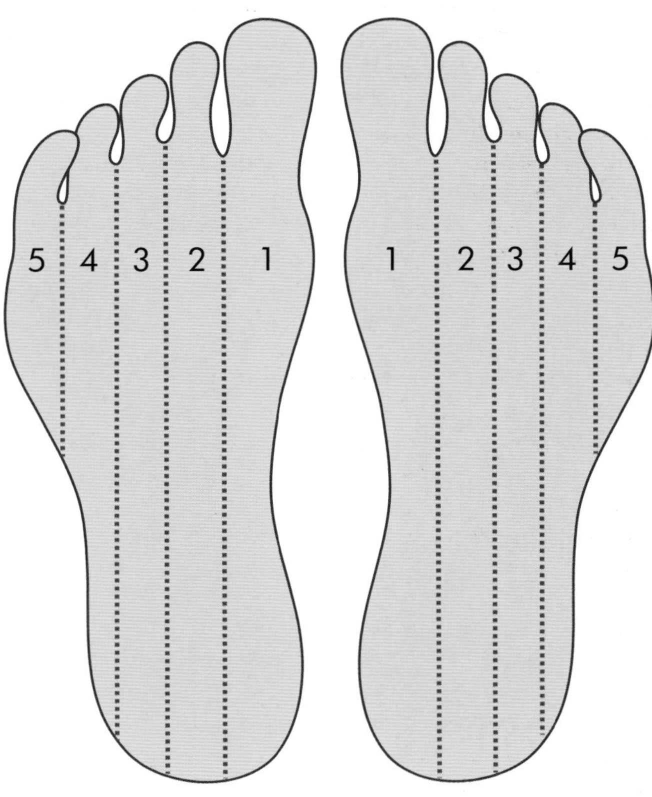

Zone 1 – big toe
Zone 2 – second toe
Zone 3 – third toe
Zone 4 – fourth toe
Zone 5 – little toe

Reflexology and energy

As we have seen, reflexology is based on the positive energies that zone therapy frees up in the body. We cannot really see this energy flowing within our bodies, but that does not mean it does not exist. We can appreciate the effect of positive energy when holding our child or a loved one.

However, it is useful to understand the effects of negative energy on the most basic structures of the body. Free-flowing energy pathways run through the body, creating homeostasis, which is the body's natural state of balance. Blockages in energy have been attributed to areas of the body not functioning well or becoming diseased.

Electromagnetic fields

An idea developed by Dr Jean-Claude Mainguy postulates that the systems of all life are governed by electromagnetic

Electromagnetic fields from mobile phones and computer screens can have a detrimental affect on your health.

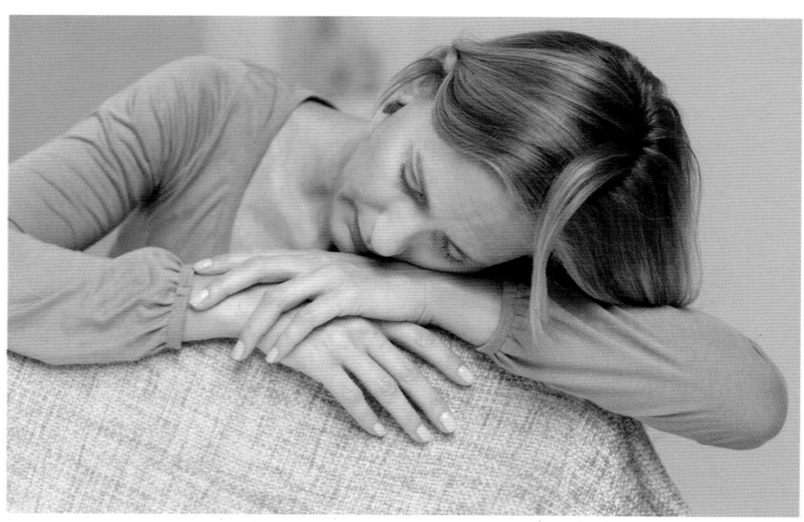

REORGANIZING THE BODY'S ENERGIES

There is a unique electromagnetic energy field around every living being. Humans have a life-force body as well as a physical one, and we absorb this life-force through fresh food, deep breathing, touch and through the feet – the life-force is an invisible blueprint of the whole body. A client may receive a reflexology treatment that incorporates healing deep within their body, whereby they are being retuned to a more orderly energy by the reflexologist's healing intention. Reorganizing the body's energies by giving reflexology and having the intention to heal represents a powerful healing tool.

fields, which can either lie within a cell or outside it. Imagine that you are like a radio, transmitting and receiving energy, and that you can be affected by low-energy electromagnetic fields. We are often exposed to electromagnetic energy, which affects the body's flow of energy, and some people suffer from symptoms of electromagnetic sensitivity, which may include nausea, sleep disturbances, dizziness, tension, fatigue, headaches and muscle pain.

The UK's Health Protection Agency is slowly recognizing that people can suffer from electro-sensitivity when exposed to electromagnetic fields from mobile phones, electricity pylons and computer screens. Zone therapy and reflexology are based on unblocking the energy pathways in the body to restore its natural equilibrium.

Becoming healthy is a matter of balancing a number of factors in your life. What you expose your body to, put into it and on it can affect your health. This book aims to show you how reflexology and a holistic approach to health can work to create the best body ecology and achieve a healthier you.

Rejuvenation through the feet

The feet lie furthest from the heart, and the circulation tends to stagnate in these extremities, especially if the calf muscles are not pumping blood properly up the body. It is important to help blood flow back up the legs to the heart, in order to avoid diseases like deep-vein thrombosis.

Waste matter, such as uric acid crystals and calcium crystals, can also build up in the bottom of the feet, because gravity pulls these toxins downwards. The aim of reflexology is not only to boost the circulation in the body, but also to disperse these crystals.

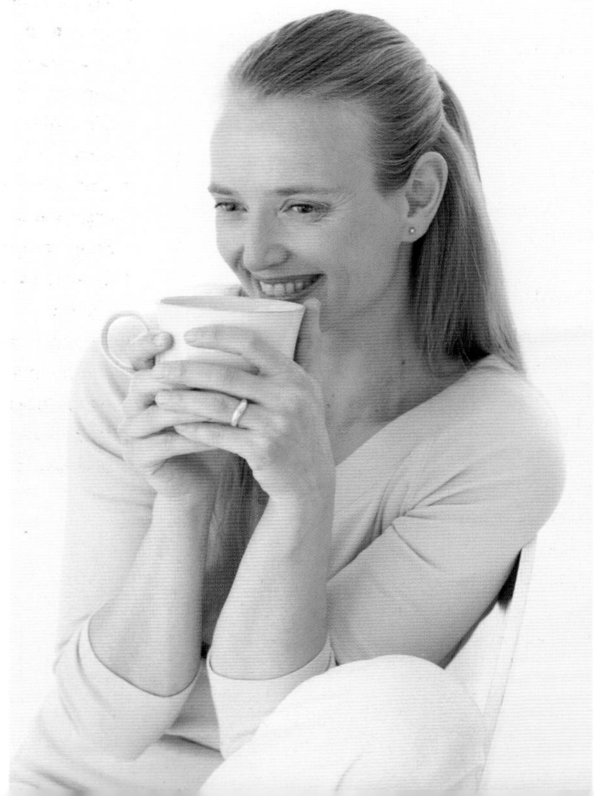

Reflexology creates a sense of balance and well-being.

Reducing stress levels

It is acknowledged that 75 per cent of all illness is stress related. Stress infiltrates our lives, causing problems when we cannot cope with it – compromising our immune systems and making us more susceptible to illness and disease.

Reflexology reduces stress by creating deep relaxation and a sense of balance and well-being. It helps the nervous system to calm down and function more normally. When you apply reflexology you stimulate more than 7,000 nerves in the feet, which can encourage the opening and clearing of neural pathways, helping the body to return it to its natural rhythms.

Creating well-being

The term 'homeostasis' refers to a balanced state in the body and the mind. Our health depends on all the thousands of parts of our body and mind working in harmony together. Too much strain on a particular area can knock our whole system out of balance. It is hard to know what to do when you feel ungrounded, unbalanced or out of sorts, but reflexology can help to create the necessary sense of balance and well-being.

THE BENEFITS OF REFLEXOLOGY

- Encourages the body to heal any current disorders.
- Relieves the effects of stress.
- Improves the immune system.
- Relieves pain.
- Encourages better circulation.
- Improves bowel movements.
- Eliminates waste products from the body.
- Clears the body of toxins.
- Improves nerve stimulation.
- Promotes general relaxation.
- Creates stronger bonds with children.
- Promotes basic hands-on-human interaction.
- Assists post-operative recovery by decreasing pain and increasing healing.

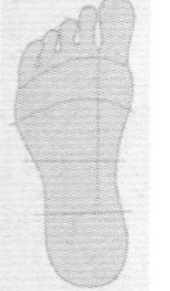

The effectiveness of reflexology

Numerous interesting research studies have looked into reflexology and its effectiveness for a wide variety of medical conditions. Generally speaking the results are very positive and show that reflexology can help on the physical as well as the emotional level. Here are a few interesting results.

Research has shown how effective reflexology is in relieving both tension headaches and migraines.

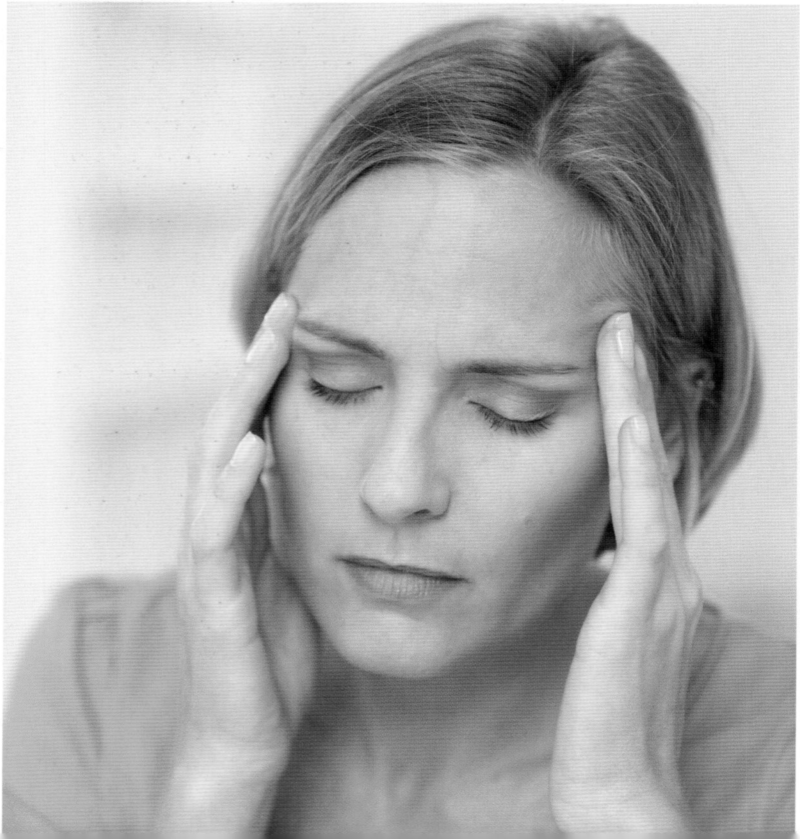

DID YOU KNOW...?

- 220 patients presenting headaches (migraine or tension) as their primary problem were treated by 78 reflexologists over a three-month period.
  Result: 16 per cent reported they were cured, 65 per cent said that reflexology had helped, 18 per cent were unchanged. [National Board of Health Council, Denmark, 1995]
- 50 female patients (aged 20–51) with dysmenorrhoea, hysteromyoma, pelvic inflammation, cysts and masses, endometriosis, menstrual disorder, infertility and 'chocolate cysts' were treated with reflexotherapy over a period ranging from ten sessions to two years.
  Result: 84 per cent found their symptoms had completely disappeared, 16 per cent that symptoms had almost completely disappeared. [Beijing International Reflexology Conference report, China, 1996]
- 42 women (aged 20–60) participated in a study to assess the impact of reflexology on chronic constipation.
  Result: the average number of days between bowel movements was reduced from 4.4 to 1.8. [FDZ-Danish Reflexology Association, 1992]
- 32 cases of Type-II diabetes mellitus were randomly divided into two groups, one of which was treated with a conventional Western hypoglycaemic agent *and* reflexology, and the other group with just the hypoglycaemic agent.
  Result: after daily treatments over 30 days, fasting blood-glucose levels, platelet aggregation, length and other factors were greatly reduced in the reflexology group, while no significant change was observed in the medicine-only group. [First Teaching Hospital, Beijing Medical University, China, 1993]

The holistic approach to health

A holistic approach to health means considering your life or lifestyle as a whole (including diet and exercise), so that you are not only looking at the symptoms of your ailment, but are also discovering the cause. For example, ask yourself, what worries or stresses do I have and how do they affect my health? Then consider the following: do you eat a healthy diet? Are you aware of digestive problems? Are you exercising enough? Are you aware of aches and pains? Is your sleep disturbed? And how is your attitude to life in general affected? All these factors could be having an impact on you and contributing to the source of your problem.

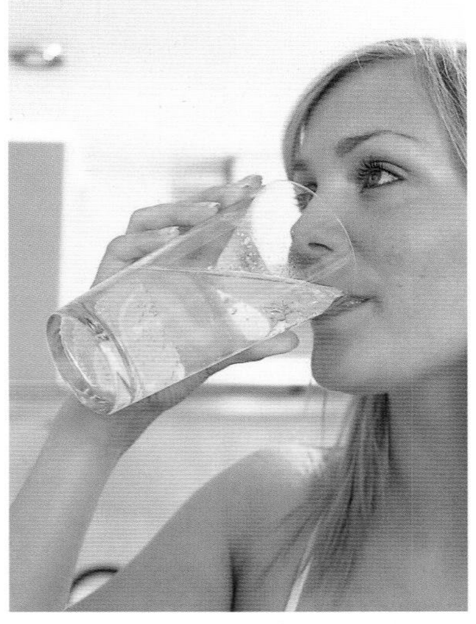

Most people benefit from drinking water throughout the day. Up to 2 litres has been recommended.

Look after your liver

The liver plays a vital role in the holistic approach to health because it detoxifies the body, helps to break down fats and produce energy and heat. If your liver is not working well, it could put you at risk of heart disease by increasing your cholesterol levels; and poor liver function will have a detrimental affect on your overall health.

Avoid refined foods, products with additives and excess sugar, because these impede the ability of the liver to metabolize hormones. The liver helps to ensure the correct functioning of the thyroid gland, which is important because an underactive thyroid has been associated with depression, weight gain, feelings of tiredness and feeling cold most of the time. The liver also deactivates and safely disposes of old hormones so that they do not return to the bloodstream.

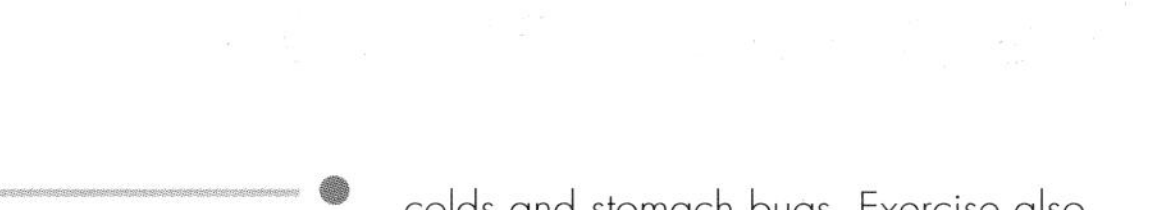

ARE YOU ALLERGIC TO A FOOD?

To find out if you are allergic to a particular food, which may be contributing to your condition, take your pulse at the wrist for 30 seconds, then double the result. Your pulse should be around 52–70 beats a minute. Eat the food you suspect you may allergic to, then take your pulse again. If it is 20 or more beats higher per minute, you probably have an allergy to that food.

Walk away from bad health

Get regular exercise – and that does not have to mean going to the gym. Walking 1.6 km (1 mile) a day can help increase the oxygen levels in your blood. This assists the absorption of nutrients and the elimination of toxins, which in turn strengthens your immune system so that you are not as susceptible to catching colds and stomach bugs. Exercise also affects your energy levels, helping you to feel more positive about life, reduce body weight and maintain a good blood-sugar balance; this in turn helps limit those cravings that we all feel guilty about after we've indulged. Exercise also reduces the risk of osteoporosis (thinning of the bones) and heart disease.

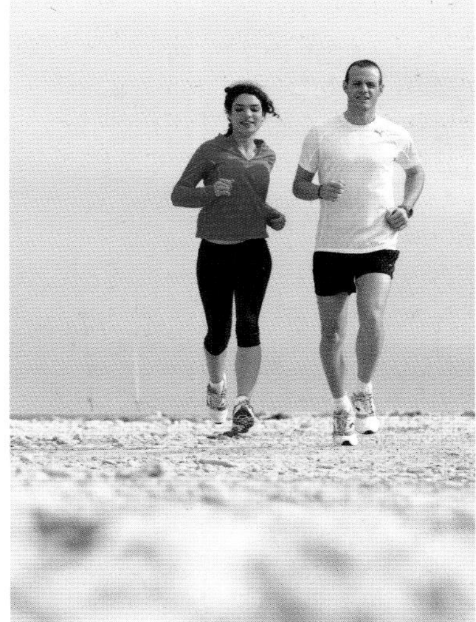

Try to find an exercise plan that suits you – and stick to it. Don't overlook the benefits of a regular brisk walk.

Building a healthier body

Knowledge is power, and being well informed can help you make healthy lifestyle choices. The basis of holistic reflexology and natural medicine is getting to the root of the problem. By understanding the impact of your lifestyle on your body, you can make informed choices. The aim of this book is to help you create the right environment to become healthier and happier.

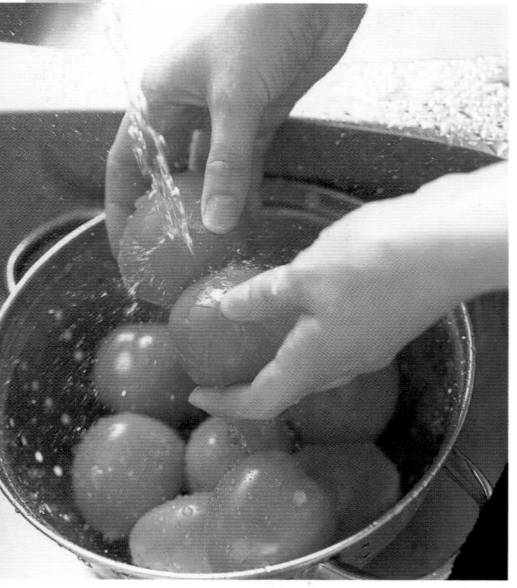

What's in your food?

Everything you choose to put into your body has an effect on every cell within it and on the development of those cells. Thinking back on what you ate over the past week, ask yourself these questions:

• What nutritional value did those foods and drinks give my body?

• Am I nourishing myself and creating a healthy environment in which my body can achieve optimum health?

The impact of food

Let us now consider the impact on our bodies of some everyday foods that we eat and one common product that we use.

• **Margarine:** This contains trans fatty acids, known as 'hydrogenated fats', which can make poor cholesterol levels worse and can stop the body making good use of the essential fats we need in order to keep our nervous system healthy.

• **Sugar:** Most concentrated forms are vitamin- and nutrient-free. Sugar can reduce your ability to fight infection by 50 per cent. And all sugars cause a rapid

Good food is the source of good health. Choose wisely and read nutritional labels to understand what you are eating.

> *Let food be thy medicine and medicine be thy food.*
>
> HIPPOCRATES (468–377 BCE)

increase in blood-sugar levels, which can disrupt the balance of your hormones, potentially making hormone-related diseases worse.

• **Caffeine:** This has been associated with raised cholesterol levels and an increased risk of osteoporosis; also with infertility and a heightened risk of miscarriage. Caffeine can make inflammatory skin conditions worse, raise the body's temperature, increase the incidence of headaches, cause insomnia, promote heart palpitations and anxiety. For some people, giving up caffeine and caffeine-related products (such as tea and cola) could make a world of difference to their health.

• **Antihistamines:** Avoid these if you are trying to become pregnant. Antihistamines and nasal decongestants dry up secretions everywhere in the body, not just in the places they are meant to act upon. They could hinder the delicate balance in the body that is needed to guarantee the correct environment to enable sperm to reach the egg and fertilize it. Vitamin C is a natural antihistamine alternative; it calms down inflammation in the body as well as boosting the immune system.

The argument for organic

Whenever you can afford it, buy organic produce. The reason is simple: non-organic meat contains high levels of antibiotics and growth hormones. Antibiotics wipe out the healthy gut bacteria that help produce the B vitamins that are important for supplying energy; the bad bacteria then multiply, increasing your risk of contracting infection and compromising your immune system. Growth hormones can disrupt the balance of hormones in your body. For instance, milk contains high levels of hormones, particularly oestrogen; to date, infertility, breast cancer, fibroids, ovarian cancer, prostate and testicular cancer, low sperm count and endometriosis have all been linked to excessive oestrogen levels.

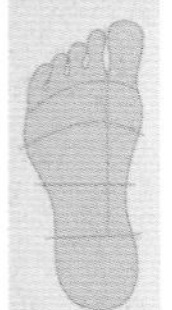

Avoid pesticides and chemicals

Pesticides are chemical or biological substances that are sprayed on crops to protect them against a range of pests, including rodents, insects, weeds, bacteria, viruses and fungi. Chemicals are used in our homes for pest control, as well as in the environment (as in crop spraying), especially if you live in an agricultural area.

Pesticides are known to affect the body's testosterone levels, and this may explain the increase in genital defects and undescended testes in male infants, as well as the increase in male infertility. They are also believed to be contributory factors in many illnesses, including headaches, cancer, depression, skin disorders, asthma,

Balance your body's hormones and prevent the absorption of harmful chemicals by choosing organic food.

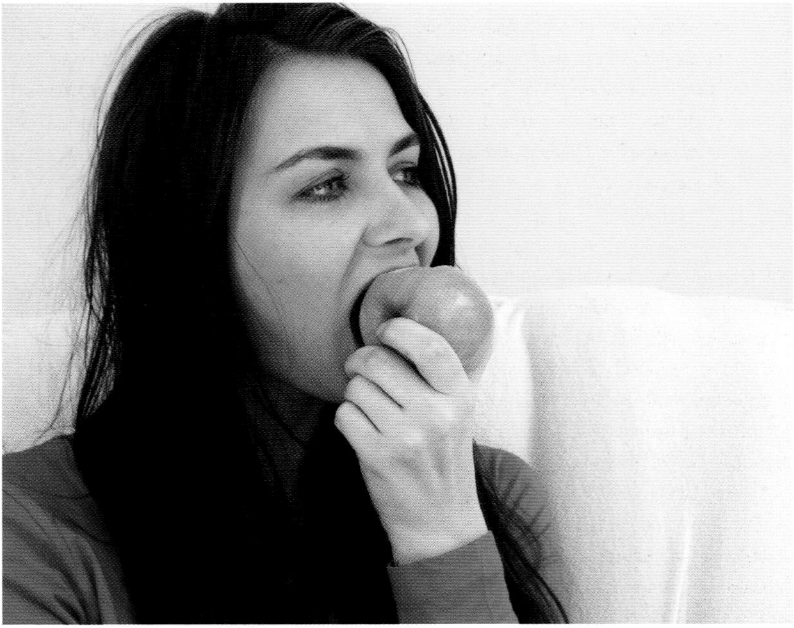

BE KIND TO YOUR SKIN

The skin is the largest organ of the body and a major organ of detoxification; it is a two-way membrane, allowing toxins both in and out through its layers. Never put anything on your skin that you would not put in your mouth.

- Avoid underarm deodorants that contain chemicals called parabens, which will be absorbed through the skin. Critics say there is a link between the use of these deodorants and the development of cancers in particular areas in the upper breasts.
- Read the label on antiperspirants, because some contain aluminium, which has been linked to dementia and Alzheimer's disease. It is possible to buy natural skin products, including antiperspirants.
- Studies suggest that the use of black hair dye is associated with cancer, because the dye enters the blood and can circulate in the body, so this product is best avoided.
- Health stores are the best place to seek advice on healthy options.

fatigue, eye conditions and disorders of the immune system. In addition, pesticides are blamed for difficulties in conceiving, associated disruptions of the hormones, miscarriages, still births and birth defects. Prevention is better than cure, and buying organic food is one good way to reduce your pesticide load.

The importance of fibre

Add lots of fibre to your diet, because it can help prevent the absorption of chemicals into the bloodstream. Good sources of fibre include organic whole grains, lentils, prunes, beans, baked beans, nuts, seeds, fresh fruit and vegetables. A lot of the nutrients in fruit and vegetables are found under the skin, so to get the most out of them, scrub them well, but leave the skin on. Vegetables are best eaten crunchy, as much of the fibre is destroyed by cooking them. Avoid refined white rice, bread and pasta, and do not overcook foods.

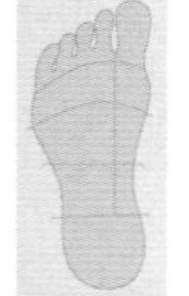

Coping with stress

Stress is any interference that disturbs your healthy mental and physical well-being, or any influence that upsets the natural equilibrium of your body or mind. It is the physiological response of the body to threat or danger: the body prepares itself for sudden action, either to run away or to stay and fight.

During times of stress the body goes through a series of changes that are designed to give you strength and speed – but these have devastating effects if you

Find positive ways of dealing with stress, so that it does not take control of your life. Take an active, energetic approach.

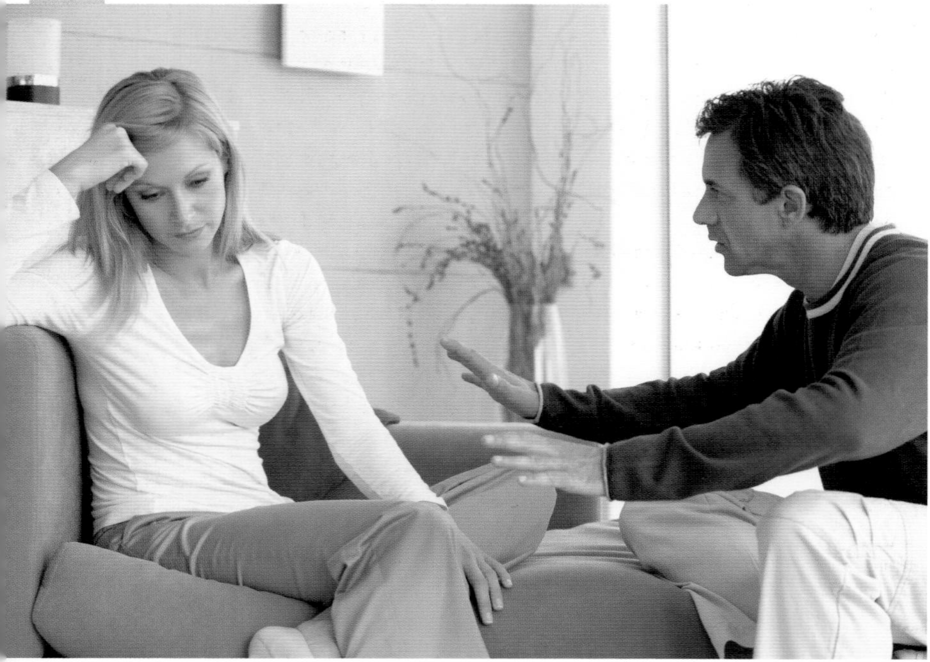

TOP TEN EFFECTS OF STRESS

Stress has a number of negative effects on the body, of which the worst are the following:

1 The body calls on fat reserves to be used up for energy. These fatty deposits stay in the blood vessels and contribute to arteriosclerosis (thickening of the artery walls). This narrows the blood vessels and puts you at risk of heart disease.

2 Your heart beats faster, increasing blood flow around the body, which can lead to high blood pressure and headaches. This puts a strain on all the blood vessels.

3 The liver pours out glucose for the muscles to use as energy. Glucose stays in the bloodstream when it does not get used up, which can lead to diabetes.

4 The adrenal glands pour out the steroid hormone cortisone. In large doses it is toxic to the brain causing depression and memory loss.

5 Blood diverts from the bladder, and if the bladder is not continually emptying, this can lead to cystitis.

6 Stress lowers the immune system so that you find it harder to fight infection and bacteria have a better chance of taking hold.

7 Tense neck and shoulder muscles lead to pain. This tightness in the muscles can restrict nerve impulses to different parts of the body. For example, tinnitus (ringing in the ears) is common during times of stress because of compression of the nerve roots.

8 Blood is diverted from the digestive system because it is considered non-essential in times of danger, so the digestive system does not function properly. This can make any digestive disorder worse.

9 Stress directly affects the hormonal system and puts the body's glands and hormones out of balance.

10 Your breathing is restricted during times of stress, so less oxygen reaches the cells and consequently there is a greater accumulation of waste products.

PRACTICAL HELP MECHANISMS

When you feel the symptoms of stress – such as palpitations, an irritable bowel, insomnia, headaches or loss of appetite – do something positive. You can use either foot or hand reflexology on a more frequent basis, and consider the following measures:

- Establish some boundaries, and learn to say 'No' when you are taking too much on board.
- If you work at a desk or have a sedentary lifestyle, get up and take some exercise regularly: walk or run up and down the stairs rather than taking the lift, so that your glucose and fat deposits get used up by the physical movement. If you do 30 minutes of aerobic exercise three times a week, you can reduce your risk of cardiovascular disease by 40 per cent.
- Adopt deep-breathing techniques throughout the day to calm the body: for instance, breathe in for five seconds, hold for five seconds, then breathe out for five seconds. Imagine your breath filling every part of your body.

are not physically active. So it makes sense, when you feel stressed, to walk, run, move or dance in order to use up the fats, hormones and sugars that the body has released.

Breathing techniques

You can practise deep breathing throughout your reflexology treatments. You can also breathe deeply when you are facing any difficult situation – at home, at work, in a plane, bus or car, in a theatre, when going somewhere unknown, facing a stressful situation or whenever you feel the need to take control of your emotions. Holding your breath is also good for relieving stress: inhale deeply through your nose with your mouth closed; hold your breath for a few seconds, then exhale slowly through your mouth. Relax your tongue as you inhale and exhale so that it flops down at the bottom of your mouth next to the gum line.

If you need to get out of a negative mindset, use positive affirmations during your breathing. An affirmation is a form of auto-suggestion whereby you visualize a positive outcome, by creating a statement of something you want to happen in your body, your relationships or your life. A good example is: 'I am making more time for myself and my loved ones.' You need to make a mental image of this desirable state and say the statement to yourself each morning in the mirror. Stress nurtures a demoralized self, and we owe it to ourselves and to our families to treat ourselves kindly, with love and self-respect. Being positive about all aspects of your life can not only change things around you but also within you. You could try repeating these affirmations to yourself throughout the day along with your deep breathing exercise.

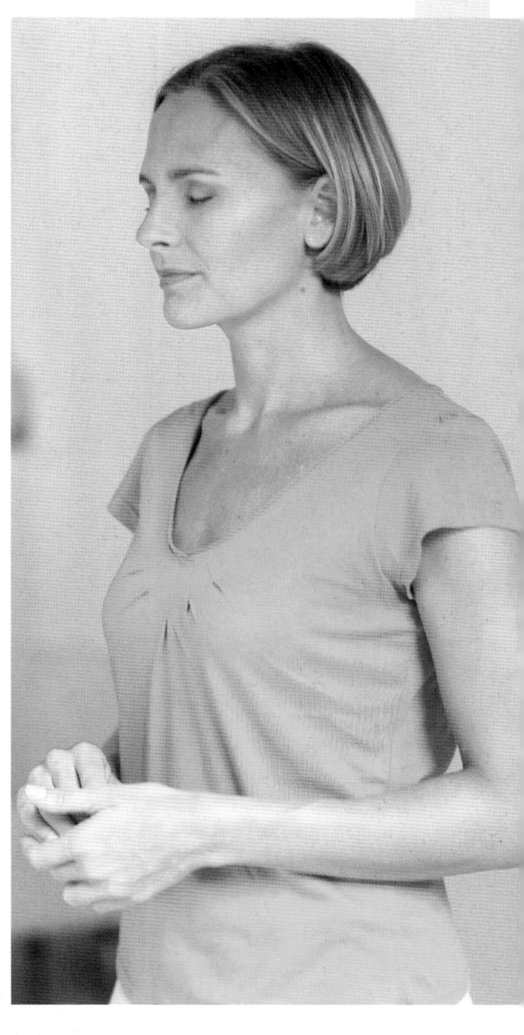

Start each day with a positive affirmation to counter the negative, destructive effects of stress.

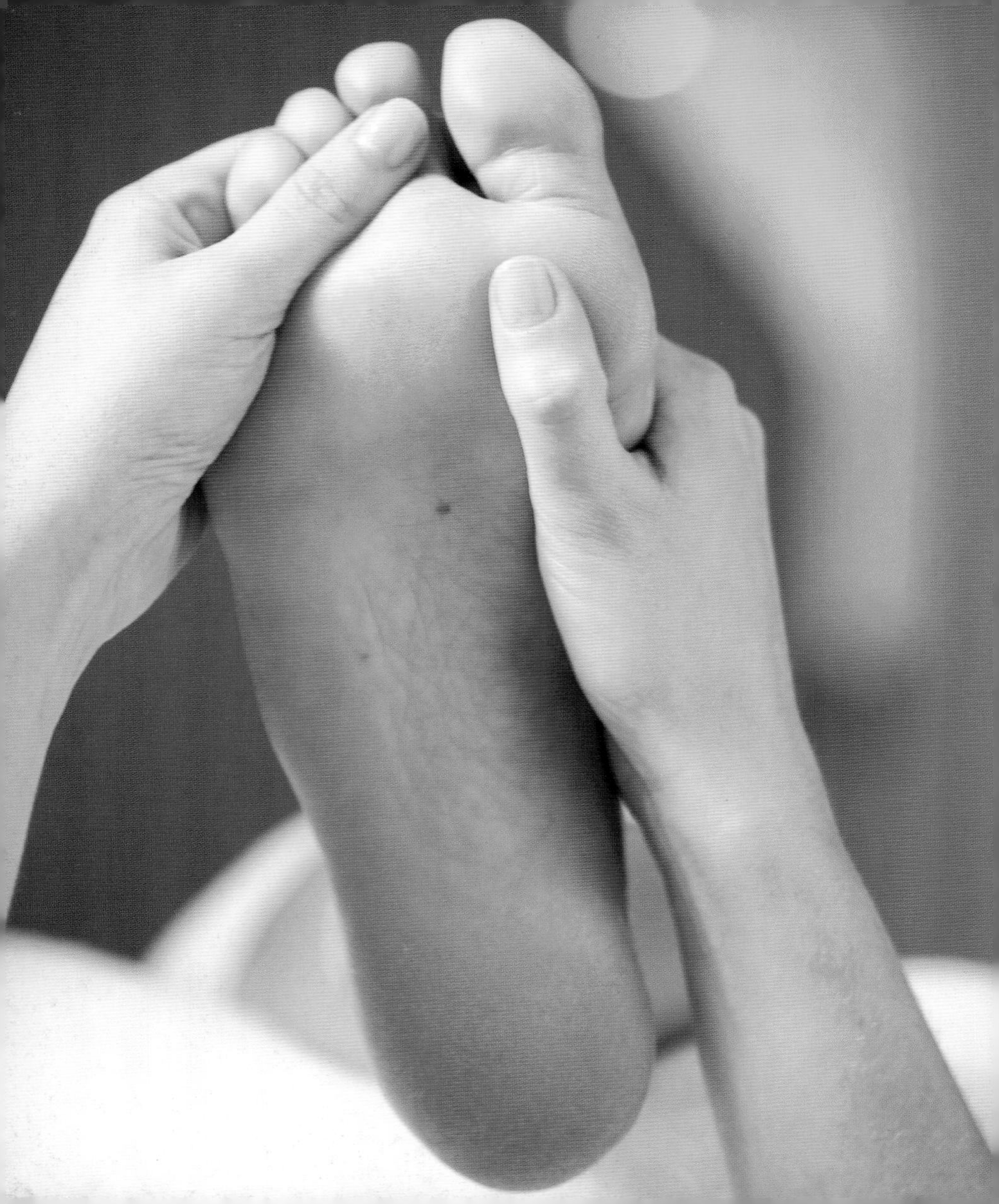

PART 2

How reflexology works

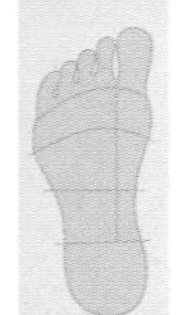

Mapping the feet

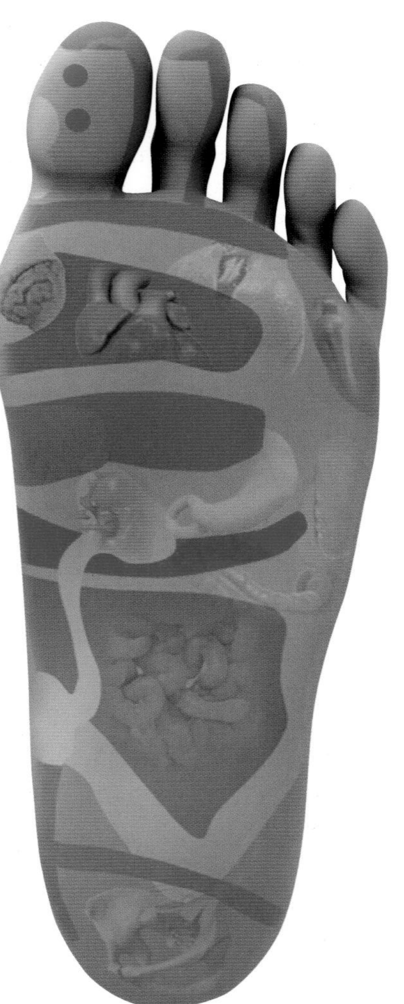

Reflexology is non-invasive, relaxing, therapeutic, and sets off all the body's healing mechanisms. It is one of the most intelligent complementary therapies around because when you understand how it works, you can identify areas of the body that are not functioning well and can help improve someone's overall physical and mental health.

The original reflexology maps of the feet were devised by Eunice Ingham (see page 14), using anecdotal evidence obtained during her reflexology work. The maps are not an anatomical representation of the body, and that is why reflexology maps differ slightly from one another, depending on their author.

Relative positions

It is important to be aware of the significant relationship between reflexes on the feet and the parts of the body to which they correspond, and reflexology maps can help you do this. The position of the reflexes on the soles of the feet generally

In reflexology all the vital organs and different parts of the body are mapped out on the feet.

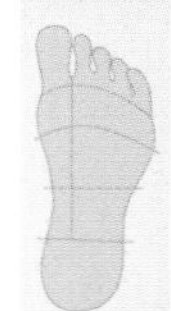

reflects the corresponding position of the different organs and parts of the body. Thus the big toes at the top of the foot represent the head, and it is there that you would apply reflexology techniques to help someone suffering from headaches. Similarly, the spinal reflex is found along the inside edge of each foot, which is also known as the medial aspect of the foot. Generally you will notice that the inside edge of the foot can be more sensitive. You can also find the reproductive organs on the medial aspect of the foot.

The right foot maps out the right side of the body, while the left foot maps out the left side. The best way to use these charts is to try and familiarize yourself with the body systems and their reflex areas, perhaps by looking at your own feet. Once you are ready to give a treatment, you can use the easy-to-follow treatment sequences described in the following parts of the book. Choose a sequence that is appropriate for you, your friend or family member, and enjoy giving the treatment as much as they will enjoy receiving it.

READING THE REFLEXES

There are a number of reasons why a particular reflex might be sensitive or out of balance, and these include an energy imbalance in the area, or congestion of energy in the related zone of the body. Often it indicates an ongoing physical problem, which the person may be well aware of and might want reflexology to help them. Reflexology can also pick up the effects of medication on different areas of the body, such as the liver or kidney reflex. You just need to learn how to 'read' the reflexes in order to identify the problem.

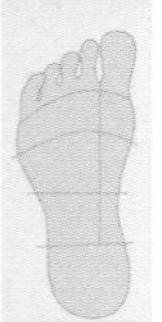

The feet: a mirror of the body

All the organs and parts of the body are generally arranged in the same order in different reflexology charts. Guidelines cross the feet to help you associate specific areas of the body with areas in the feet – for instance, you can find the organs of respiration between the shoulder line and diaphragm line. All the many reflexology points are located within these guidelines. The major guidelines are:

TRANSVERSE ZONES: PLANTAR ASPECT

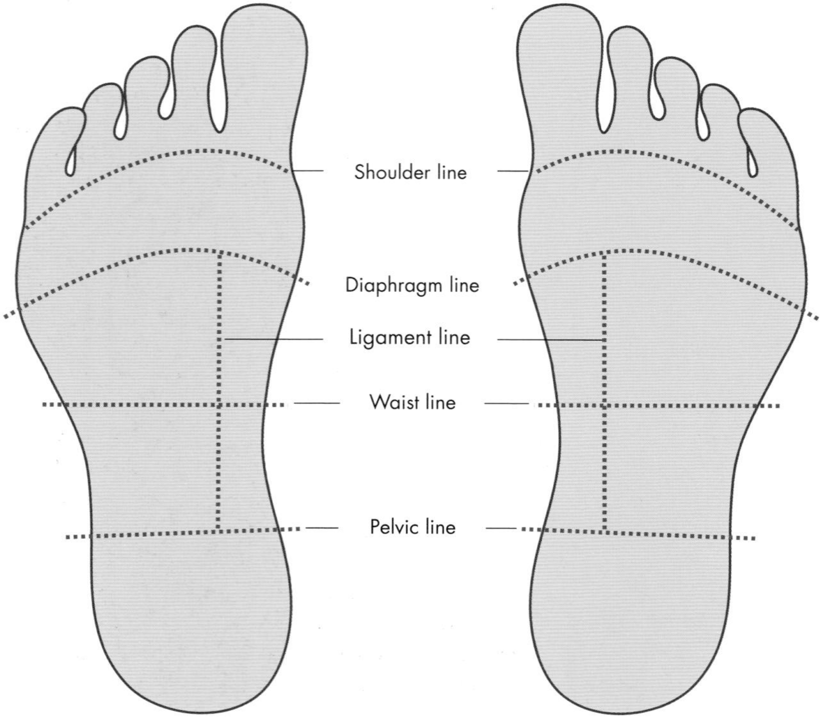

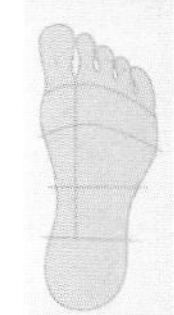

• **The shoulder line:** This transverse zone is found just below the bases of the toes; above this line you can find the head, occipital, pituitary, inner ear, teeth, jaw, sinus, eye, Eustachian tube, outer ear, throat and shoulder reflexes.

• **The diaphragm (or solar plexus) line:** This is found under the base of the metatarsals. A distinguishing feature is that the colour of the skin on the metatarsal area changes – the skin is darker around the metatarsals (diaphragm line) and lighter below. In between the shoulder line and the diaphragm line you can find the lungs, thyroid, oesophagus, hiatus hernia, pancreas and gall bladder reflexes.

• **The waist line:** This is found by running your finger along the lateral side of the foot and feeling a small bony protrusion about midway. Then draw a line across the foot (this area often forms the narrowest part of the foot). In between the diaphragm line and the waist line you can find the kidney/adrenal, stomach, liver, spleen, transverse colon, hepatic and splenic flexure reflexes and part of the small intestines.

• **The pelvic (or heel) line:** This is found by drawing an imaginary line from the ankle bones on either side of the foot over the base of the heel. In between the waist line and the pelvic line you can find the ascending and descending colon, part of the small intestines and bladder. The sciatic area runs transversely across the middle of the pelvic line.

• **The ligament line:** This alone runs from the top of the foot to the bottom, rather than across it.

Aspects of the feet

Throughout this book the different views or 'aspects' of the foot are referred to as follows:

• **Dorsal aspect:** the view of the top of the foot as you look down at it.

• **Plantar aspect:** the view of the sole or underside of the foot, which you place on the ground.

• **Medial aspect:** the inside edge of the foot, running from the big toe to the heel.

• **Lateral aspect:** the outside edge of the foot, running from the little toe to the heel.

Familiarizing yourself with the various aspects of the feet will help when you come to the techniques given in Parts 4, 5 and 6, where you will sometimes work on one aspect first, followed by another – for example, the medial aspect and then the lateral aspect.

Plantar foot map

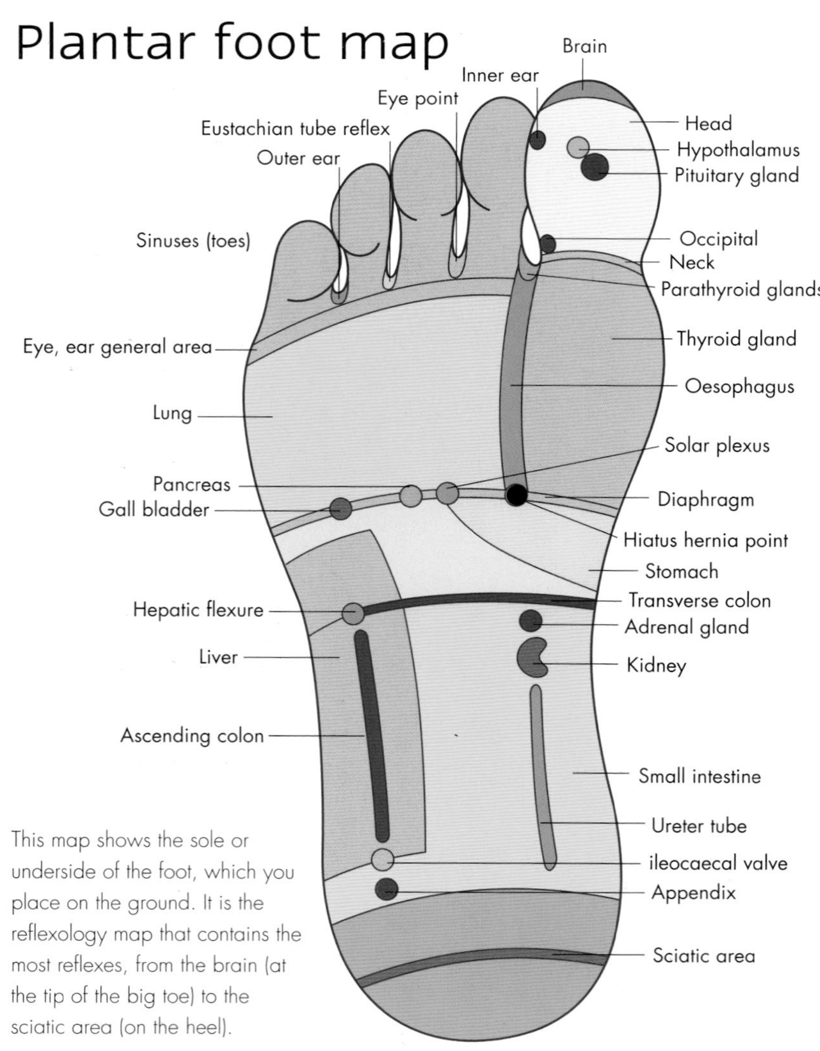

This map shows the sole or underside of the foot, which you place on the ground. It is the reflexology map that contains the most reflexes, from the brain (at the tip of the big toe) to the sciatic area (on the heel).

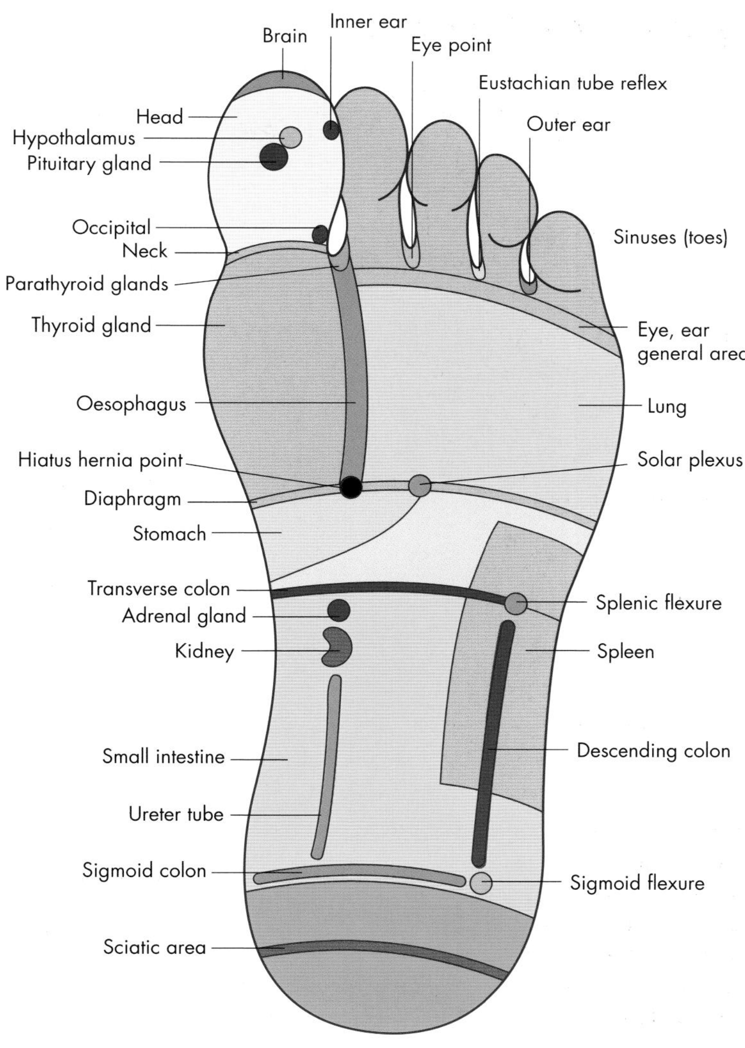
Brain
Inner ear
Eye point
Eustachian tube reflex
Outer ear
Head
Hypothalamus
Pituitary gland
Sinuses (toes)
Occipital
Neck
Parathyroid glands
Thyroid gland
Eye, ear general area
Oesophagus
Lung
Hiatus hernia point
Solar plexus
Diaphragm
Stomach
Transverse colon
Splenic flexure
Adrenal gland
Kidney
Spleen
Small intestine
Descending colon
Ureter tube
Sigmoid colon
Sigmoid flexure
Sciatic area

LEFT FOOT

Dorsal foot map

This map shows the top of the foot as you look down at it. It includes the reflexes for the teeth, jaw, throat and upper lymphatics (on or between the toes) and for the breast and shoulder (on the foot in front of the little toe).

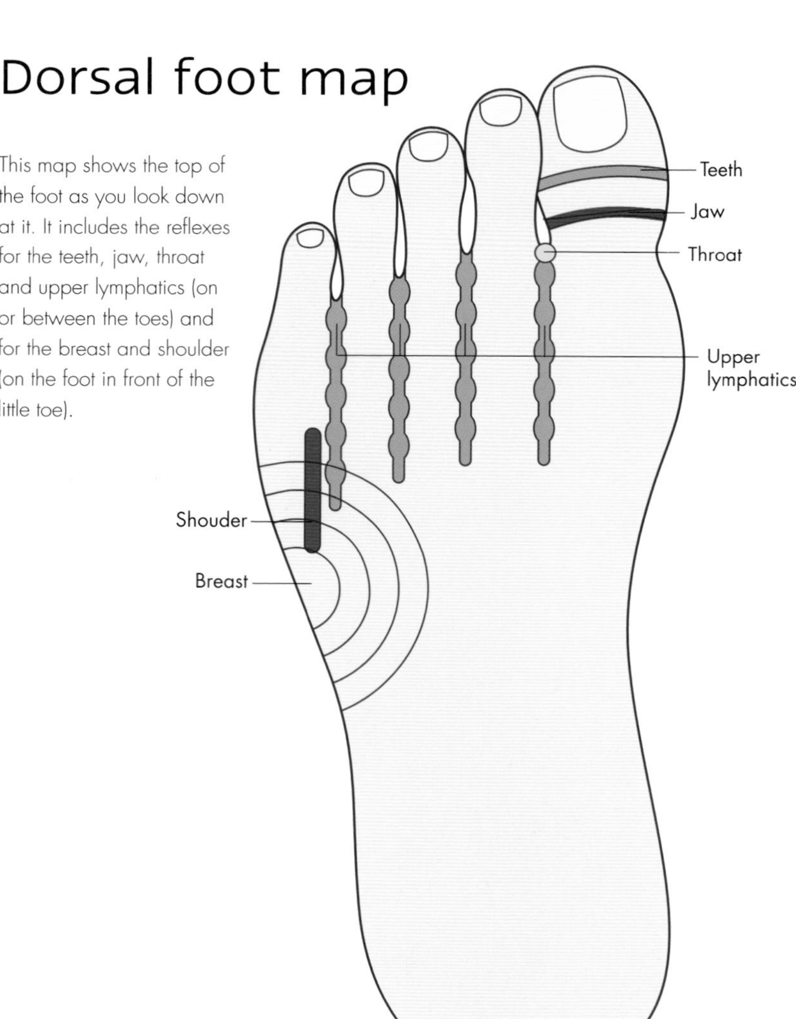

LEFT FOOT

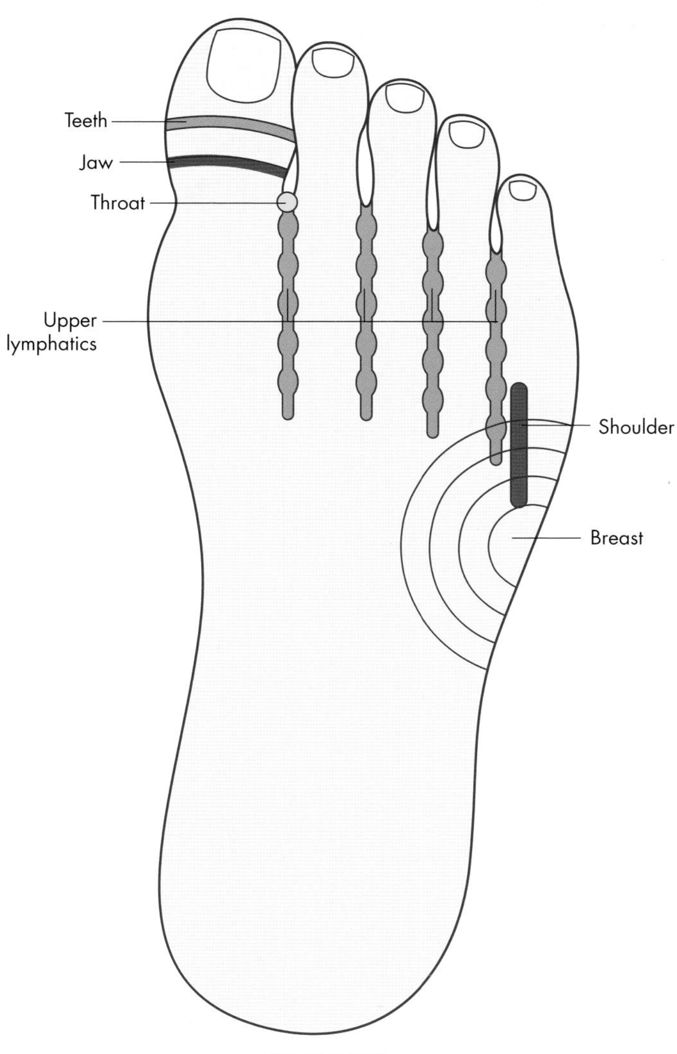

RIGHT FOOT

Medial foot map

This map shows the inside edge of the foot, running from the big toe to the heel. It contains the reflexes for the cervical, thoracic and lumbar vertebrae, the bladder and the uterus (in women) and prostate gland (in men).

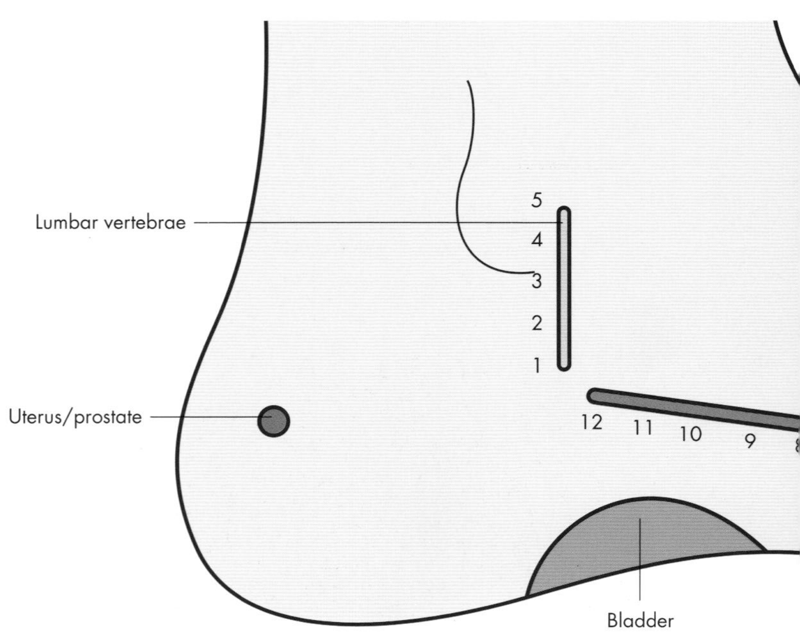

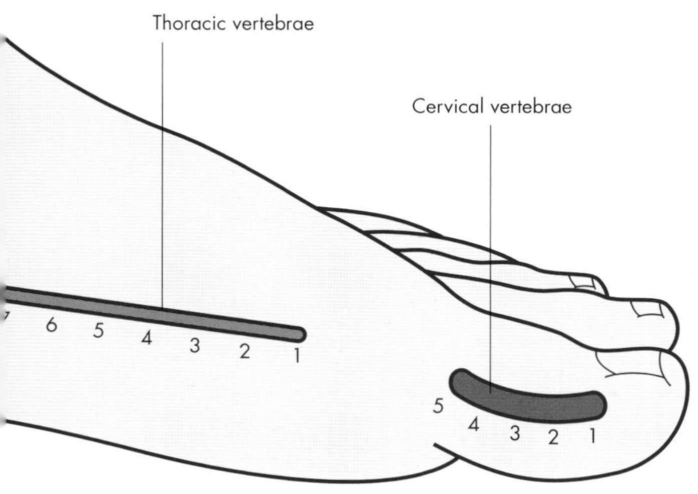
Thoracic vertebrae
Cervical vertebrae
6 5 4 3 2 1
5 4 3 2 1

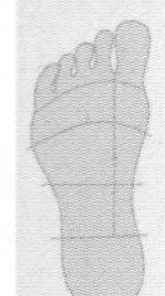

Lateral foot map

This map shows the outside edge of the foot, running from the little toe to the heel. It contains the reflexes for the wrist, elbow and shoulder, the knee, hip and sacrum, and the ovaries (in women) and testes (in men).

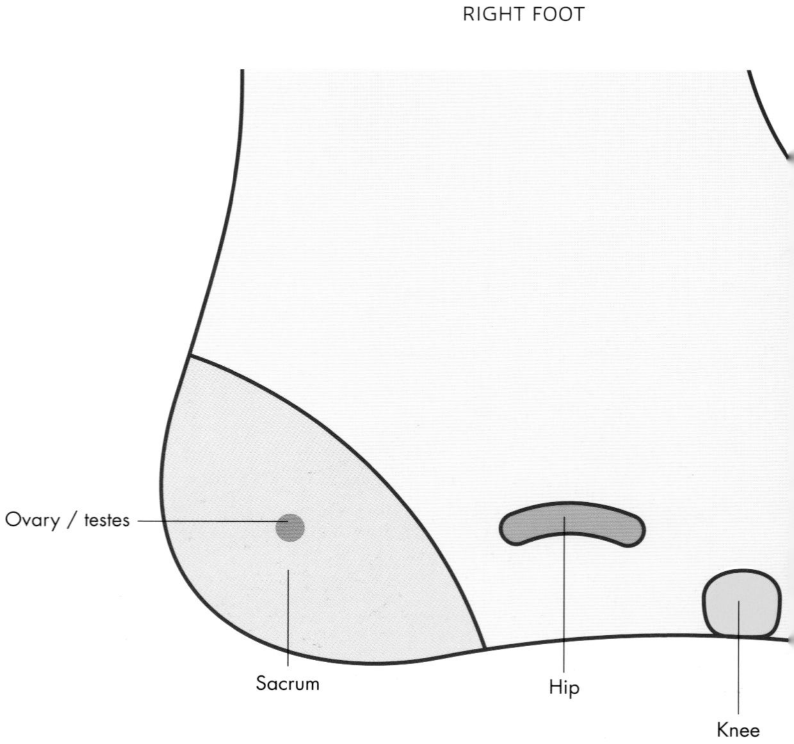

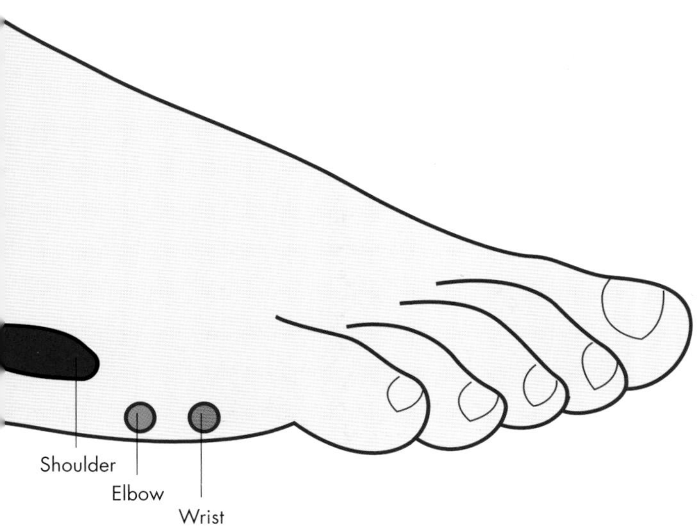
Shoulder
Elbow
Wrist

Using reflexology to read the feet

A trained reflexologist will be able to use a reflexology sequence on the feet to find reflex points or areas that are sensitive or out of balance. These correspond to specific parts of the body and indicate a problem in the related body area.

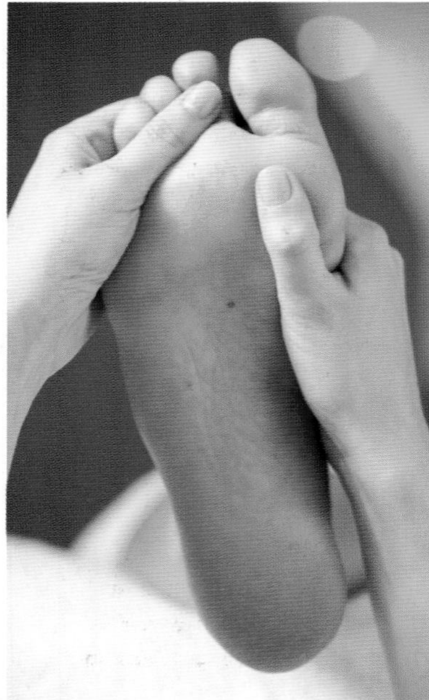

Use reflexology on the feet to determine a client's state of health.

Crystals in the reflexes

A reflexologist discovers congested areas by finding crystals in the feet. These crystals are made up of uric acid or calcium and build up in the nerve endings in the feet. If, say, the lungs become weak, their normal muscular activity slows down and the extremities of their nerve endings become blocked. This blockage may only be small, but it could be enough to reduce the circulation to the lungs so that they do not get an ample supply of fresh blood, oxygen and nutrients while simultaneously having their toxins removed.

By applying pressure to these crystals, the reflexologist will break them up, so that they dissolve and are carried away in the blood. The more crystals you find, the longer you should work on them, so that they can be broken down by reflexology. Sensitivity in a reflex can warn of a weak area in the body and, if the imbalance is treated and corrected with reflexology, illness can often be avoided.

Using the right amount of pressure (see page 95) is important, because if you apply too much, it could cause pain and give a false reading. Use the charts (see pages 40–49) to establish which parts of

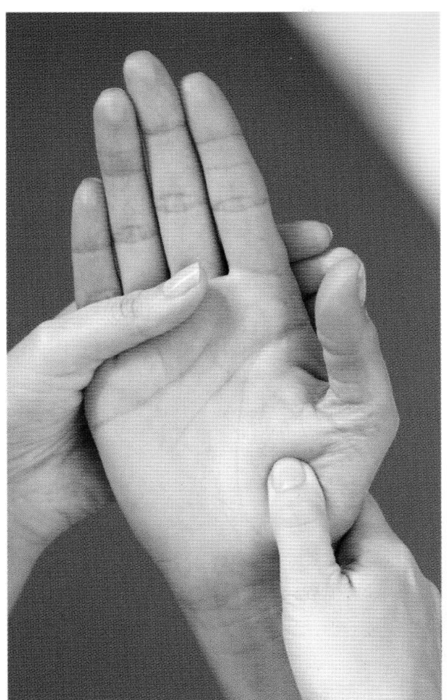

Reflexology on the hand can pick up both past and furture problems.

the body a sensitive reflex area relates to. Then work over it several times, taking small steps as you cross the area and returning again at the end of the treatment. In this way you will ensure that you are disbursing as many crystals as possible.

PAST, PRESENT AND FUTURE PROBLEMS

Reflexology is like a time orb – it can pick up both current problems and the memory of an old problem, now long gone. Would you believe that if someone had a hysterectomy 20 years ago the reflex would still be sensitive now? This is because the body remembers injuries and operations, just as we do. You can also pick up a past condition that has been suppressed and resolved, such as childhood asthma. Finally, reflexes on the feet and hands can highlight any areas of weakness or vulnerability that may give rise to future problems. In this way you can use reflexology as a preventative therapy that focuses on treatment, diet, lifestyle and emotional well-being to create good health.

Cross-reflexes

If the feet are too sensitive, swollen or injured to treat, it is best to use a cross-reflex instead. Cross-reflexes work on the 'zone therapy' theory of Dr William Fitzgerald (see page 16). There are energy zones that run up and down the body, with corresponding paths travelling up from the toes and legs to the head, and from the fingers and arms to the head. The cross-reflexes have a mirror-effect on the body, so that treatment on the feet can affect the hand and arm area, and vice versa.

An example would be a client who has sprained an ankle, with pressure building up in the area of the sprain. Naturally the ankle would be too injured to work on, so you would apply reflexology massage on the wrist to prevent soreness, swelling or other possible complications. For a broken leg you would select the corresponding area on the arm and work that, in order to improve circulation to the injured leg and hasten the healing process.

Principal cross-reflexes

By understanding the theory of cross-reflexes, you can treat areas of the body that you could not normally work on. Additionally, you can work on your own hands as an effective treatment, or as homework in between reflexology sessions. The principal cross-reflexes are as follows:

- Fingers/toes
- Foot/hand
- Sole of foot/palm of hand
- Top of foot/back of hand
- Ankle/wrist
- Calf/inner part of forearm
- Shin/outer part of forearm
- Knee/elbow
- Thigh/upper arm
- Hip/shoulder.

If you are treating someone with a broken lower leg, choose the cross-reflex which is the lower arm. Supporting the arm, gently massage the area of the corresponding part of the arm that relates to the injury.

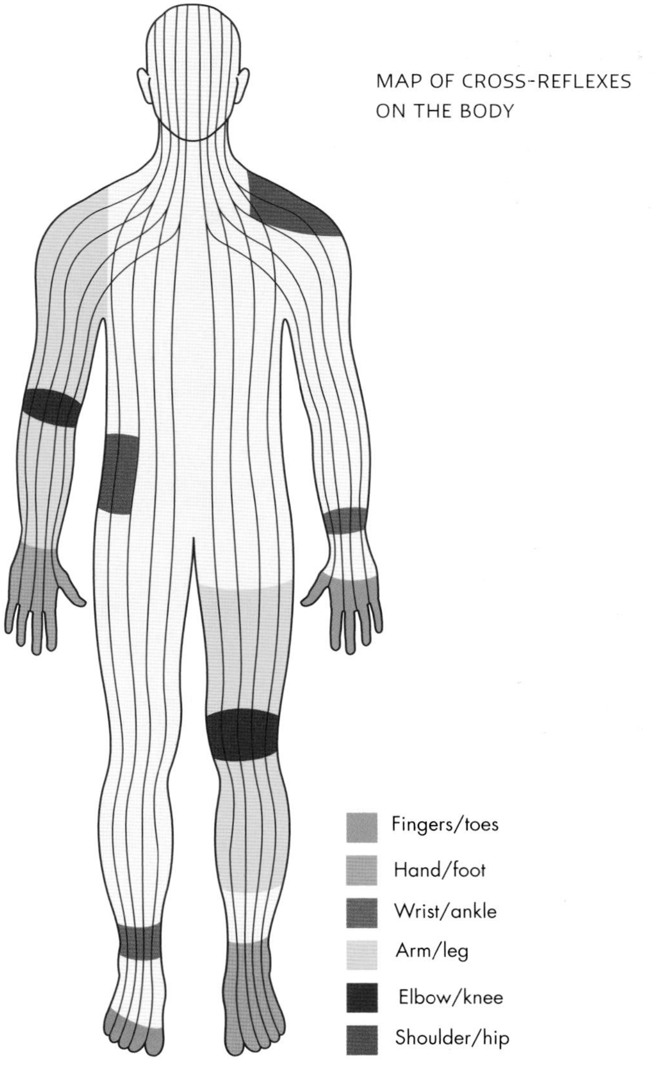
MAP OF CROSS-REFLEXES
ON THE BODY
Fingers/toes
Hand/foot
Wrist/ankle
Arm/leg
Elbow/knee
Shoulder/hip

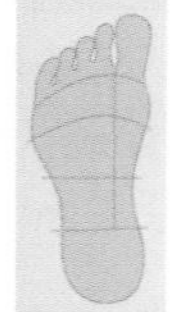

Anatomy of the foot

The feet can reveal a host of stories to a reflexologist. Their structure, as well as the reflexes, can show up both emotional and physical weakness and strengths. The feet support the weight of our body and, if we allow the muscles in our body to weaken, this can affect the muscle tissue in our feet. Any impairment or change to the functions of the body can displace our centre of gravity. A good example is the way that back, knee and foot problems develop during pregnancy, when the body's centre of gravity and disposition of weight change as the nine months go by.

The average foot contains 26 bones, 100 ligaments, 20 muscles and an intricate network of nerves and blood supply. Connective tissue, blood vessels and nerves join the bones together, covered by layers of skin. The foot has two important functions – weight-bearing and propulsion – which require a high degree of stability. In addition, the foot must be flexible, so that it can adapt to uneven surfaces. Problems affecting the foot's structure could affect posture.

REFLEXOLOGY AND FOOT CIRCULATION

At the most basic level, reflexology improves the circulation. Stress, tension, poor posture and badly fitting shoes all restrict blood flow and create a sluggish circulatory and lymphatic system. This could mean that an infection like athlete's foot or a foot or leg ulcer may take weeks to clear. When blood flow or lymphatic circulation is poor, it is hard for oxygen-rich blood, nutrients and white blood cells to reach various areas of the foot to fight infection, digest germs, remove toxins and waste products. Regular reflexology can help to develop healthy feet as well as improving overall body circulation.

Bones of the feet

The forefoot includes five metatarsal bones and the phalanges (the toes).

- **The first metatarsal** bone bears the most weight and plays the most important role in propelling the body. The second, third and fourth metatarsal bones are the most stable.
- **The sesamoids** are two small oval-shaped bones close to the head of the first metatarsal, on the plantar surface of the foot. They develop inside a tendon, where it passes over a bony prominence. They are held in place by their tendons and are supported by ligaments.
- **The tarsal bones** are mostly in the mid-foot. Five of the seven tarsal bones can be found here (the navicular, cuboid and the three cuneiform). It meets the forefoot at the five tarso-metatarsal joints.
- **The talus and the calcaneus** make up the hindfoot. The calcaneus is the largest tarsal bone and forms the heel. The talus rests on top of it and forms the pivot of the ankle.

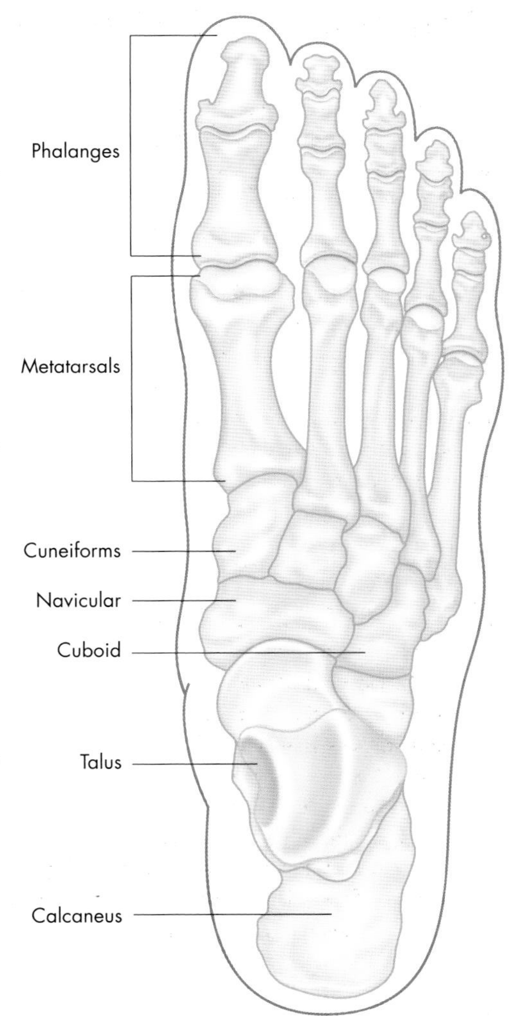

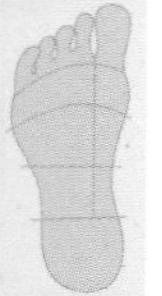

Arches of the foot

The three arches of the foot are maintained by the shapes of the bones, muscles, tendons and ligaments.

- **The transverse arch**, underneath the foot, is composed of the cuneiforms, cuboid and the five metatarsal bases and helps with balance.
- **The lateral longitudinal arch** is lower and flatter than the medial arch; it is composed of the calcaneus, cuboid and the fourth and fifth metatarsals.
- **The medial longitudinal arch** is the highest and most important; it is composed of the calcaneus, talus, navicular, cuneiforms and the first three metatarsals.

ARCHES OF THE FOOT

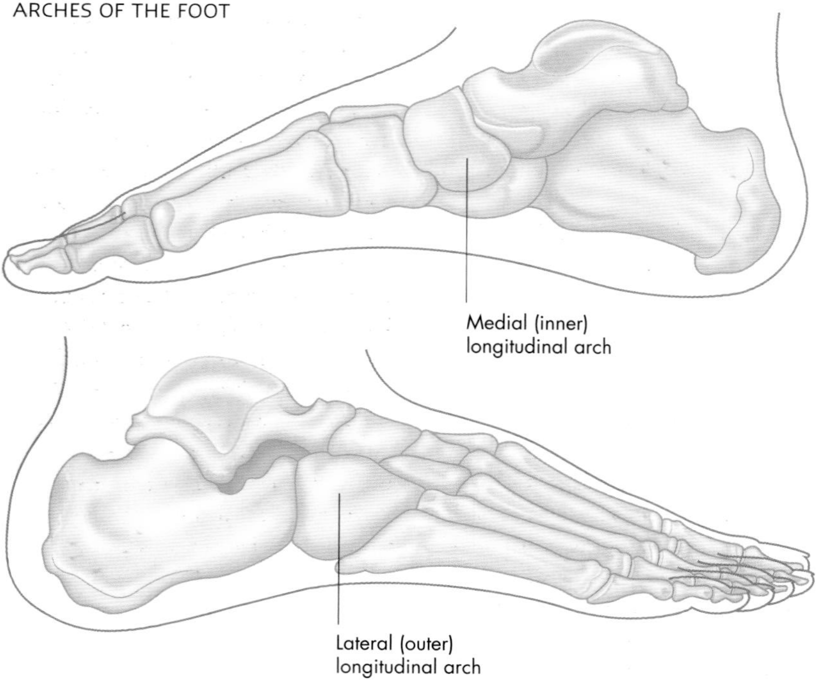

Medial (inner) longitudinal arch

Lateral (outer) longitudinal arch

Healthy arches

Foot problems can displace your centre of gravity, which can affect the whole of your spine. Foot disorders like bunions not only affect your ankles, knees and hips (because of difficulty in walking), but the over-compensation in posture can actually cause headaches and tinnitus. A good foot structure forms the foundation for your spine and helps keep your spinal alignment healthy and functioning well. A healthy foot has healthy arches, which play important roles in the body:

- Bearing the weight of the body and distributing this weight across the feet.
- Absorbing shock when you are running or exercising.
- Acting as a lever to propel the body forward in motion.
- Balancing the body and keeping all the vertebrae aligned.

High arches

High arches are normally hereditary, which means that if your mother or father had them, you may also have been born with them; some people with spina bifida also suffer from high arches. It may mean that the toes do not make correct contact with the ground when standing, which could develop into a claw foot; and overall the foot usually lacks manoeuvrability and may feel stiff. Corns and calluses are a common problem because of the pressure exerted on areas of the toes and the front of the feet. This condition can, however, be corrected by surgery.

Flat feet

Some people are born with flat feet, which means that they have no arches; other people develop them as a result of walking injuries, incorrect walking or obesity. The resulting problems can affect the whole body: the ligaments in the feet become overwhelmed and collapse, which then affects all the bones in the feet and ankles; and the soles no longer have a shock-absorbing effect on the body, which may lead to foot pain, burning soles, general fatigue and a painful spine. The arches normally protect the 7,000 nerves in the feet as well as the blood vessels, so the whole weight of the body presses down on them. The best thing to do if you suffer from flat feet is see a podiatrist, who will create tailor-made insoles to wear in your shoes and will suggest muscle-building exercises.

Anatomy of the body

This section of the book will give you a basic understanding of how the body works. To appreciate the effects of reflexology, you need to have some knowledge of the body's structure and the workings of the body's systems. You need to be a health detective. Ask yourself questions such as: what happened before my body reacted in this way? What did I do recently that could have affected me? What did I eat or drink? What have I come into contact with, or what products have I put on my body?

Overview of the body

The human body consists of several levels of structure that are all associated with one another:

- **The chemical level** is the lowest level, and includes all chemical substances that are essential for maintaining life; the chemicals are put together to form the next level of organization.
- **The cellular level** comprises the basic structural and functional units of the body.
- **The tissue level** is made up of groups of similar cells and the intercellular material that performs a specific function; when individual cells are joined together, they form a tissue (examples are muscle tissue, connective tissue and nervous tissue); each cell in the tissue has a specific function.
- **The organ level** occurs in many places in the body, where different kinds of tissues are joined together to form a higher level of organization and perform a specific function; organs usually have recognizable shapes – for example, the heart, liver, kidney, brain and stomach are all organs.
- **The system level** consists of an association of organs with common functions; for instance, the digestive system – which breaks down and digests food – is composed of the mouth, saliva-producing glands, pharynx (throat), oesophagus (gullet), stomach, small intestine, large intestine and rectum, plus the liver, gall bladder and pancreas.
- **The total organism** comprises all parts of the body functioning with each other, to make one living individual.

How you look and feel, and the state of your health, depends on everything that you put into and on your body – and sometimes there may not be an obvious cause for a problem. For example, if someone has a severe peanut allergy, there would be an immediate reaction and the body's chemical levels would be affected as the person coped with the

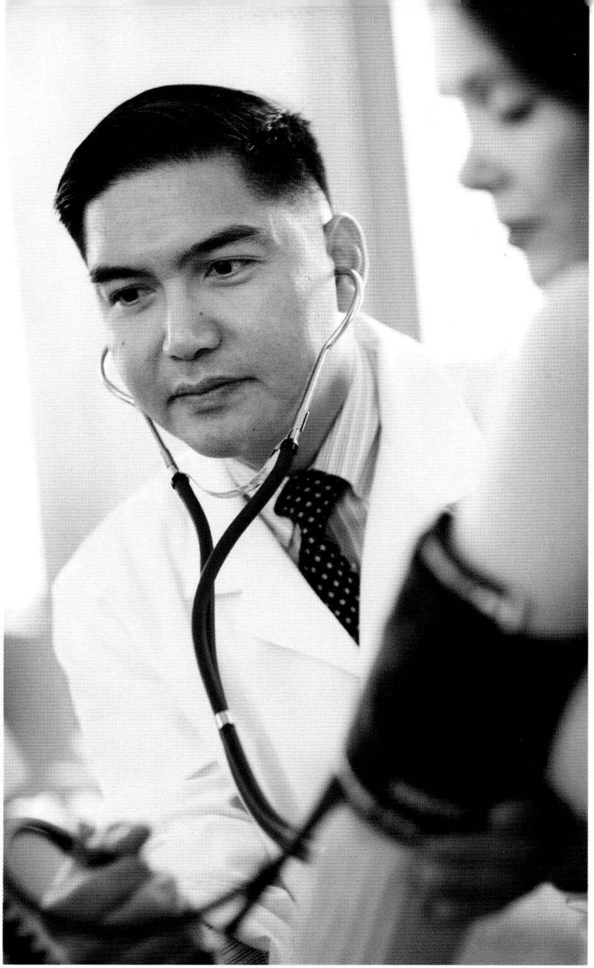

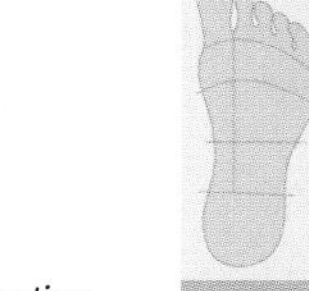

A health detective will apply an holistic approach to your health.

allergen. However, hair loss could be caused by a less obvious reaction to chlorine in a swimming pool. You should always try to find what it is that is affecting all levels of the body. Understanding the body's anatomy and physiology will help you make decisions to create and maintain good health.

The cells of the body

Cells are the essential building blocks of life. The human body is made up of cells, which subsequently form fluid, tissues and organs. Blood is made up of a fluid connective tissue that consists of plasma and different types of cells.

A SIMPLE CELL

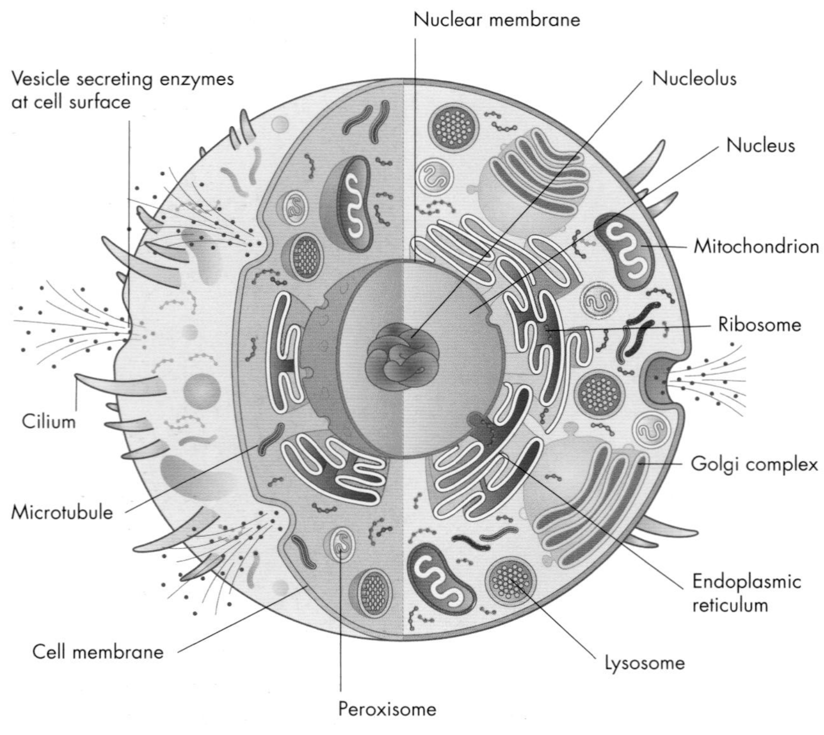

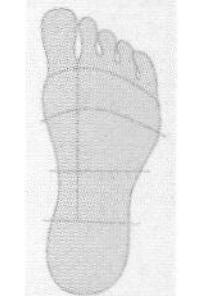

Cells live independently from each other and can reproduce themselves. Each cell has a different structure and function – for example, a sperm cell has a whiplike tail to propel itself up the cervix. DNA (deoxyribonucleic acid) is the material from which the chromosomes of a cell's nucleus are formed, governing cell growth and inheritance. Certain diseases are passed down through generations within the cells, so looking at your family history can give you an indication of the diseases to which you may be predisposed.

Cell structure

All living organisms on Earth are divided into cells. These contain smaller pieces, including proteins and organelles, and larger pieces called tissues and systems. Cells are small compartments that hold all of the biological equipment necessary to keep an organism alive on Earth.

Each cell is surrounded by a cell membrane, which is like a filter and lets some substances in and out of the cell, while other substances are blocked from entering. For instance, the cell membrane allows in oxygen and nutrients from the blood to provide it with energy, and then passes out waste products and carbon dioxide back into the bloodstream to be excreted from the body. The nucleus of the cell governs all its functions, while the cytoplasm is the cellular material in which the organelles are suspended.

Mitochondria are the energy powerhouses of cells, where nutrients are broken down to release energy for cell repair, defence mechanisms and other processes that maintain the body.

REFLEXOLOGY AND THE CELLS

Reflexology can assist by increasing the circulation in the transportation of energy to all the cells of the body and in removal of the waste products, thereby helping to prevent disease. Remember that everything you do in life has an effect on the cells of your body.

The skin

The skin covers and protects the contents of your body, as well as holding everything together. It gathers sensory information from the environment through nerve endings close to the surface and plays an active role in protecting you from disease. Skin also helps to keep the body at just the right temperature.

Skin may develop tumours or be affected by an inadequate blood supply. It can become infected with bacteria, parasites, viruses and fungi, and may be irritated by chemicals or other substances with which it comes into contact. So don't put anything on your skin that you would not put in your mouth!

Skin structure

The epidermis is the outside layer of the skin and comprises layers of cells, with a basal layer that is always forming new cells through cell division. The new cells move towards the surface (which takes around one to two months) and, as they do so, the outermost layer of flat, dead cells is worn away. The epidermis varies in thickness, and is thicker on the soles of the feet and palms of the hands (1.5 mm) and thinner on the eyelids (0.05 mm).

The dermis is the layer underneath, and is composed entirely of living cells. It consists of bundles of tough fibres, which give your skin its elasticity and strength. Its most important function is respiration. There are also blood vessels here, feeding vital nutrients to these areas. The nerve endings in the dermis protect you by telling the brain if your skin is in contact with too much heat, cold, pressure or pain.

REFLEXOLOGY AND THE SKIN

Reflexology can help to revitalize the condition of the skin by encouraging an adequate blood and nerve supply that reaches all parts of it. It can also reduce the incidences of skin-related conditions such as acne, by stabilizing the production of sebum and keeping bacteria levels under control.

The skin contains sebaceous glands, which produce an oily substance known as sebum that helps to make the skin waterproof and prevent it drying out. The acid mantle on the surface of the skin is made up of sebum and sweat, creating a protective coating against bacteria and preventing infection and disease.

Cell division

Body cells can detect how crowded they are – this is called cell density. When cell density decreases, cell division occurs to make new cells; when it increases, the rate of cell division slows down. This process is usually strictly controlled in the body, but occasionally the control mechanism fails and cell division continues at an abnormally high rate. This is how the tumours in cancer occur.

Cell division is important in skin repair after a cut or other injury. On the cut surface, cell division is stimulated and new cells fill the gap.

THE SKIN

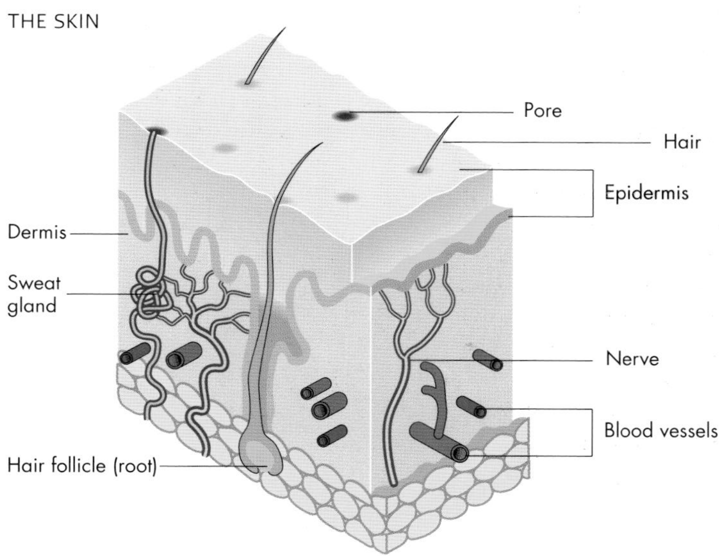

The skeleton

The bones that make up the skeleton are very strong and light. They are at risk of fractures and postural deformities, which may be caused by environmental or congenital factors or by disease. Bones provide protection to the internal organs, as well as supporting the body's structure. They also store most of the calcium, magnesium, phosphorus and other minerals that the body needs. The bones of your skeleton are very much alive, growing and changing all the time, just like other parts of your body.

Skeletal structure

A baby's body has about 300 bones at birth and, as they grow, the bones get bigger and eventually fuse to form 206 adult bones. Cartilage, a special material that is soft and flexible, is slowly replaced by bone, with the help of calcium that is absorbed from the intestines. This process becomes complete at around the age of 22, following which there is no further growth in the length of bones.

More than half the bones in the human skeleton are found in the hands and feet; each hand has 27 bones. While some bones (such as the femur, or thigh bone) are very large, the smallest (the stirrup bone in the ear) is the size of half a grain of rice. A bone's strength or size is determined by its function.

The skeleton consists of two parts:

- **The axial skeleton**, including the skull, vertebral column, sternum and ribs, supports the head, neck and torso.
- **The appendicular skeleton**, including the shoulder girdle, upper and lower limbs and pelvic girdle, supports and attaches the limbs to the rest of the body.

REFLEXOLOGY AND THE SKELETON

Reflexology can help the distribution and absorption of vitamin D and minerals into the bones, to promote a healthy skeleton. It can also ease the aching joints associated with arthritis, improving mobility and helping to heal fractures.

The spine

The spine or backbone lets you twist and bend and holds your body upright. It also protects the spinal cord, a large bundle of nerves that sends information from your brain to the rest of your body. It is the central support for the body, and consists of separate irregular bones known as vertebrae. These comprise spongy bone surrounded by a layer of compact bone. In between each vertebra is a layer of cartilage (the 'disc') that keeps the bones from rubbing against each other.

There are 26 vertebrae in the spine, seven cervical vertebrae in the neck, 12 thoracic vertebrae in the ribcage and five large lumbar vertebrae that take the weight of the body. There are also five fused bones in the pelvis called the sacral vertebrae or sacrum, as well as the coccygeal vertebrae, four bones forming the coccyx. Although each vertebra can move only a little bit, the total spine is very flexible. A healthy spine is curved, enabling it to balance the human body on just two legs.

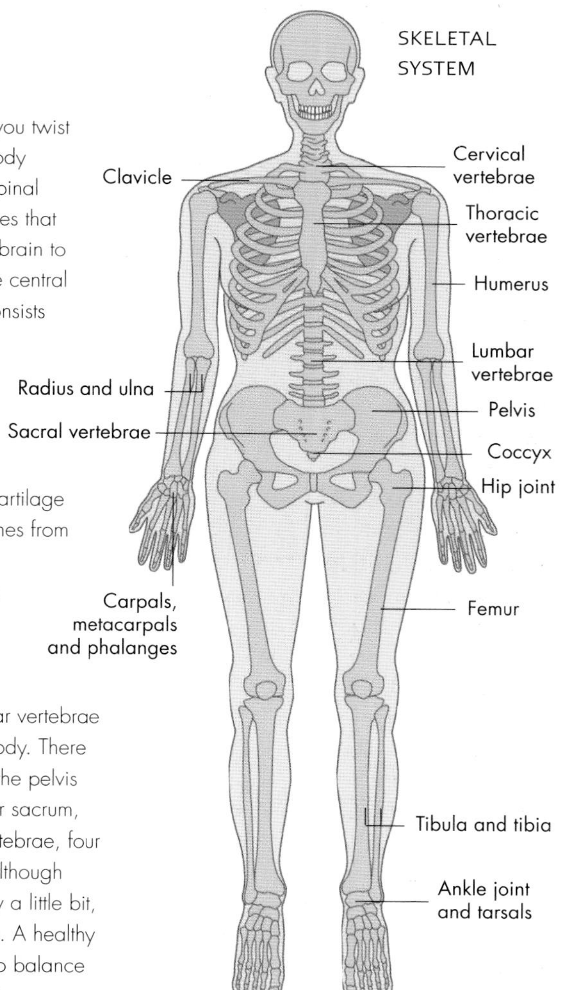

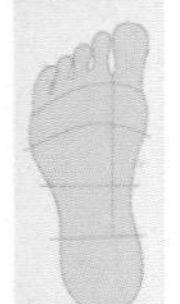

The circulatory system

The circulatory system is responsible for transporting materials throughout the body. It conveys nutrients, water and oxygen to the billions of body cells, and carries away waste such as carbon dioxide. Blood is the body's fuel and is delivered by the circulatory system – it is like a postal system throughout the body, delivering essential nutrients and oxygen to power the cells while taking away debris.

Components

The circulatory system is made up of muscle and vessels that help control the flow of blood around the body. The main parts of this system are the heart, arteries, veins and capillaries.

The heart is really a special muscle and is the circulatory system's engine, pumping blood around the body. It is usually located a little to the left of the middle of your chest, and is about the size of a fist. The right side of the heart receives blood from the body and pumps it to the lungs, a process known as pulmonary circulation. The left side does the exact opposite: it receives blood from the lungs and pumps it out to the body, a process known as systemic circulation.

Arteries and veins are the circulatory system's pipes, transporting blood around the body. Arteries are blood vessels that carry oxygen-rich blood away from the heart, while veins carry blood back towards the heart. Capillaries are tiny blood vessels, thinner than human hairs, that connect arteries to veins. Oxygen, nutrients and waste products pass in and out of the blood through the capillary walls.

Heartbeat and pulse

When we are young, our heartbeat is faster, but as we get older it gradually

REFLEXOLOGY AND CIRCULATION

Reflexology can help increase the circulation, thereby preventing a sluggish blood flow that could result in clotting. The relaxation aspect of reflexology treatment can help to prevent high blood pressure, angina, heart attacks and strokes.

slows down. Have you ever considered how blood comes back up your legs to the heart to become reoxygenated? This occurs through muscular action – the action of your calf muscles as you move keeps the blood flowing. So exercise can keep the blood circulating around your body, from your fingers or toes to your heart and back again.

Feel your pulse by placing two fingers at pulse points on your neck or wrists. The pulse you feel is blood stopping and starting as it moves through your arteries. As a child, your resting pulse might have ranged from 90 to 120 beats per minute; as a healthy adult, it slows to an average of 72 beats per minute. Your body has about 5.6 litres (10 pints) of blood circulating through it three times every minute. In one day, the blood travels a total of 19,300 km (12,000 miles).

MAJOR BLOOD VESSELS

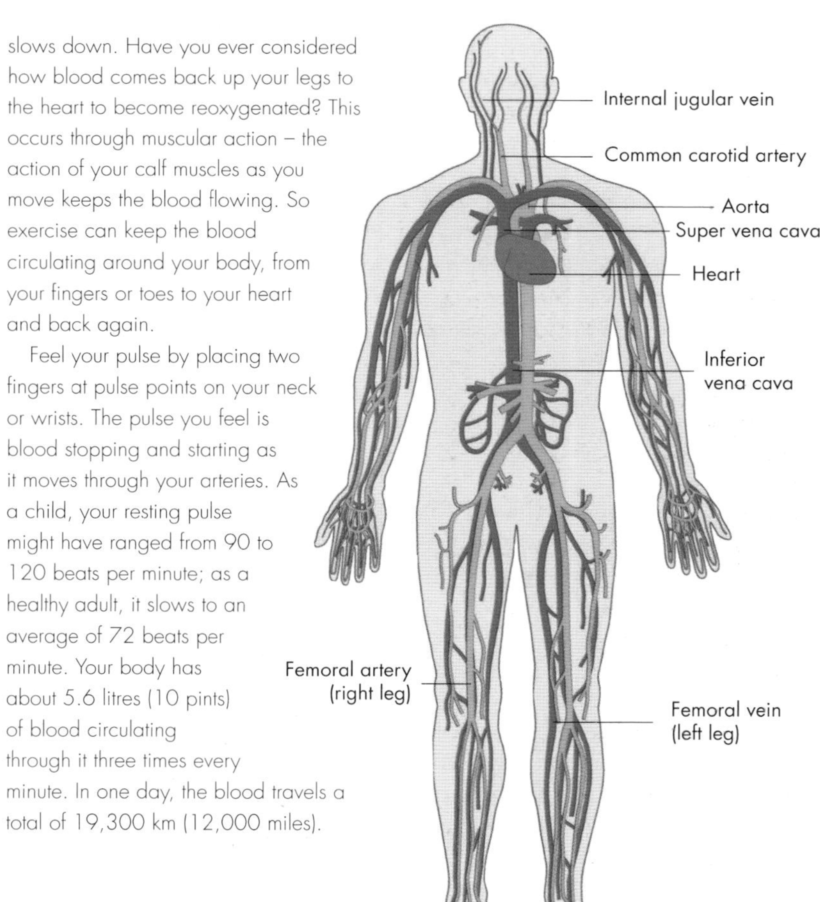

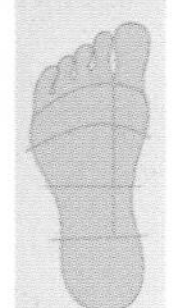

The digestive system

The digestive system is a series of hollow organs joined in a long, twisting tube from the mouth to the anus, and is responsible for eating, digestion and excretion. Digestion is the process by which food and drink are broken down into their smallest parts, so that the body can use them to build and nourish cells and provide energy.

When we eat, most of the foods are not in a form that the body can use as nourishment. Our food and drink must be changed into smaller molecules before they can be absorbed into the blood and carried to cells throughout the body. The digestive system contains a number of organs responsible for changing food chemically in order to enable their absorption by body tissues. The process involves breaking food down into simple soluble substances that are absorbable. Ask yourself each time you eat: 'What nutritional value does this food have for my body?'

REFLEXOLOGY AND DIGESTION

After a reflexology treatment it is common to have a bowel movement, which cleans out the colon. Sometimes this waste can be responsible for raising cholesterol and oestrogen levels in the body. Removing waste products efficiently leads to better health and well-being, and proper absorption of the nourishment from food.

Components

The series of structures that transform the foods we eat into substances that can be used by the body for growth, repair and energy include the mouth, salivary glands, oesophagus, stomach, liver, gall bladder, pancreas, small and large intestines and anus. After digestion, the intestinal walls absorb the nutrient molecules, which are then circulated around the body. The food that does not get digested becomes waste matter and is excreted as faeces.

Digestion incorporates both physical and chemical processes. The physical processes include chewing to reduce food to small particles, the churning action of

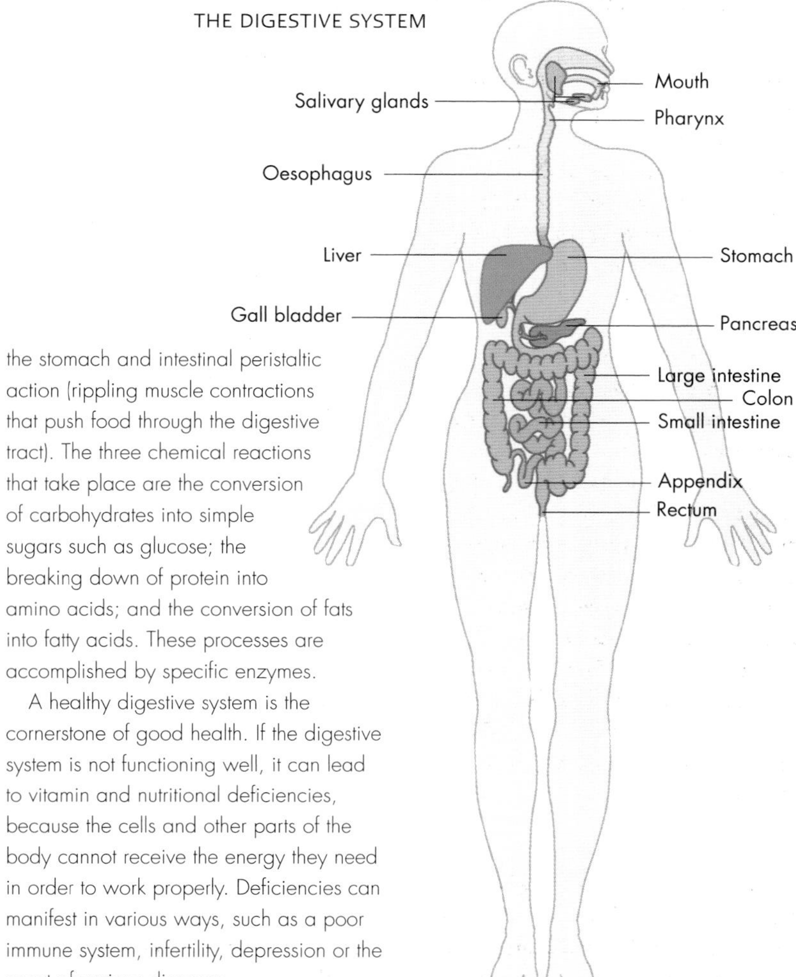

the stomach and intestinal peristaltic action (rippling muscle contractions that push food through the digestive tract). The three chemical reactions that take place are the conversion of carbohydrates into simple sugars such as glucose; the breaking down of protein into amino acids; and the conversion of fats into fatty acids. These processes are accomplished by specific enzymes.

A healthy digestive system is the cornerstone of good health. If the digestive system is not functioning well, it can lead to vitamin and nutritional deficiencies, because the cells and other parts of the body cannot receive the energy they need in order to work properly. Deficiencies can manifest in various ways, such as a poor immune system, infertility, depression or the onset of various diseases.

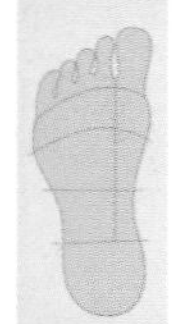

The nervous system

The nervous system coordinates the activities of the muscles throughout the body, monitors the organs, sends messages to and from the senses and initiates actions. Communication between the billions of nerve cells occurs through chemical and electrical signals, and that is why drugs, alcohol and electromagnetic frequencies can affect us. The nervous system relays messages to and from the brain, and in this way the body reacts and protects itself.

Components

There are two main parts of the nervous system in the human body, called the central nervous system and the peripheral nervous system. The central nervous system is made up of the brain and spinal cord, while the peripheral nerves connect the central nervous system to the rest of the body. The peripheral nervous system is made up of the following divisions:

- **The somatic system or sensory division**, which consists of sensory nerve fibres that relay information about inner-body sensations and events occurring in the outside world.
- **The autonomic system**, which is responsible for unconscious activities in the body, such as digestion and breathing; it consists of the parasympathetic and sympathetic systems.

The sympathetic division prepares the body for stress, which is the primitive 'fight-or-flight' response. When this division is activated, you may be aware of a racing heart or faster breathing and your digestive system may play up. The parasympathetic division focuses on maintaining and creating homeostasis, which is the body's natural state of balance. Reflexology aims to switch on the parasympathetic nervous system response.

The hypothalamus area at the base of the brain connects the autonomic and the endocrine systems (see page 72). It works with the pituitary gland to help regulate the body's temperature, food intake and water/salt balance, blood pressure, blood flow, the sleep/wake cycle, sexual behaviour and the activities of hormones.

REFLEXOLOGY AND THE NERVES

Reflexology helps to open up neural pathways, assisting in the control of stress levels and has an analgesic affect, reducing pain by releasing endorphins (natural painkillers) into the system.

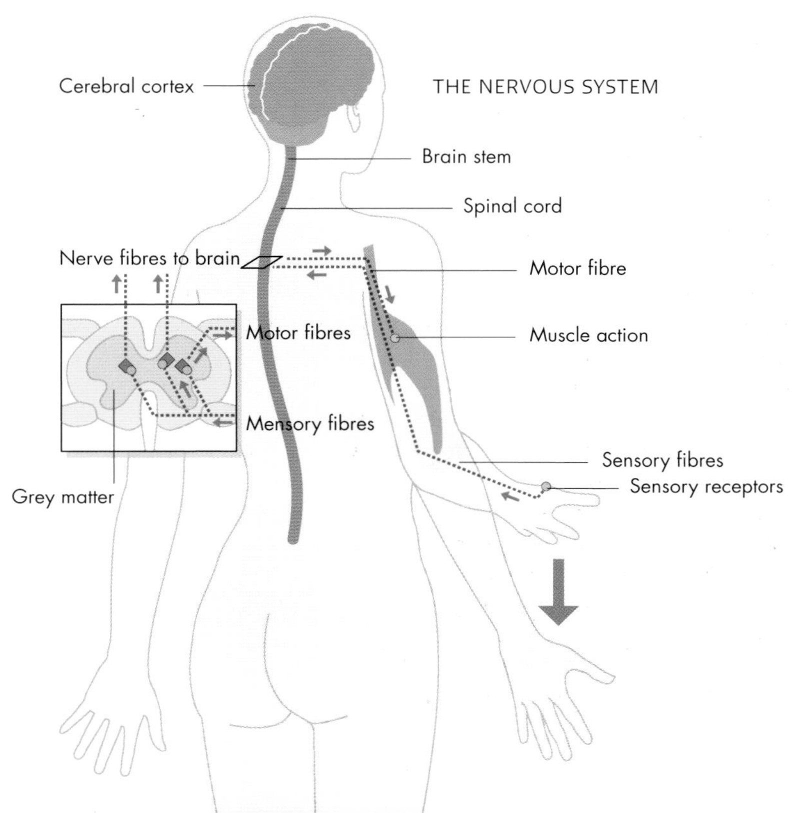

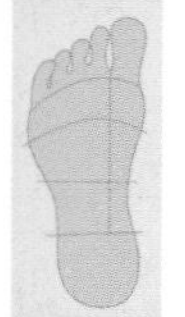

The endocrine system

The endocrine system is made up of ductless glands that secrete hormones directly into the bloodstream. Hormones are the body's internal chemical messengers, which carry information that control the rate at which the body functions and how the glands and organs work. They also control our behaviour.

Each gland produces a specific hormone that fulfils a particular task – this includes regulating metabolism, blood-sugar levels, our response to stress and when ovulation occurs.

Components

The major glands and functions of the endocrine system include:

- **The pituitary gland:** This is connected to the hypothalamus (see page 71); its functions include regulating height and growth, controlling the adrenal cortex, regulating blood pressure, controlling sexual development, controlling ovulation, stimulating sperm production and the production of oestrogen and testosterone; it also regulates the production of breast milk and initiates labour.
- **The thyroid gland:** This controls energy levels, weight and the absorption of calcium in our bones.
- **The parathyroid glands:** These maintain healthy bones.
- **The adrenal glands:** These regulate blood pressure and the level of salts in the body, especially sodium chloride and potassium; they also provide hydrocortisone, which helps reduce inflammation and pain, and the hormone androgen, which stimulates the development of male characteristics;

REFLEXOLOGY AND THE HORMONES

Reflexology can help with the distribution and balance of the hormones in the body. The treatment works non-invasively on the endocrine glands to help regulate the production of hormones. An effective treatment can help increase energy levels, stabilize moods, help control eating habits and alleviate menstrual or menopausal issues.

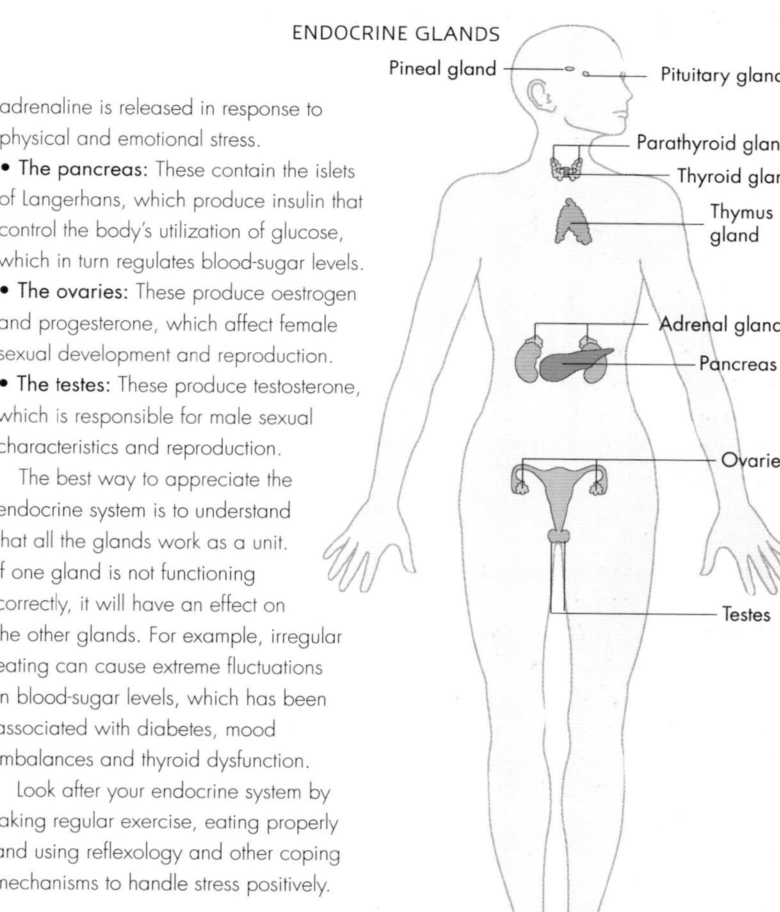

adrenaline is released in response to physical and emotional stress.

- **The pancreas:** These contain the islets of Langerhans, which produce insulin that control the body's utilization of glucose, which in turn regulates blood-sugar levels.
- **The ovaries:** These produce oestrogen and progesterone, which affect female sexual development and reproduction.
- **The testes:** These produce testosterone, which is responsible for male sexual characteristics and reproduction.

The best way to appreciate the endocrine system is to understand that all the glands work as a unit. If one gland is not functioning correctly, it will have an effect on the other glands. For example, irregular eating can cause extreme fluctuations in blood-sugar levels, which has been associated with diabetes, mood imbalances and thyroid dysfunction.

Look after your endocrine system by taking regular exercise, eating properly and using reflexology and other coping mechanisms to handle stress positively.

The lymphatic system

The lymphatic system is entwined with the circulation of the blood, and is a system of vessels that drains a colourless liquid called lymph from all over the body back into the bloodstream. It plays a major role in the immune system and defends us against disease and infection; it is the body's own security system, constantly guarding the body.

Components

The lymphatic system consists of thin tubes that run throughout the body carrying lymph. Lymph is generally moved by exercise and deep breathing, and obstruction of lymphatic flow results in oedema – swelling of the tissues due to the collection of excess fluid. Lymph circulates around the body and contains a number of white blood cells. Plasma comes from the capillaries (see page 66) and bathes the body tissues, then drains into the lymph vessels and empties back into the blood circulation.

Lymph nodes are scattered around the body and contain scavenging white blood cells that ingest bacteria, as well as other foreign matter and debris. These nodes filter lymph, destroying harmful micro-organisms, tumour cells, damaged or dead tissue cells and toxins. Lymph from most tissues and organs crosses lymph nodes to become filtered, before draining into the bloodstream. Swollen lymph nodes normally indicate disease. There are lymph nodes in the armpits, neck, groin, abdomen, pelvis and chest.

The lymphatic system also includes the spleen, tonsils, adenoids and thymus gland. The job of the spleen is to filter the blood to remove old, worn-out blood cells and destroy them; these are then replaced by new red blood cells made in the bone marrow. The spleen also filters out

REFLEXOLOGY AND LYMPH

Regular reflexology can help boost the lymphatic system, which means that the body will have an increased ability to fight off illness and disease. It promotes a reduction in the number of colds and helps you stay healthier for longer.

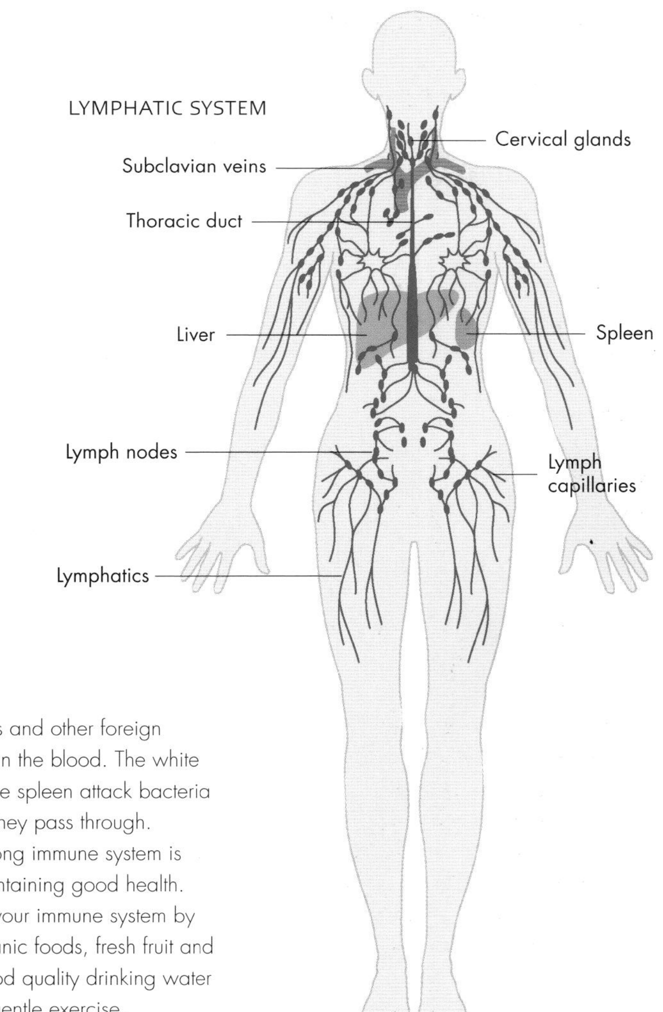

bacteria, viruses and other foreign particles found in the blood. The white blood cells in the spleen attack bacteria and viruses as they pass through.

Having a strong immune system is essential in maintaining good health. You can boost your immune system by consuming organic foods, fresh fruit and vegetables, good quality drinking water and by taking gentle exercise.

The respiratory system

The body's cells require oxygen in order to function properly, so the respiratory system is the body's breathing equipment. It contains the lungs, air passages, pulmonary (lung) vessels and breathing muscles. Haemoglobin (an oxygen-carrying compound) found in red blood cells continually removes dissolved oxygen from the blood and binds with it to transport it around the body. Carbon dioxide is removed by the respiratory system and is a waste product of the body's tissues.

Components

External respiration starts at the nose and mouth. The nose moistens and warms air entering the nostrils. This warming of air is very important for asthma sufferers who find that going out into the cold air triggers an attack; by breathing through the nose instead of the mouth, they can avoid this type of attack because, as the nose warms the air, it prevents the sudden rush of cold air into the lungs.

The trachea (windpipe) extends from the neck into the thorax (chest cavity), where it divides into right and left main bronchi (air passages), which enter the right and left lungs. The left lung is smaller, because it

REFLEXOLOGY AND THE LUNGS

Reflexology can help to improve the function of the diaphragm and lungs, increasing the quantity of air being breathed in and of waste products being breathed out. It also assists in the distribution of oxygen around the body. Reflexology can help aid recovery from respiratory conditions such as asthma, bronchitis, emphysema, influenza and the common cold. A helpful tip is that a relaxed person takes deep breaths, while a nervous person takes shallow breaths. If you take deep breaths while working on the solar plexus reflex on the hand, this can help to relax you.

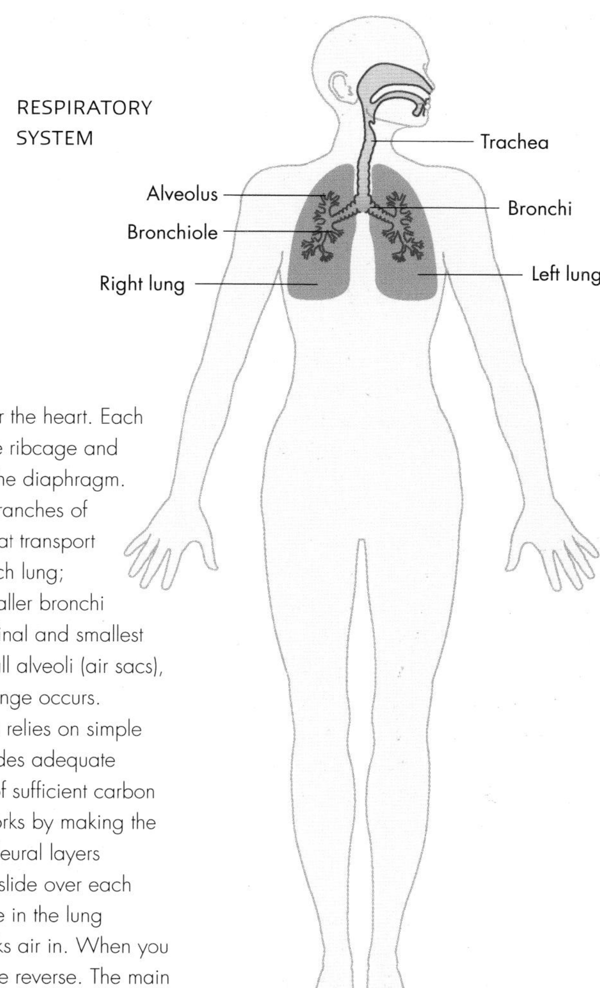

has to allow space for the heart. Each lung is enclosed in the ribcage and supported below by the diaphragm. The bronchi are the branches of the respiratory tube that transport air into and out of each lung; they break up into smaller bronchi and bronchioles (the final and smallest tubes) and end in small alveoli (air sacs), where gaseous exchange occurs.

Gaseous exchange relies on simple diffusion, which provides adequate oxygen and gets rid of sufficient carbon dioxide. Breathing works by making the ribcage bigger: the pleural layers surrounding the lungs slide over each other, and the pressure in the lung decreases, which sucks air in. When you breathe out, it does the reverse. The main muscle of breathing is the diaphragm.

The urinary system

The body is made up of about 65 per cent water, which is therefore our most important nutrient. Certain tissues – like the white blood cells, skeletal muscles and skin – contain the largest amount of water. We lose around 1.5 litres (2½ pints) of water a day through the intestines, skin, breathing, sweat and as urine.

Water is the solution that many chemical reactions need in order to take place in. It also helps to supply nutrients and hormones between the body cells and distributes heat around the body. During our daily activities we are exposed to harmful substances, and the kidneys use water to help dilute these so that we can stay healthy. We need to drink around 2 litres (3½ pints) a day to maintain the healthy functioning of the kidneys.

REFLEXOLOGY AND THE KIDNEYS

Reflexology helps the urinary system with the distribution of water around the body by improving its circulation. The treatment can also aid the functioning of the kidneys and the removal of waste and sodium. Reflexology can be effective in reducing water retention and combating urinary-tract infections.

Components

The urinary system consists of the kidneys, from which urine is formed to carry away waste material and blood; the ureters, which carry urine from the kidneys; the bladder, which stores the urine until it can be disposed of; and the urethra, through which the bladder is emptied to the outside. This system uses a combination of filtration and excretion to dispose of harmful waste products such as alcohol and urea from our body.

Under the influence of hormones, the two kidneys produce urine and keep the body's inner chemistry in balance. They excrete excess sodium, which is associated with raised blood pressure; as sodium levels in the body rise, fluids become less concentrated by retaining more water, and this can cause fluid retention and oedema.

The ureters transport urine from the kidney to the bladder. Ureteritis is an inflammation of the ureter, which may be caused by a blockage of the ureter by a stone or by the spread of infection from the bladder. The bladder itself is a hollow, muscular organ that collects and stores urine. The urethra is a slender tube that passes from the bladder to the outside of the body. The male urethra is much longer than the female urethra (it runs the length of the penis) and passes through the prostate gland.

Natural remedies

Chamomile tea is a natural diuretic – it helps to reduce water retention. Dandelion tea cleanses the blood and is also diuretic, making it the ideal tea to drink during a detoxification programme. Salt in the diet is associated with high blood pressure; a good alternative is Solo sea salt, which contains 46 per cent less sodium than normal salt.

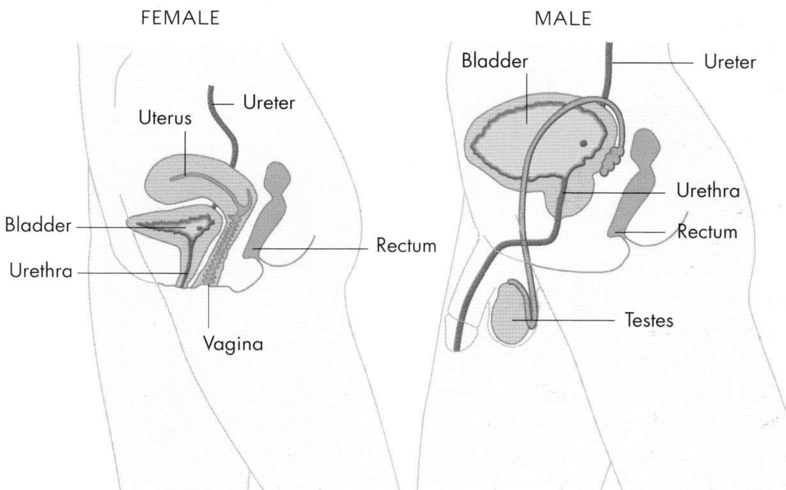

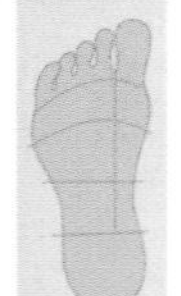

The reproductive system

The primary biological function of humans is to produce babies so that we can continue the species. We do this by the fusion of a male sperm cell and a female ovum. This fusion may be the result of sexual intercourse, assisted conception or IVF (*in vitro* fertilization) and is known as fertilization.

Male reproductive system

The organs of the male reproductive system are essentially those that enable a man's sperm to reproduce with a woman's ovum. The sperm and male sex hormones are made in the testes, which are a pair of ovoid glands suspended in a pouch called the scrotum. During erection, sperm pass via the vas deferens into the seminal vesicle. The prostate gland in men is located at the base of (under) the bladder and surrounds the urethra, and looks like a ring donut. The function of the prostate is to produce milky secretions that form part of the seminal fluid. These secretions increase the volume of the semen, which is ejaculated from the erect penis.

Female reproductive system

This system includes all the organs that enable a woman to ovulate, have sexual intercourse, nourish and develop a fertilized ovum, support it until it has grown into a fully grown fetus and give birth. A woman's reproductive organs can be found in the pelvic cavity, with the exception of the vulva, which comprise external genitalia. The ovaries are two

REFLEXOLOGY AND THE REPRODUCTIVE SYSTEM

The human reproductive process is complex, but fascinating. In order to accomplish pregnancy, the processes of ovulation and fertilization have to be in balance, but for so many couples trying to have a baby something can go wrong. Reflexology and a holistic approach to health can balance the hormones, create healthier sperm and enhance regular ovulation.

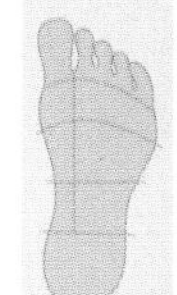

egg-shaped glands that secrete female sex hormones, including oestrogen and progesterone, which control the woman's reproductive cycle. Each month a woman of child bearing years should release an ovum from one of the ovaries, which is carried along the Fallopian tube to the uterus. The uterus is a hollow muscular organ in the pelvic cavity, situated behind and above the bladder in front of the rectum, and provides a suitable environment in which the fetus can grow. If fertilized by a sperm, the ovum begins to divide and implants into the lining of the uterus, to develop into an embryo. At birth the baby is forced out of the cervix, the narrow passage that forms the neck of the uterus. The function of the female reproductive system begins at puberty with the start of menstruation and ends at the menopause.

FEMALE REPRODUCTIVE SYSTEM MALE

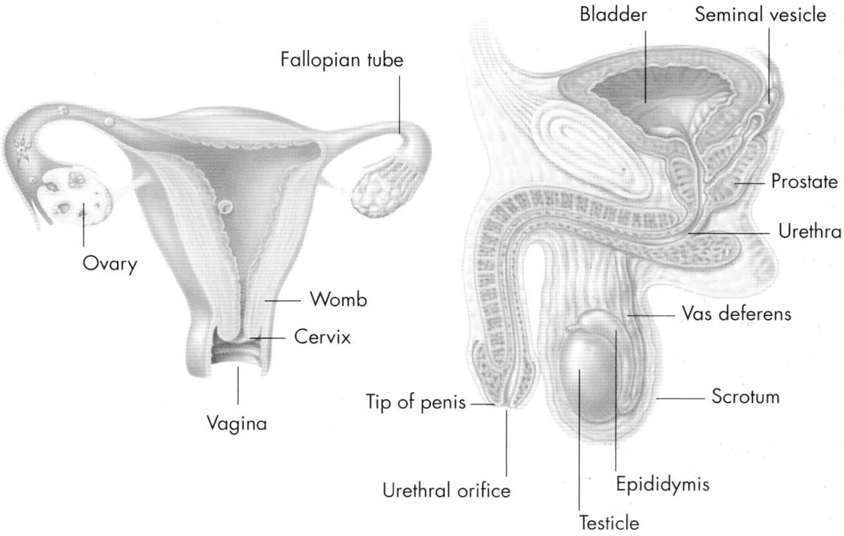

Fallopian tube
Ovary
Womb
Cervix
Vagina

Bladder
Seminal vesicle
Prostate
Urethra
Vas deferens
Scrotum
Tip of penis
Urethral orifice
Epididymis
Testicle

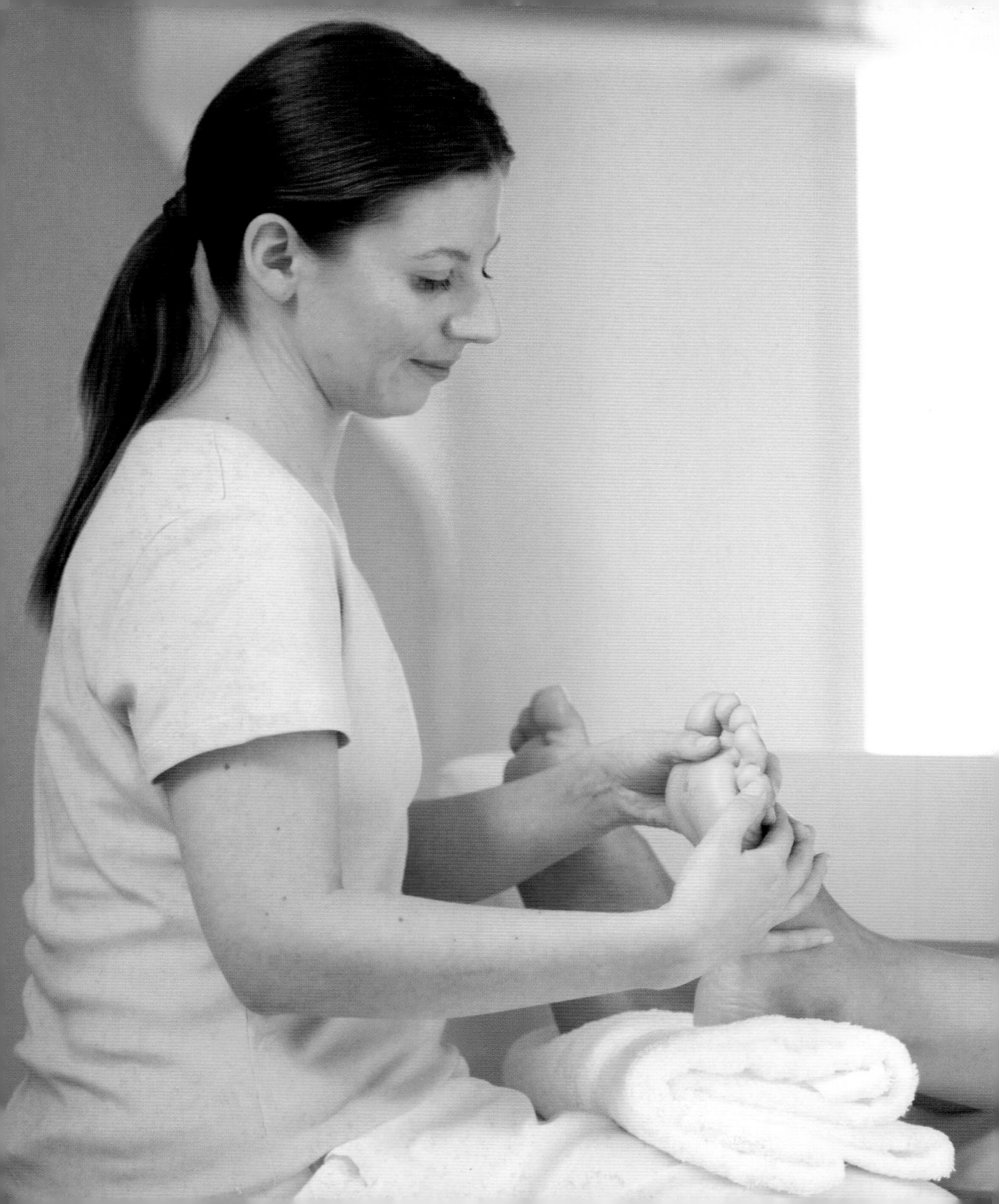

PART 3

Reflexology preparation

What the feet reveal

Our feet reveal our state of health, and often the problems we suffer with our feet relate to problems in the body. How we lead our lives, what we eat and drink, how we exercise and how we feel may all be reflected in what a reflexologist finds on the feet. For example, tense feet may indicate tension in the body, while limp feet may point to poor muscle tone. Cold, bluish or reddish feet may indicate poor circulation. Someone with sweaty feet (especially if they are also smelly) may have a problem with their hormones. Puffiness and swelling around the ankle can be related to a number of internal problems and should be examined by a doctor.

Not looking after your feet can result in corns, blisters, ingrowing toenails and bunions, which can affect posture and metabolism. Conversely, some reflexologists feel that a poor metabolism and posture can cause these conditions. Foot problems are suffered by as much as two-thirds of the population. It is important to be aware of some of the most common foot conditions, so that you can refer the sufferer to a chiropodist.

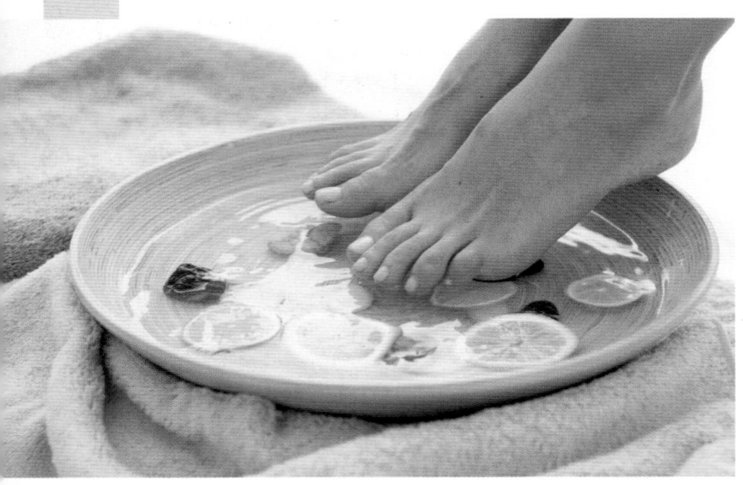

Your feet can reflect your state of health, and can also reveal physical problems in other parts of the body.

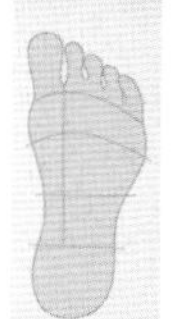

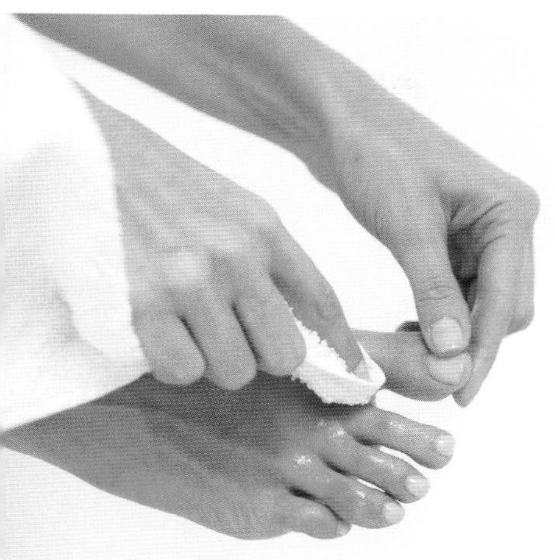

Drying thoroughly in between the toes is a practical way of avoiding the fungal condition athlete's foot.

Athlete's foot

This fungal condition affects the skin at the base of, or between, the toes. The skin becomes itchy and sore, and sometimes there is cracking, peeling of the skin or flaking, especially between the fourth and fifth toes. There may also be white soggy areas, and the feet may have a distinctive, unpleasant smell. Causes include inadequate ventilation of the feet; going barefoot in public baths or showers where infection spreads; not drying adequately in between the toes; or using an infected towel or bathmat.

Athlete's foot sometimes clears up without medication, but most fungal infections will respond to antifungal drugs prescribed by a chiropodist. Aftercare includes changing the socks or stockings frequently, drying carefully in between the toes, avoiding shared towels and wearing well-ventilated shoes. When applying reflexology, avoid the contagious area or, if it is very bad, treat the hands instead.

Verruca

A verruca appears as a raised area of skin, due to an increase in the size of the cells of which the skin tissue is composed. Also known as a plantar wart, it is thought to be caused by a virus.

Advice for treating a verruca naturally includes rubbing a garlic clove on it, then covering it with duct tape, which inhibits its oxygen supply. Or cover it with a small piece of the inside of a banana skin, and tape this into position so that it does not fall off overnight; repeat nightly for two to three weeks for the best results. To avoid cross-infection when treating someone with a verruca, cover the contagious area with

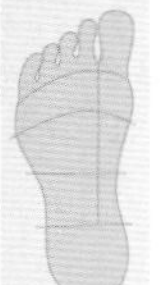

a plaster or avoid it altogether and refer the sufferer to a chiropodist.

Bunion

A bunion is a thickened, fluid-filled bursa or sac overlying the joint at the base of the big toe (or occasionally the fifth toe). It may be painful and inflamed. The cause might be persistent pressure or friction from an outside agent, displacement of the foot due to high-heeled shoes, inherited joint weakness or an injury to the joint.

Treatment for bunions includes wearing properly fitting footwear, a protective pad to ease the discomfort or, as a last resort, surgery to remove them.

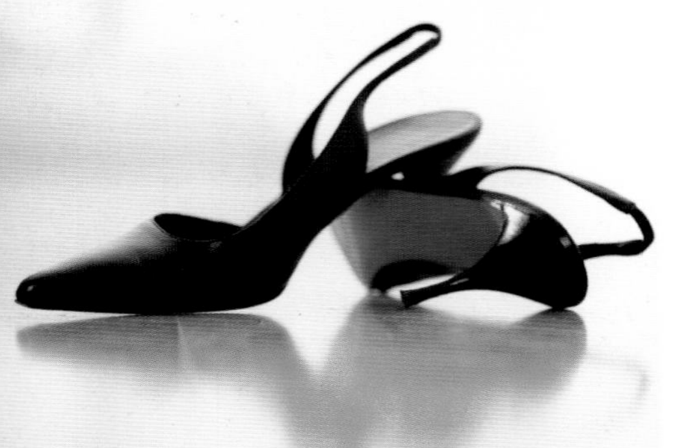

High-heeled shoes can cause the calf muscle to shorten, so you may find it painful to wear flat shoes.

Ingrowing toenail

A lot of young people in their teens and twenties are affected by this painful condition of the big toe, in which one or both edges of the nail penetrates the adjacent skin. The nail becomes embedded in the soft skin tissue, which may lead to bleeding, infection and inflammation. It usually results from cutting the toenail too short or cutting down the sides of the nail. Tight, ill-fitting shoes, heredity or poor personal hygiene can also cause it.

If the condition is chronic, a chiropodist will trim a small section of the nail to relieve pressure from the ingrowing toenail. If the condition is acute (meaning that it is red, swollen and possibly infected), surgical removal of a section or of the whole of the nail plate may be necessary.

Corn

A corn is a concentrated area of hard skin and is the most common skin problem on feet. It is cone-shaped and has no root. It often develops as a means of protection: at the focal point of pressure the skin hardens and thickens. A hard corn is a plug of hard skin, usually found on the tops of the toes and sole of the foot, especially on the ball; it shows that the

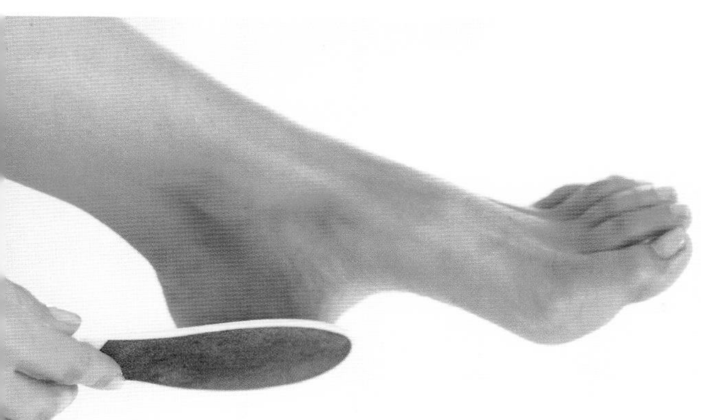

Rubbing away hard skin should be a regular part of your bath-time routine.

skin is being rubbed and pressed too much. A soft corn can be found between the toes and sometimes underneath the nails; it is caused by too much pressure, combined with excess sweat and is sometimes painful.

Corns can be prevented by wearing roomy shoes. A podiatrist can remove a hard corn easily and fit a pad or insole to ease the pressure, which should stop it coming back. The treatment for soft corns is drying the skin out by applying surgical spirit every day. If the corn is painful, it can be removed by a podiatrist or protected by a small removable pad.

Callus

A callus is an area of thickened, sometimes hornlike skin and is yellow or dark-brown and discoloured. It often appears on the big toes, tops of the toes, heels or ball of the foot, because they are weight-bearing. If aggravated by persistent pressure, it can become painful. Foot calluses are common because we subject our feet to a great deal of pressure on a daily basis.

The causes are tight, ill-fitting shoes, regular prolonged pressure or friction, such as jogging, extended standing or uneven body weight. Treatment includes wearing properly fitting shoes, paring away thickened areas of skin or placing a moulded insole in the shoe. Using a pumice stone and moisturizing the foot twice a day can help to get rid of a callus. Add moisturizing your feet to your bath-time routine.

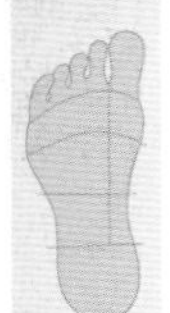

What the nails reveal

Did you know that nails grow faster when hormone levels fluctuate, such as during pregnancy or just before menstruation? On average, nails grow about 3 mm (⅛ in) per month, but nail growth can be slowed or stopped during periods of severe illness. When a nail starts to regrow it is thinner, so there is a line running across it known as a Beau's line, caused by an interruption in the protein formation of the nail plate.

Nails are mostly made from a fibrous protein called keratin, which is also found in the hair. Often people who suffer from alopecia (hair loss) find that their nails become thin too, or even drop off. It is the fat and water molecules between the layers of keratin that makes nails flexible and shiny.

Looking after the nails

Nail hygiene is important, so if you go for a pedicure, make sure that you choose a reputable salon with spotless instruments. Viral infections such as hepatitis B and C and warts can be transmitted by improperly sterilized instruments.

When applying nail varnish, it is recommended that you always use a clear base coat first, to prevent the nails yellowing. Lemon juice is an excellent natural way to remove stains on the nail body: simply mix the juice of one lemon with half a cup of warm water and soak for 20 minutes.

White spots on your nails could be a sign indicating that you are consuming too much sugar.

THE NAILS AND DIET

The nails are a reflection of the nutrition that goes into the body:

- Cuts and cracks in the nails may indicate that you need to drink more liquids. Try to drink at least eight glasses of water each day.
- Dry and brittle nails may indicate a lack of vitamin A and calcium in the body. Vitamin A is found in liver, cheese, eggs and rich, oily fish (especially sardines and pilchards). Calcium is found in milk, yoghurt, sardines, canned salmon, purple sprouting broccoli and cheese.
- Excessive dryness, very rounded and curved nail ends and darkening of the nails may indicate a lack of vitamin B12. Vegans are at a higher risk because B12 is only found in foods of animal origin, such as meat, fish and eggs.
- If the nail bed is pale, this may be a sign of anaemia, which is caused by a lack of red corpuscles in the blood – iron deficiency is the most common cause. Increase your intake of lean meat, sardines, liver, oily fish, dried apricots and leafy green vegetables.
- Nails that are spoon-shaped, concave or have ridges may indicate a diet that is deficient in iron. This is a disorder known as koilonychias, and a doctor will be able to perform a haemoglobin test to confirm iron levels. Good sources of iron are liver, oily fish, dried apricots and leafy green vegetables.

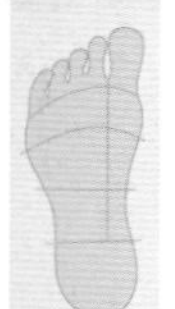

Treatment basics

The effects of a reflexology treatment are often experienced immediately after the session. For example, a client may notice that their headache has disappeared or a frozen shoulder has become much more mobile. But it may take three to five treatments to bring about complete (or considerable) improvement in a client's condition or complaint.

Generally, disorders that someone has suffered from for many years will take longer to improve. This means that a reflexologist and a client will commit to a treatment plan that spans a few months. The problem is that we live in a quick-fix society. Most people tend to expect immediate results, and a single treatment may not correct a problem that has been developing for years. A longer course of treatments is recommended for all conditions, ranging from twice a week to once a month.

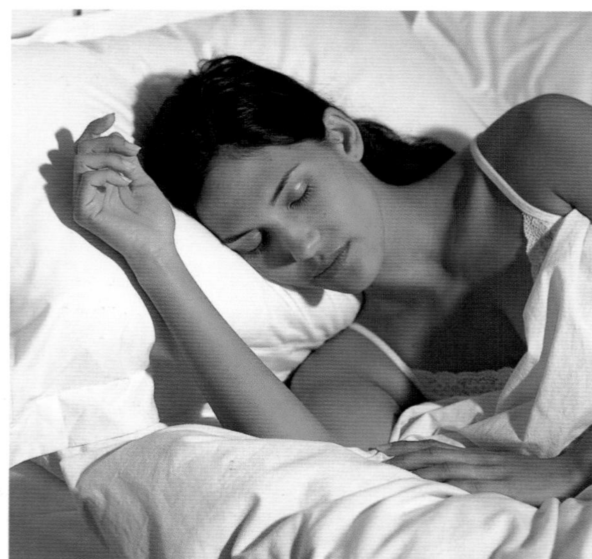

Reflexology is a powerful therapy that can help restore disturbed sleep patterns.

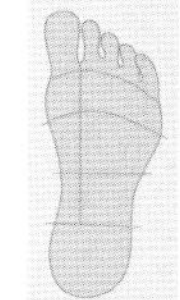

Understanding illness

Reflexology stimulates the body's own healing processes, and it can sometimes disrupt the body's ecology because it alters its internal environment. This often causes changes in body and mind as a result of treatment. Generally people find that after reflexology they sleep better, are more able to cope with life and see a reduction in the symptoms that were bothering them.

Reactions to treatment differ just as much as people themselves differ. Our lives, diet, exercise, emotions and health all affect the reactions we may experience following reflexology treatment. Generally, you can use reflexology on most people successfully; however, it is advisable not to treat those with the following contra-indications to foot reflexology:

- Contagious disease
- High fever
- Gangrene
- First trimester of pregnancy
- Deep-vein thrombosis.

Each condition that we suffer from lives with us and has its own pattern during the day. Illness is catalyzed by what you do – for example, the cup of coffee that aggravates a headache; skipping breakfast, which sets off irritable bowel syndrome; the new hand cream that activates dermatitis. However, the key to understanding illness is to focus on what you did before you were aware of the illness or before it got worse.

Reflexology works on emotional and mental levels as well as the physical body. It is common that treatment can release an emotional block, possibly stirring up repressed feelings. However, these emotions are normally only temporary.

CAUTION

- Avoid working on parts of the feet, ankles and legs where you see varicose veins, because you could further damage the veins.
- Always work around any areas of dermatitis or eczema; clients suffering from these conditions often prefer that you use oil rather than powder.

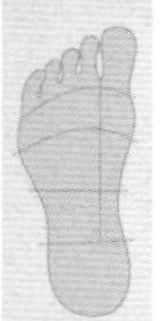

Reactions to reflexology

The first few reflexology treatments should always be given with a light touch, because this will reduce any possible healing crisis reaction, which some people may find uncomfortable.

Healing crisis reaction

Reflexology promotes the body's own healing mechanisms, so some type of response should be expected. Most people experience a sensation of well-being and feel energized, rejuvenated or deeply relaxed. But sometimes reflexology can bring about a 'healing crisis reaction', whereby symptoms may appear worse before they get better. This is a cleansing process as the body rids itself of toxins. You should look at this from a positive perspective; it can be an important turning point in the pattern of the illness.

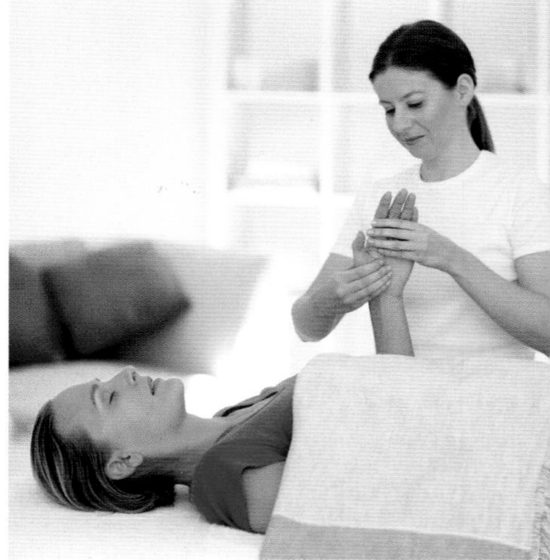

A gentle treatment will be less lilkely to cause a healing crisis reaction.

Clients who have a lot of impurities in their system, or who are going through an emotional time, are more likely to experience a healing crisis reaction. However, this usually passes within 24 hours and can be eased by drinking 2 litres (3½ pints) of water the day before, the day of the treatment and the day after. This helps to flush toxins out of the body and reduce the intensity of a healing crisis reaction. Such clients may also find treatment quite painful in some areas – in which case, reduce the pressure to avoid causing discomfort.

Hypersensitive response

Less common reactions during a treatment are known as a 'hypersensitive response' and may include sudden sweating, unusual chilliness, feelings of nausea,

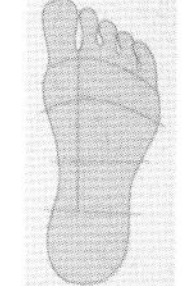

POTENTIAL TREATMENT REACTIONS

This list shows you the range of reactions that someone may experience following reflexology treatment:

- A temporary worsening of symptoms
- Feeling very relaxed
- Sleeping more soundly than usual
- Feeling cold
- Needing to sleep a lot
- Experiencing increased energy
- Feeling hot
- Increased urination/defecation
- A little diarrhoea
- Feeling emotional/upset
- Skin reactions
- Feeling irritable/restless
- Runny nose
- Feeling on a high
- Increased sweating from the hands and feet
- Nausea/dizziness
- Feeling thirsty

You might find that a client feels cold suddenly while receiving reflexology treatment. It is a good idea to cover them with a blanket before you start the session. And don't be surprised if someone falls asleep during treatment – this is perfectly natural.

faintness or distress. If necessary, you can stop the treatment at any time and open the window, give the client some water and generally meet the needs of the person you are working on.

Normally, however, people respond very favourably to treatment and often cannot believe what a positive effect reflexology has on their health, their emotional well-being and their interpersonal relationships. Whatever reactions your client experiences, they are a necessary part of the healing process and will generally pass within 24 hours.

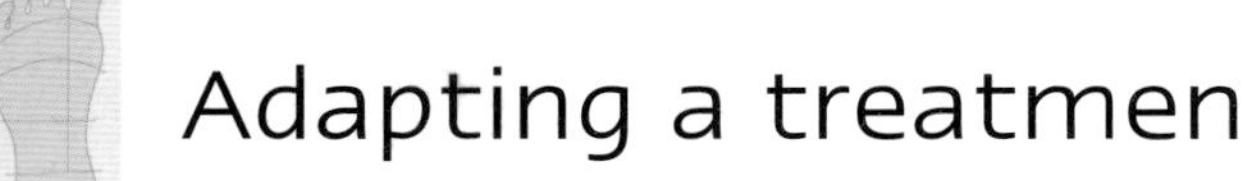

Adapting a treatment

Reflexology is cumulative, which means that the more treatments someone has, the greater effect it will have on their body. Most people have a course of treatments, and the pressure used during these sessions will alternate from soft to hard, depending on the conditions that are being worked on. There are, however, cases where you should adapt your treatment because of age or health issues.

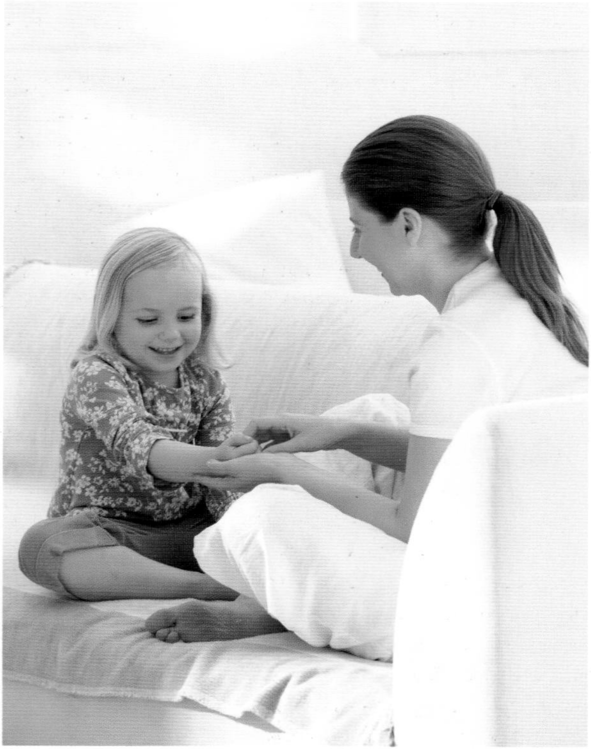

Giving your child a reflexology treatment can reinforce the bond between you.

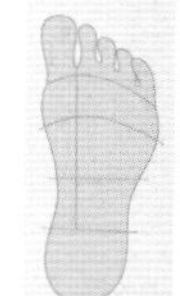

Sometimes you need to adopt a drip-feed method and work more lightly over a longer period of time, because for certain people it is better to avoid the discomfort of a healing crisis reaction (see page 92).

Treating children

The effects of reflexology on children are quite soporific, and treatments can help to reintroduce a bedtime routine with younger children, if necessary. Children's energies tend to be clearer and therefore they react to treatments more quickly. I always recommend lighter treatments for children under 16 – and don't forget to gain parental consent before you treat a minor.

Setting the scene before the treatment is important. The music and lighting that you use should be thought about carefully: light, classical music often works well to relax a child. You can have books or toys available, or ask a parent to come with a child's favourite toy. You will probably have to adjust your equipment, with more pillows, so that a child will be comfortable. A good method is to use oil on a child's feet. Your movements should be slow and relaxing – and how about telling a little story as you give treatment to a young child? You could make up a story about a little caterpillar munching its way through the garden as you use the walking technique (see page 130) with your thumb and fingers. For more about reflexology treatment for specific ailments in young children, see pages 322–335.

Treating older people

Reflexology aims to provide what the body needs – whether that is more energy, a more efficient body system, a better memory or a happier nature. As we get older our internal body energies are affected by poor posture, an inadequate diet, pollution, illness, negative thoughts, worries and stress. This leads to stagnation of the energy flow around the body and may create more toxins. Reflexology aims to eliminate toxins from the body. The more toxins the body contains, the greater chance there is of someone having a healing crisis reaction.

On older people, use a lighter pressure with a slow, gentle rhythm. Don't overwork any of the reflexes – which means only staying on a particular reflex for around five seconds and then moving on to the next part of the sequence. Spend more time on relaxation techniques at the

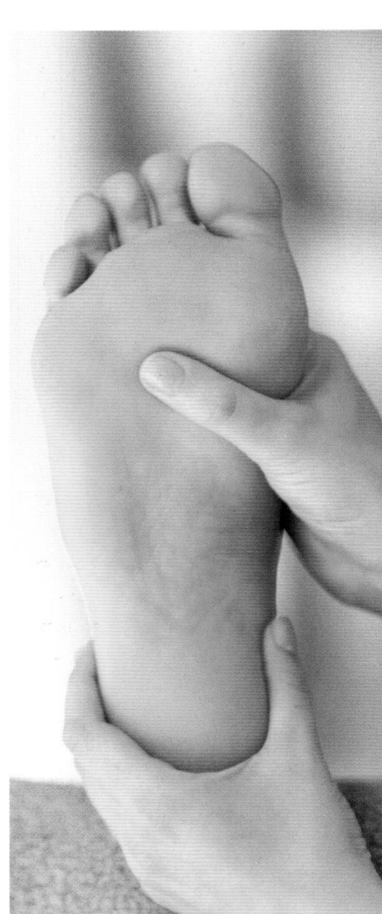

You can treat a client twice a day with gentle pressure if needed.

beginning and end of treatment; you may want to spend ten minutes of your actual treatment time on this. For more about reflexology treatment for the golden years, see pages 336–345.

Reducing pain

If someone is suffering from a painful condition, reflexology can help to reduce the feeling of pain by stimulating the production of endorphins, the body's natural painkillers. Endorphins are produced by the pituitary gland (see page 72) and are ten times more powerful than the drug morphine. Working lightly can encourage the brain to produce endorphins, while minimizing the possibility of aggravating the pain. You should pay special attention to the pituitary reflex (see page 42) and revisit this point for an extra 20 seconds just before you close the foot up with toe rotation.

Treating the terminally ill

In the case of terminal illness, you want reflexology to make any pain more bearable and the person you are treating more comfortable. Focus your treatment on helping the client with the stress surrounding their disease, any issues with sleep patterns, and on reducing any side-effects of the medication they are taking.

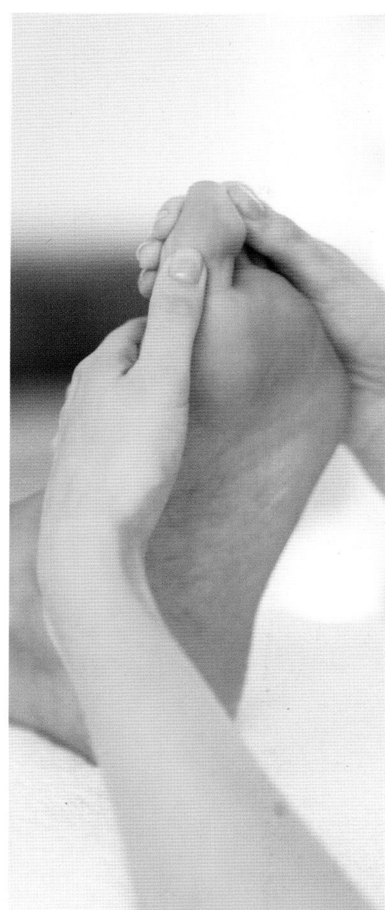

Always use a lighter pressure for clients on medication as their responses may be dulled because of the medication.

Many terminally ill people find that reflexology sessions help them to breathe more easily and retain greater control of their bowels and bladder. It can be a very uplifting experience to see how much terminally ill clients improve, both physically and emotionally, from the treatments. Try starting your treatment with two minutes of deep breathing while you work the solar plexus reflex point (see page 42). Always put aside enough time to talk to your client before or after treatment – this offers them space to discuss any spiritual needs.

Treating clients on medication

If someone is taking prescribed medication, always apply gentle pressure, just to be safe, because the medication may have dulled their responses to reflex points. Keep the rhythms of the treatment smooth and flowing. Commonly people do have side-effects to medication, ranging from swelling of the ankles to increased blood pressure that began after they started taking their prescription. If clients are experiencing side-effects, focus your treatment on the presenting condition and refer them to their doctor to discuss the side-effects.

At the most basic level, reflexology increases the body's circulation and this

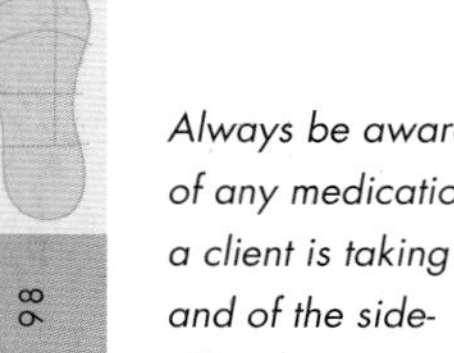

Always be aware of any medication a client is taking and of the side-effects it may provoke.

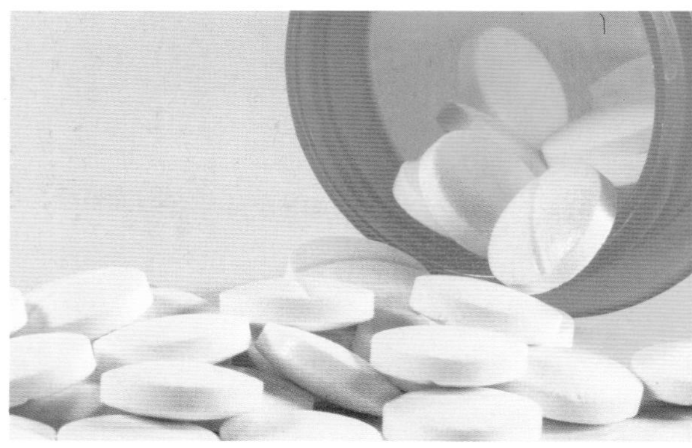

can sometimes make drugs more effective – if there are any changes, notify their doctor. There are some theories that reflexology treatment can eliminate the need for life-saving drugs, but this has not been proven. Pay special attention to the liver and kidney reflexes (see page 42), which need help in detoxifying the body. Keep revisiting these reflex points lightly throughout the treatment.

Treating pre- and post-operative clients

Some fascinating research conducted on orthopaedic wards in Welsh hospitals has looked at how reflexology can help speed up recovery after surgery. There are many studies that show that reflexology can shorten post-operative healing time, reduce pain and assist in shorter hospital stays. Since reflexology aims to build up the immune system, it is helping to reduce the risk of hospital-acquired infections.

Start your course of treatment around ten weeks before the operation and focus on balancing your client's emotional levels. This is important because it is well known that having a positive outcome to an operation speeds up the body's ability to heal itself. When giving treatment before surgery, lightly pay special attention to the areas that will be operated on. Treatment should be given at least two to three times a week for the month leading up to the operation. Afterwards, start the treatments as soon as possible, aiming to treat every day for the first week and twice a week after that.

To reduce bruising and pain after surgery, give your client fresh pineapple each day as a mid-morning snack. Pineapple eaten in between meals has powerful anti-inflammatory properties. Also, show your client the adrenal-gland reflexes on the hand (see page 357) and ask them to stimulate and massage these reflexes throughout the day, to help reduce pain and inflammation.

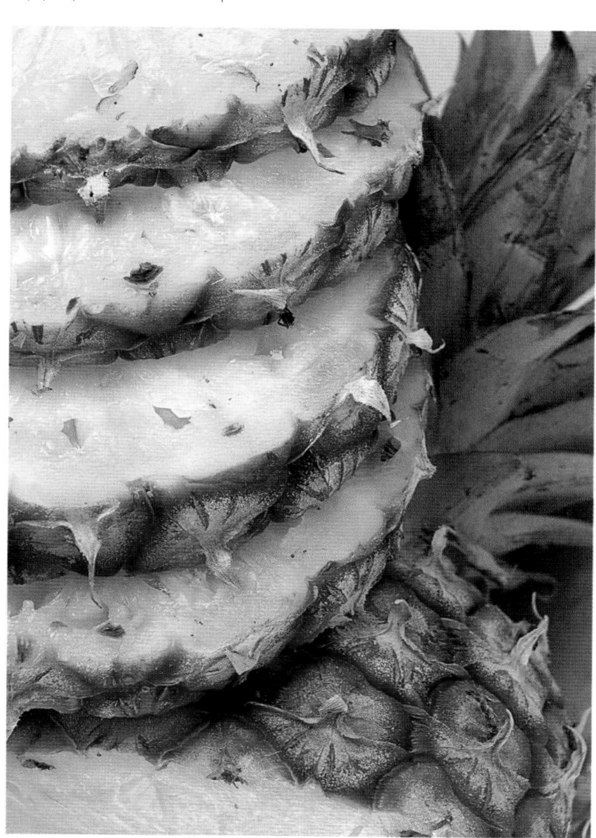

Bromelain, the enzyme found in pineapple, can help reduce inflammation and bruising.

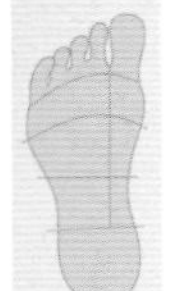

Where to treat

A professional reflexologist normally offers treatments at a clinic, in their home or runs a mobile practice, and generally uses a massage table or a special reclining chair. However, it is not necessary to invest in either of these pieces of equipment. Having a limited budget will not prevent you from giving a good, professional reflexology treatment. Having a reflexologist visit at home is wonderful for the client, because it means that they can relax comfortably afterwards.

Sitting comfortably

Always make sure that both you and your client are sitting comfortably throughout the treatment and that you have easy access to the feet. Here are four basic positions that you can use when giving a reflexology treatment.

Having a treatment while lying in a bed is very relaxing, and the client can go to sleep afterwards.

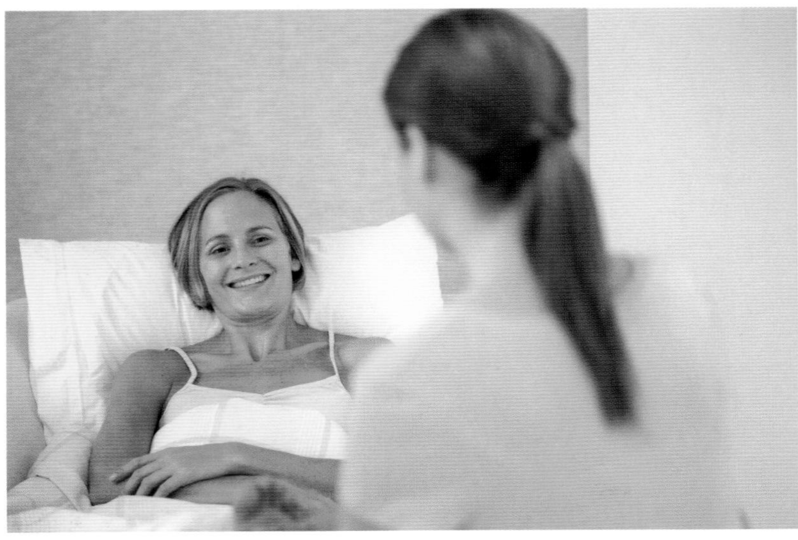

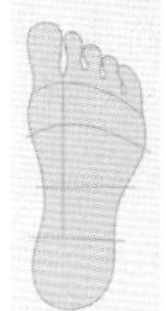

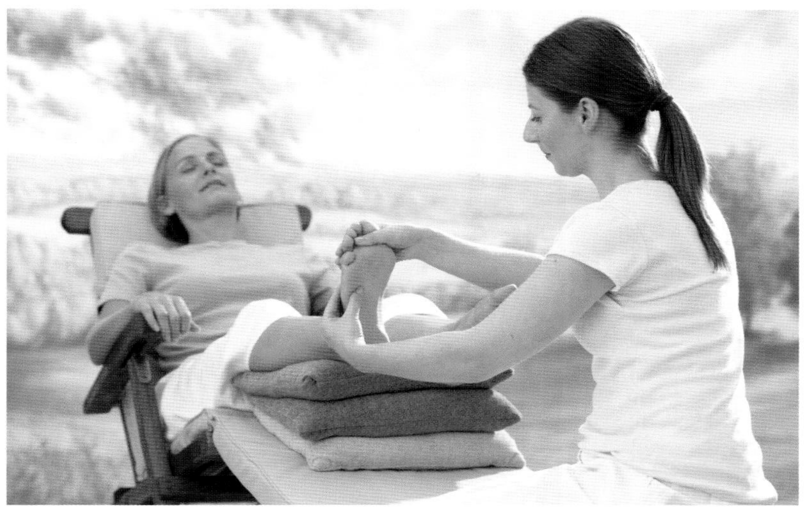

Treatments can be relaxing in any setting, as long as both reflexologist and client are comfortable.

1 Using a bed

You can either use a massage table, or a bed with a low stool at the end to gain easy access to the feet. Put two pillows under your client's head for comfort, and so that you can observe their facial expressions during the session. Eye contact is important, because most people will react in some way when a sore reflex point is worked on. Put another pillow under their knees to support the lower back, and two pillows under the feet, so that they are at a comfortable height for you to work on. You can place a towel just under the client's feet for hygiene reasons, and to cover the feet with when you are not working on them.

2 Using a garden chair

If you don't have a sun lounger or reclining chair, a good alternative is an ordinary garden chair covered in a white sheet.

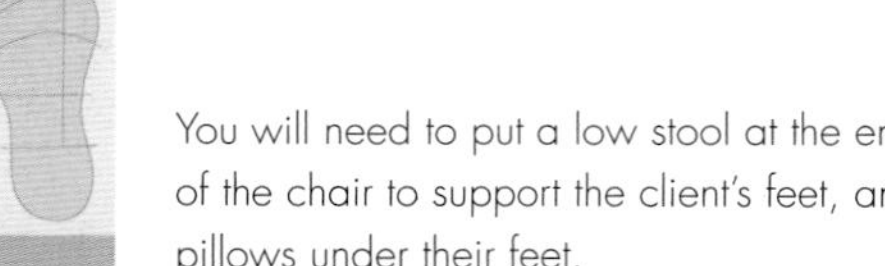

You will need to put a low stool at the end of the chair to support the client's feet, and pillows under their feet.

3 Using an armchair

The best way to treat the elderly and less mobile is to use a low stool at the end of an armchair. Make sure that their feet are well supported and that they are comfortable. You may have to sit cross-legged on the floor, but do try to keep your back straight throughout the session.

4 Using a sofa

Giving a treatment on a sofa is so relaxing for the client – it is great place to treat, because it takes just a minute to set things up, so it is very handy for impromptu sessions. Use a pillow to support your client's head, then place a number of pillows under the knees and another under the feet. Place a chair at the end of the sofa and make sure that the client's feet are at the right height for treatment.

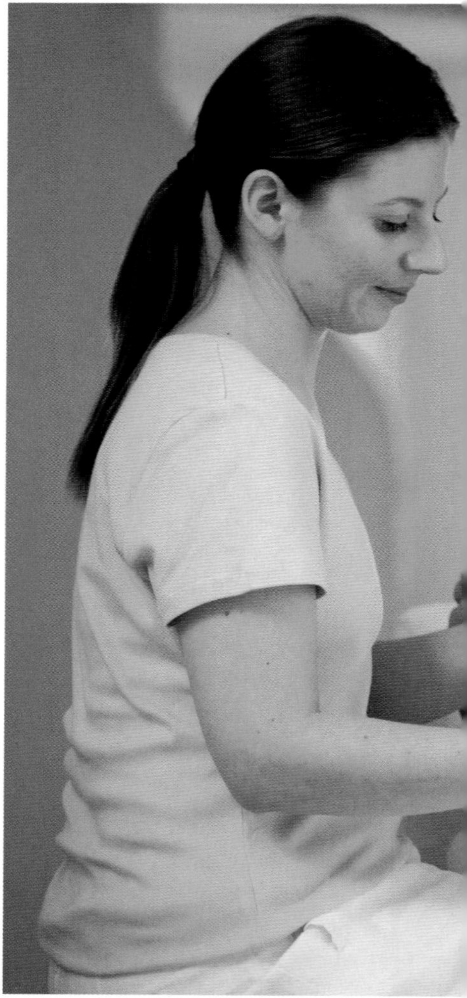

It is important for the reflexologist to keep a good posture during the treatment to avoid backache.

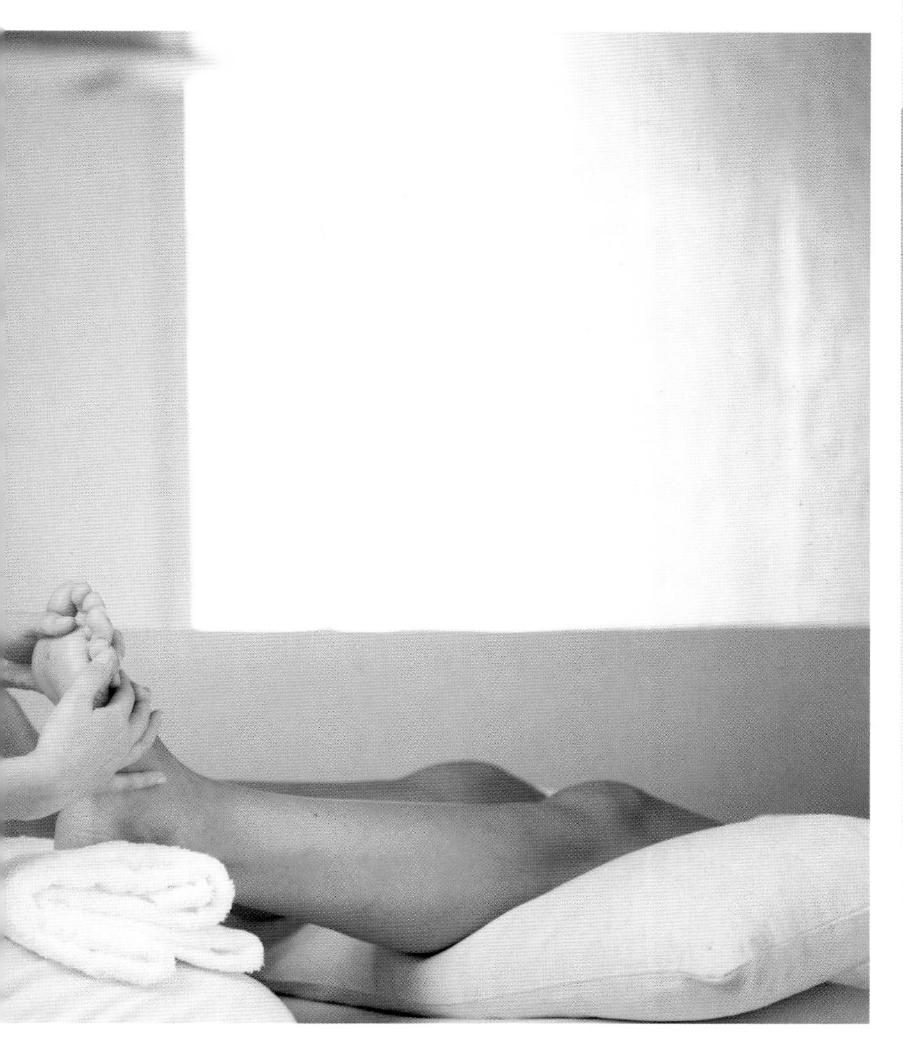

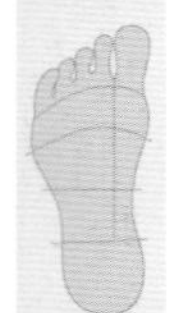

Setting the scene

Setting the scene in a professional and thoughtful way will help to give your client confidence in your treatment. The environment that you create for treatment is called the 'healing space'.

Music

Soft music can often help to create a relaxing environment, so choose something soothing that you have previously heard all the way through – not a piece that will surprise you with a sudden change of pace. 'Environmental music' is not always a good idea, because it can aggravate phobias. Think about how a client with a fear of drowning would react to a tape of the sound of water; or a client with hay fever to music depicting a summer glade.

Scent

A great way to perfume your treatment room is to burn relaxing essential oils or light a scented candle for 30 minutes before the treatment. Remember to blow out the candle or burner at least five minutes before treatment commences, because you do not want any heavy fragrance in the air that could aggravate respiratory conditions.

If someone you are treating has asthma, don't perfume the room, but ventilate it well before you give the treatment. Avoid cut flowers in your treatment room, because their pollen could set off a client's hay fever or allergies.

Lighting

It is very important to consider lighting: keeping light levels low will help to create a relaxing, professional environment. You may want to use floor lights so that the bulbs don't shine in your client's eyes. You certainly do not want lights to shine in the eyes of an epileptic – epilepsy is common and affects around one in 2,000 people; it occurs as a result of short circuitry in the brain, and lighting has been associated with seizures.

Water

Have a glass of water close by, so that you can offer it to your client after the session. Water helps to flush out from the body any toxins that have been released during treatment. Most people feel a little thirsty after a reflexology session.

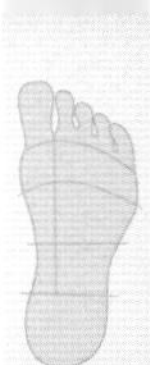

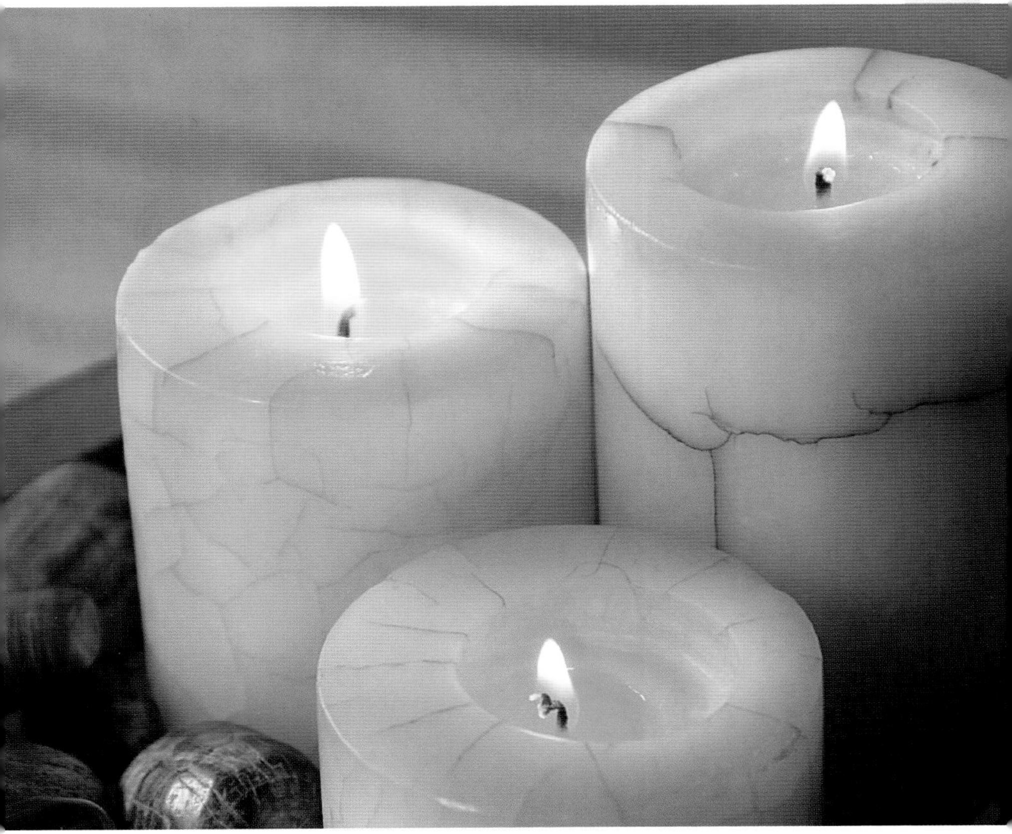

Scented candles are a splendid way to help create a relaxing atmosphere before a reflexology treatment.

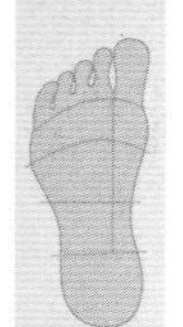

Preparing yourself

The image that you present can indicate what sort of treatment you will give. If you want to take a professional approach, then you need to look the part. Always dress in a white T-shirt or shirt and smart trousers or skirt, to give the impression of professionalism and help others respond to you in this way.

Hygiene

Keep your nails short and clean, otherwise they may dig into your client's skin when you give a treatment. Always wash your hands before and after treatment so that they are clean and fresh. If you have long hair, tie it back so that it does not fall over your client's feet during the session. Take off any rings or bracelets before you start.

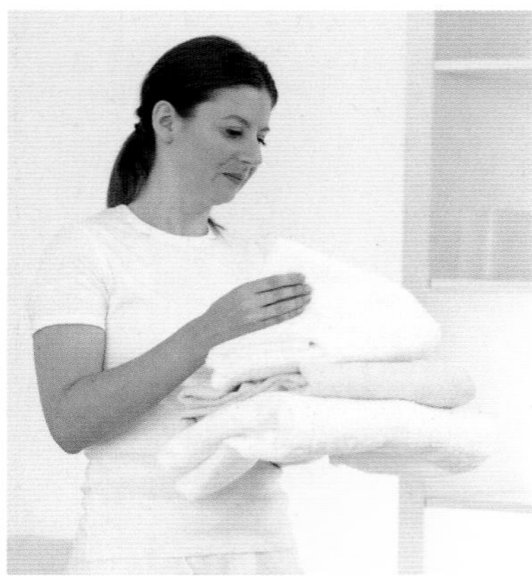

Professional standards in dress, health and hygiene, and client safety and care are all-important.

Breathing and posture

Breathe deeply throughout the session as you work, because this provides oxygen for your muscles, enabling you to give a great treatment and your mind to concentrate on working the reflexes. The wonderful thing about giving reflexology is that you, too, can benefit from it. If you have good posture, your breathing is steady and you are centred throughout the treatment, then these techniques can give you a physical and emotional boost.

Create boundaries

Establish treatment boundaries by turning off mobile phones and televisions and getting rid of any distractions. Focus your attention wholly on the person you are treating, and avoid conversations about yourself, your worries and your day. Your attitude, image, environment and intentions are all important, both before and during treatment, because you will be affecting your client on numerous levels.

PREPARATION CHECKLIST

- Is the environment warm and well ventilated?
- Is the lighting calming?
- Have you switched off the phones and television?
- Have you found somewhere comfortable to treat your client?
- Have you checked the suitability of your treatment area by sitting or lying there yourself?
- Are you using a clean pillow and towel, for hygiene reasons?
- Are you dressed so that your client can respect the value of your treatment?
- Are your fingernails clean and filed short?
- Have you removed any jewellery that may interfere with the treatment?
- If you have long hair, is it tied back so that it does not fall over the client's feet?
- Do you have non-allergic plasters available, to cover verrucae with, if necessary?
- Do you have a blanket to cover your client with during treatment?
- Have you suitable music to play during the session?
- Have you powder and oil ready to use (see page 109)?
- Have you read through your treatment plan (see page 113), so that when you have your client next to you, it will all become familiar?
- Have you a glass of water ready to give your client afterwards?
- Do you have a glass for yourself?

Preparing your client

Bathing your client's feet in water before a treatment is a pleasurable experience, because it relaxes all the muscles in the feet and makes it easier to access the reflex points. You can also soften the feet by wrapping them in hot towels and letting the heat soak through to the feet. Baths are an important ritual in many cultures, and you can create a wonderful-smelling footbath as a caring act before the treatment.

Footbaths with stones

Place a selection of large stones in a footbath and cover them with hot water. Leave to stand for five minutes so that the stones retain the heat and the water cools down a little. Test the temperature of the water with the tip of your elbow, then ask

A footbath with warm stones and cloves can help relieve the symptoms of arthritis.

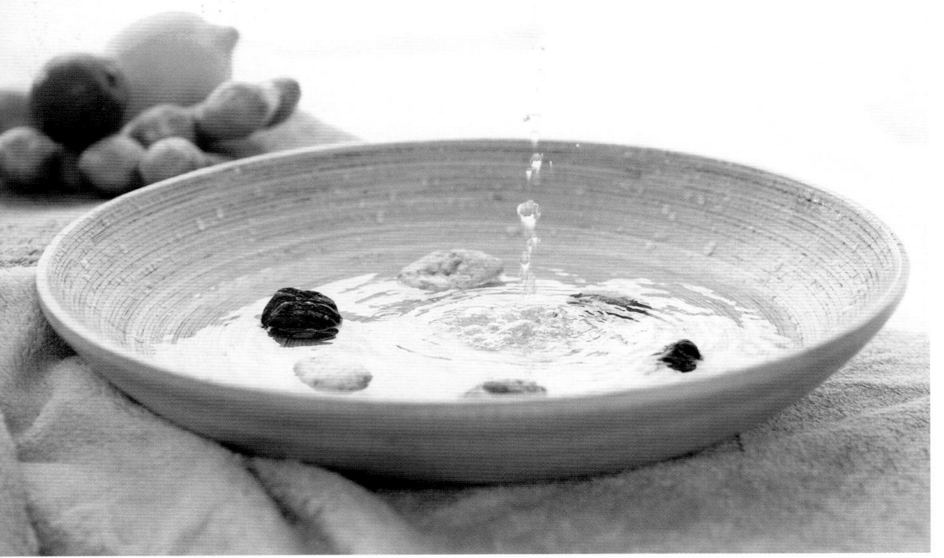

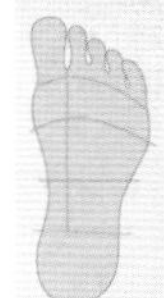

your client to place their feet in the footbath for a couple of minutes.

You can add a fragrant herb or flower that you feel will help your client: put it in a small muslin bag, tie the bag with cotton, then drop it into the warm water for its soothing effect. Alternatively, create any combination of herbs or flowers that you feel will work for your client. Floating a few flowers or rose petals on the surface of the water looks wonderful. Try the following suggestions:

- **Ginger** is good for boosting the circulation, muscle stiffness and foot exhaustion.
- **Jasmine** is beneficial for its overall relaxing properties; it is excellent for relieving depression, stress, fatigue, premenstrual syndrome and irritability; it can also help to reduce skin itchiness.
- **Lemongrass**, traditionally used as a remedy for skin complaints, was burned to kill germs and used as an insect repellent; it has properties that can help with headaches and poor circulation and speed up the healing process.
- **Clove** has antibacterial properties and warms the skin; it can help reduce swelling and provide temporary relief from arthritis, rheumatism, sprains and bruises.
- **Lime** can ease varicose veins, poor circulation, cellulite, respiratory problems and infections; lime slices placed on top of the footbath look attractive and smell really fresh.

After the footbath thoroughly dry your client's feet and apply powder to them. This enables your thumbs to glide around the feet while you alternate pressure on the various reflexes.

MASSAGE MEDIA

A range of products is available for massage, from powders and creams to oils. I like to use cornflour, because the treatments flow better and you can use firm pressure without your thumb slipping. Cornflour is a safe alternative to talcum powder, and generally looks and feels like talc. There has been some concern that talc may be associated with causing cancer, so cornflour is an ideal substitute.

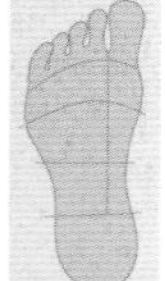

SCENTED REFLEXOLOGY POWDER

A great idea is to create your own scented reflexology powder. This is simple, cheap and fun to do. Think about the kind of scents you like and what images they evoke. Choose the scent with which you want to fragrance your powder. You will need: one small to medium container; cornflour; dried products to create the scent; scales; paper and pen; a large muslin square; cotton with which to tie the muslin.

1 Fill your container with regular cornflour.
2 Gather your chosen dried fruit, cocoa beans, dried orange peel, dried flowers, herbs or spices. Be inventive and weigh different amounts of each product, to create your very own reflexology powder.
3 Write down your combinations and weights, so that you can create the scent again at a later stage.
4 Wrap your ingredients in a small muslin bag tied with a piece of cotton. Push the bag into the middle of cornflour, then leave it to scent the powder for 48 hours.
5 Name your signature reflexology powder scent.

Enjoy creating your own personal signature scent.

Once you have created your signature scent, place the powder on your hands and rub it directly on the feet, then you can start your treatment. Another scent suggestion is to place a vanilla pod and a star anise into a container filled with cornflour and leave it to infuse for 48 hours.

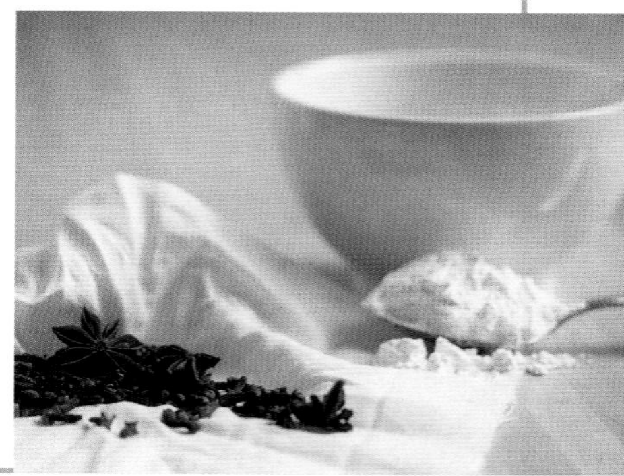

Oils and creams

Some people find they have an allergy to powder, or that it makes them sneeze or cough during treatment. If a client has eczema on the feet, it is better to use oil so that you don't dry out these areas.

It is preferable not to use a nut oil such as almond oil, because of allergies that you may not even be aware of. However, grapeseed oil has a fine texture and is easily absorbed by the skin. If you want moisturizing oil for ageing or dry skins, use evening primrose oil in a 20 per cent dilution with grapeseed oil. Professional reflexologists do not use essential oils on the feet, simply because they are not trained in aromatherapy, and essential oils, being powerful, may be contra-indicated by a client's condition.

Towels and blankets

During the treatment you will need two clean, dry towels. Place one under the client's feet on a support pillow, for hygiene reasons. The other towel is to cover the feet with and keep them warm. Place the feet 30 cm (12 in) apart before you start, covering both with a towel and removing it when you begin the relaxation techniques. Place the towel over the left foot to keep it warm while you are working on the right, and vice versa.

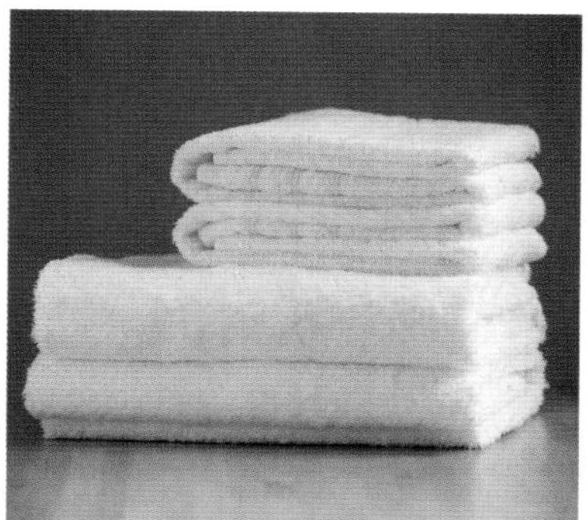

Before you start a treatment, wrap your client's feet in hot towels to make them feel warm and relaxed.

When you end the treatment, cover both feet again with the towel in a nurturing way and hold for 20 seconds.

During treatment clients often lose body temperature and become very cold, because all the body's energy has been directed within for healing. Before you start a session, cover your client with a blanket, even in warm weather, to prevent them becoming cold. A good tip is to put your towels over a hot radiator before giving a treatment – that says you care about your client. It is often such small details that create a special atmosphere. Feeling cold can also be a reflection of someone's low energies on an emotional and physical level.

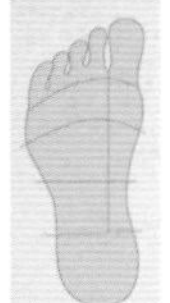

The reflexology session

Most clients will have heard of the wonderful health benefits of reflexology. However, it is important to give a definition of reflexology before you start treatment. You can use the illustrations in this book to show how you work on the feet, as well as how certain reflexes correspond to certain areas of the body.

Explain how long the treatment will take, and that you will speak to the client afterwards about any reflexes that are out of balance. Show them on their hands the techniques you will be using on their feet. Reassure your client that you will ease up if any area feels sensitive, and that if they fall asleep during treatment, that is fine.

Taking a medical history

Finding out someone's medical history is just as important as understanding why they wish to receive treatment, because it can shed light on their current condition. All conditions have a symptom pattern; this means that there are certain things a client does to aggravate the disease and other things that can make it better. For example, coffee can make inflammatory skin conditions such as eczema worse. Knowing this, you could adapt your treatment to pay particular attention to the liver and kidney reflexes, as well as suggesting that your client avoid coffee and see whether their eczema gradually calms down.

Taking a medical history will also enable you to check for any contra-indications. Treatment should not be given in the first trimester of pregnancy, in cases of high fever, gangrene or an infectious disease like tuberculosis. At other times a very light treatment is needed or it may bring about a healing crisis reaction (see page 92), a bruise or create pain afterwards.

THE IMPORTANCE OF CONFIDENTIALITY

Whether you are treating clients, friends or family, you need to take a medical history. This should always be given in confidence, and you should mention this before you start, to create a relationship of trust and professionalism from the outset.

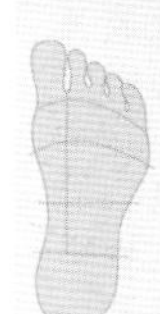

Treatment plan

Use the information from a client's medical history to provide the basis of your treatment plan. Work out how often your client should receive treatments: it may involve daily, three-times-a-week or weekly sessions. Focus your treatment on the areas where stress is most evident in the body, and plan out the reflexes that relate to these body areas.

Pressure

Always warm your hands before you place them on the feet. Your treatment pressure should range from gentle to firm, depending on who you are working on. A gentle grip on the feet will feel comforting

Understanding a client's symptom pattern can help you identify the underlying cause of their problem.

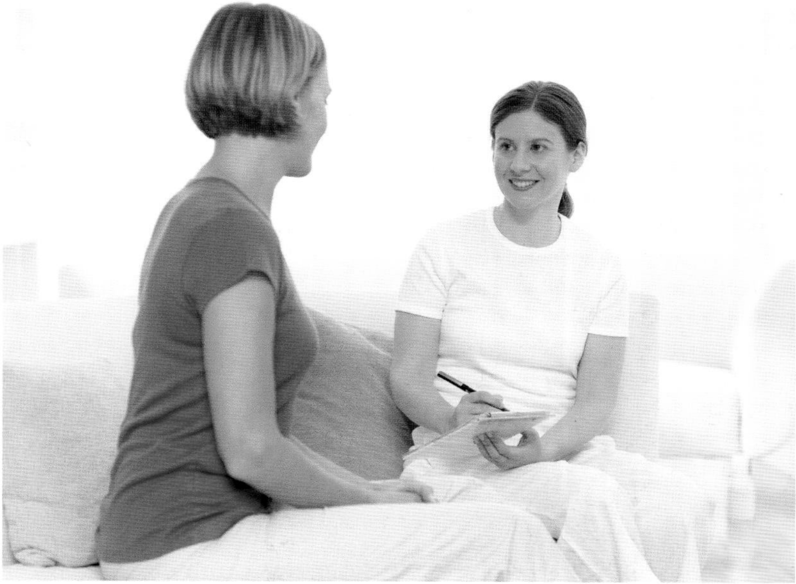

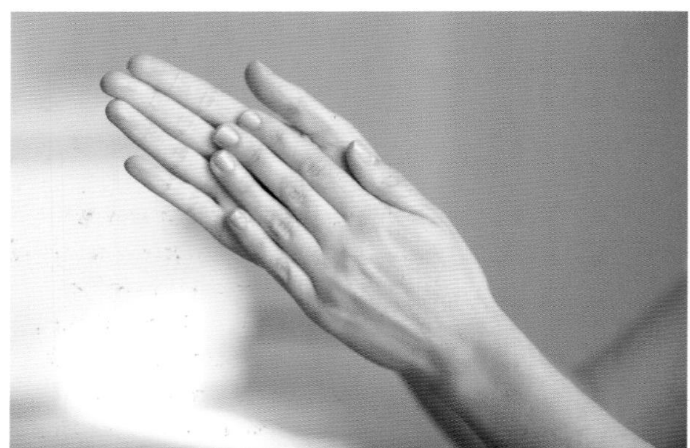

It is important to warm your hands before you give a treatment.

to your client while you are treating them. If you apply excessive pressure, you could damage your thumbs or cause pain to the client. Throughout the treatment adjust your pressure as necessary to avoid causing any discomfort.

Watch your client's reactions, because if an area is painful to them, this may indicate that the related body part is not functioning properly. If the client expresses any discomfort, reduce the pressure immediately and continue to lightly stimulate the reflex point or area for ten seconds, by which time the discomfort should have subsided.

If you are treating someone who is unwell, elderly or young, use a lighter pressure. If a client has previously had a healing crisis reaction to treatment, work at a much lighter pressure during the next session. If someone is on painkillers or recreational drugs, be aware that these can desensitize the reflexes on the feet, so it is important not to use firm pressure. A good tip to keep your own hands strong and healthy is to hold your thumb as close to your hand as possible throughout the treatment. This decreases the risk of wrist and muscle injuries.

Touch sensations

The sensations you can expect to feel during a treatment will vary according to your client's health at the time. If a part of their body is not functioning well, the reflex area will feel sensitive. The client's reactions may vary from a dull ache or discomfort to feeling something sharp being pressed into the foot; this is just a crystal being disbursed (see below). The sensations your client experiences should become less painful as treatments continue and the affected area of the body becomes stronger.

If an area feels sensitive, stay on it and make little gentle circles with your thumb until the discomfort goes away. If you feel any crystals, remain on that area until you have broken down as many as possible. However, it may take a number of treatments to break down all the crystals that you feel. Use the following list to tick off sensations as you feel them:

- Bubbling or popping, like bubble wrap
- Crystals that feel like sugar or sand when you break them down
- Soft spongy areas
- Areas that feel empty
- A sensation of lumpiness
- A granular feeling
- Hard areas.

A visualization for healing

You are about to begin your treatment. Focus on where you are now in your mind and body. It is important that we live happily, with a strong spirit of optimism; we need to be able to direct our minds continually in a bright, positive and beneficial direction and help those around us do so too. We should strive to develop a state of life where we feel a sense of joy, no matter what happens.

Close your eyes and direct a bright, positive light from the centre of your body. Let this energy radiate out through your arms, legs, toes and fingers. You are now ready to begin your treatment.

RECOMMENDED TIMINGS FOR YOUR SESSION

Setting the scene	5–10 minutes
Taking a medical history	5–20 minutes
Relaxation techniques	5 minutes
Basic foot-reflexology treatment	15–30 minutes
Relaxation techniques at the end	5 minutes
Feedback after the treatment	5–10 minutes

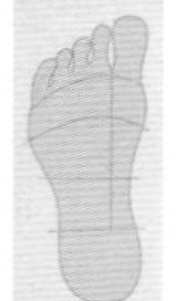

Aftercare

During your treatment certain reflexes may have been painful for your client, or you may have felt crystals in the foot. This means there has been, is or may be an imbalance in the corresponding part of the body and indicates a reflex that is out of balance.

Sometimes you can expect sensitivity in a reflex – for example, if someone has been suffering from headaches, then the head, occipital and neck reflexes will be out of balance. However, if you don't know the reason, you need to investigate using a holistic approach. What aspects of your client's lifestyle have affected their well-being, their health or the functioning of a part of their body?

Investigating problems

Start by explaining to your client that you expected to find certain reflexes out of balance, because of the problems they had told you about. For example, if they are suffering from heartburn, you expect to find that the oesophagus reflex is sensitive. Certain reflexes should be sensitive depending on a client's medical history. For reflexes that were out of balance for no apparent reason, ask your client the following questions:

1. During treatment there was a lot of sensitivity in this particular reflex – can you think of any reason why?
2. Have you ever had, or do you currently have, a problem in this area?
3. Are you on any medication that you have not told me about?
4. Are you doing any sports, or is there something in your lifestyle that could aggravate this area in any way?

Once you have an answer to these questions, you could make some simple lifestyle suggestions that will help your client enhance their energy levels, reduce stress or improve their diet – these might include exercise, hot baths before bed, or eating more fruit and vegetables. However, you cannot wrap up everything neatly in a box, and some points will go unanswered. Ask your client to be aware of the weak area and not to aggravate it. Always remember to refer them, when appropriate, to a doctor, voluntary worker or statutory support service, or to another complementary therapist.

End the session by covering your client's feet with a towel, washing your hands and offering them a glass of water to flush away any toxins that have been released during the reflexology treatment.

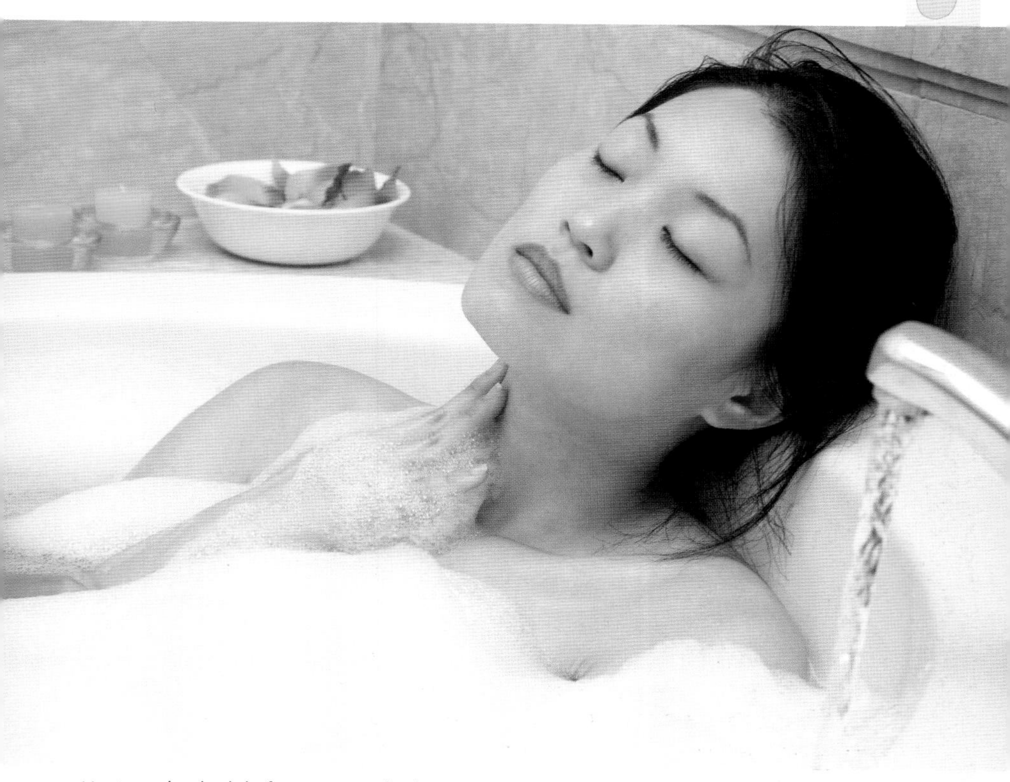

Having a hot bath before going to bed can help alleviate the problem of disturbed sleep patterns.

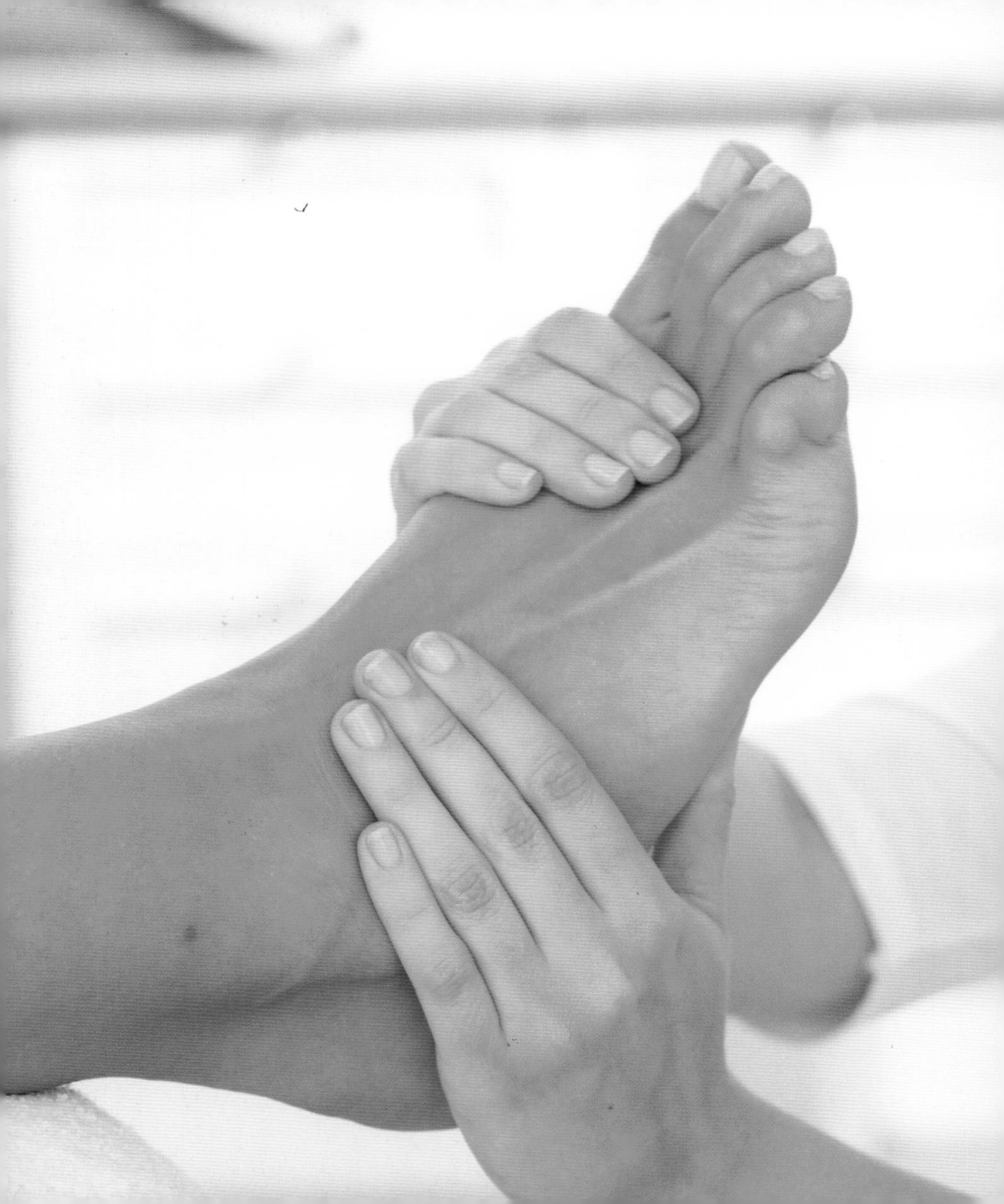

PART 4

Treating the feet

Working on the feet

This part of the book shows you how to apply an effective foot reflexology treatment. You should make the treatment as pleasurable an experience as you can, for both you and your client, but you don't necessarily have to plan it in advance; spontaneous treatments on friends and family can be very successful. The treatment time will vary from ten minutes (when treating a young child) up to an hour (when treating an adult).

Giving treatment with the right intention can be calming and balancing for you, as well as providing vital energy. The 'right intention' is simply the desire to heal the person you are working on. If you want to attain this state of mind, body and soul, start your treatment with inner energy breathing (see page 123) and spend a little time breathing along with your client. As you do so, feel the energies washing down over you, enveloping your body in healing white light.

Dispersing the crystals

Reflexology is one of the most intelligent of all the complementary therapies because, as you give the treatment, you will find clues to the state of your client's health. These clues come in the form of crystals on the reflex points or areas, or places where the client feels discomfort. These tell you that there is, has been or could be a problem in the related body area. Sometimes you can expect this, because you know about the client's health, but at other times you can surprise them by picking up health issues they haven't yet mentioned to you.

Your job is to disperse the crystals that you find in the feet during treatment, using your thumbs and fingers. This stimulates the body's own healing powers to help restore good health. After the treatment you can refer the client to their doctor or an appropriate specialist who can help with diet, posture, counselling, and so on. Do remember that reflexology does not diagnose or cure.

Start your treatment with confidence in your own abilities, because to become good at anything you have to begin with a small step and believe in yourself.

Your intention to heal the person you are working on is an important aspect of the process.

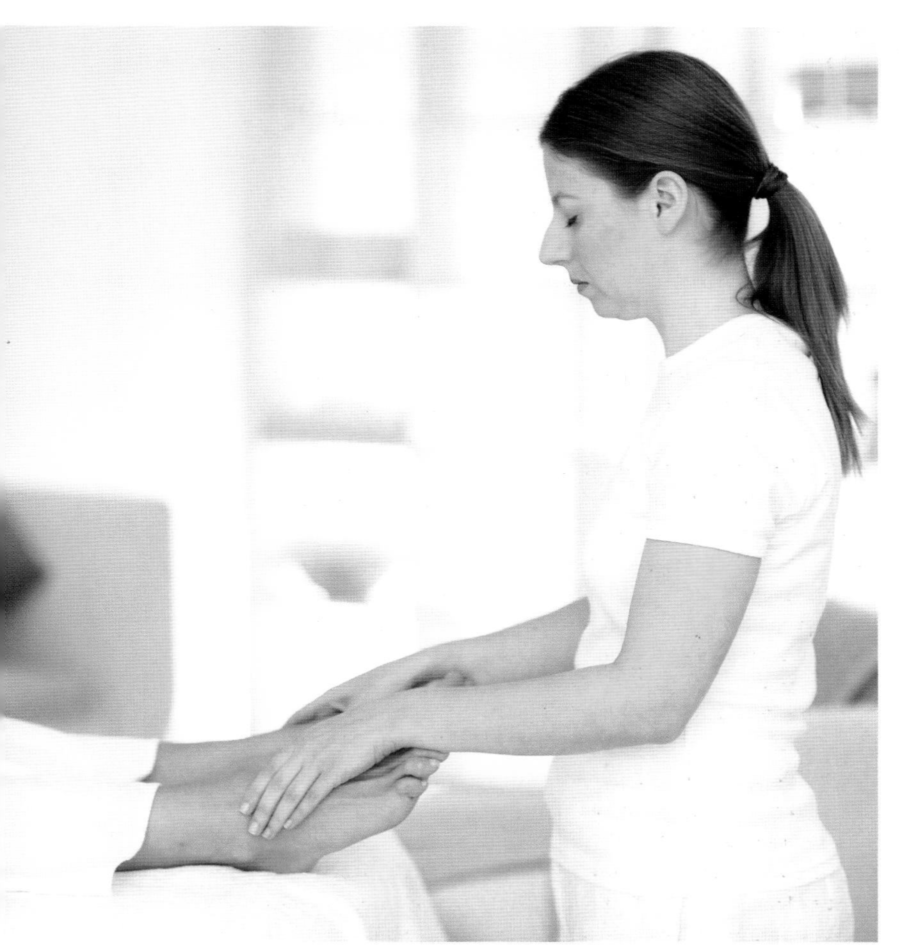

Relaxing the feet

Here and on the following pages are a range of movements that have been designed for comfort and to melt away tension – not only in the feet, but also in the whole body.

They can all be used both to start and end a treatment. Some clients, like the elderly, will appreciate you spending more time on these movements, because they help to reduce pain and discomfort and increase the circulation. These relaxation techniques can also be used on their own for young children, as part of a nightly bedtime routine to help them sleep better. You can spend as little time or as long as you wish on them. Use your intuition and try to meet the immediate needs of the person you are treating.

Your aim is to work first on the right foot and then on the left foot. Use a soft, confident touch and try to make your movements flow from one to the next. Approximate time guidelines are given to help ensure the effectiveness of each one.

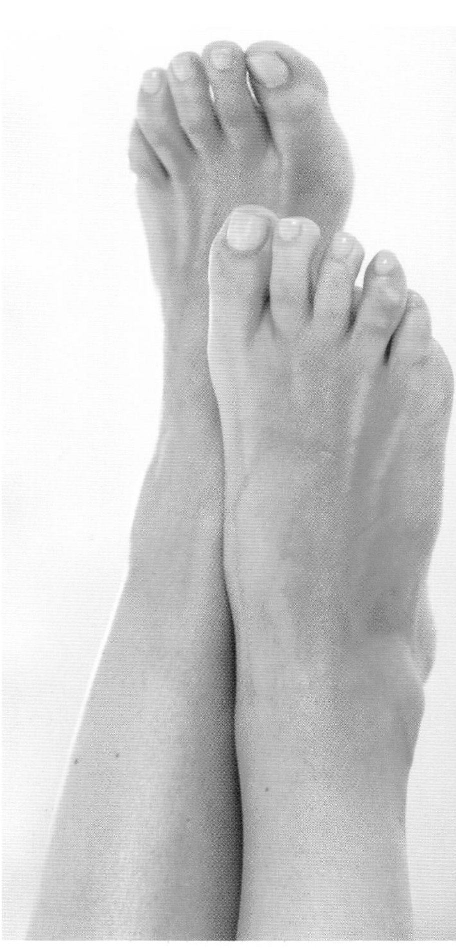

When you give a treatment, focus first of all on relaxing the feet.

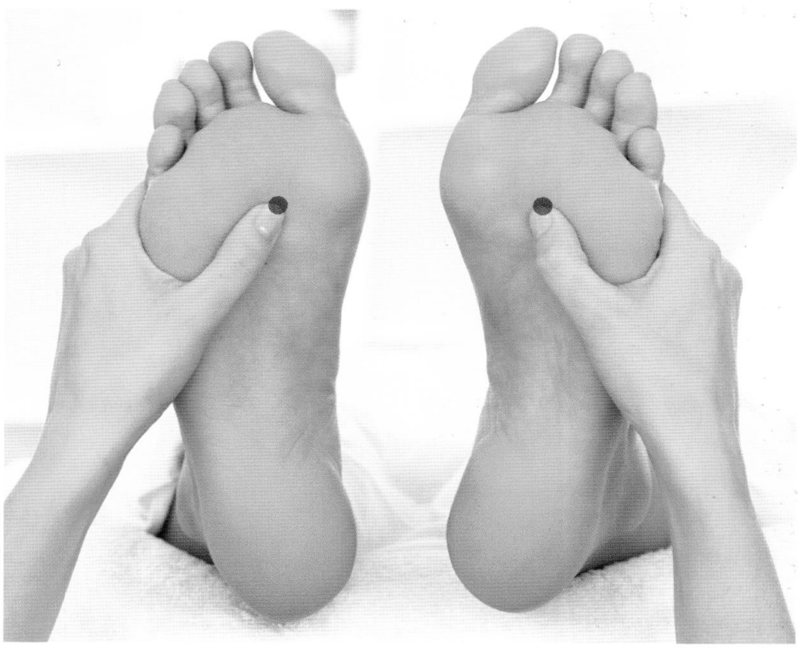

INNER ENERGY BREATHING

Place your left thumb on the solar plexus reflex point on the right foot, and your right thumb on the solar plexus reflex point on the left foot. Centre yourself for a moment by closing your eyes, and focus on the energies running down from your head to your fingers and toes.

Ask your client to take a deep breath in for five seconds while you make small circles on the solar plexus reflex. They should then hold their breath for five seconds as you continue to work on this reflex. Then ask them to breathe out for five seconds and reduce pressure on the solar plexus reflex. As your client breathes in and out, so should you. Take in the calming breath to create your intention and energy for the treatment. Repeat this movement four times.

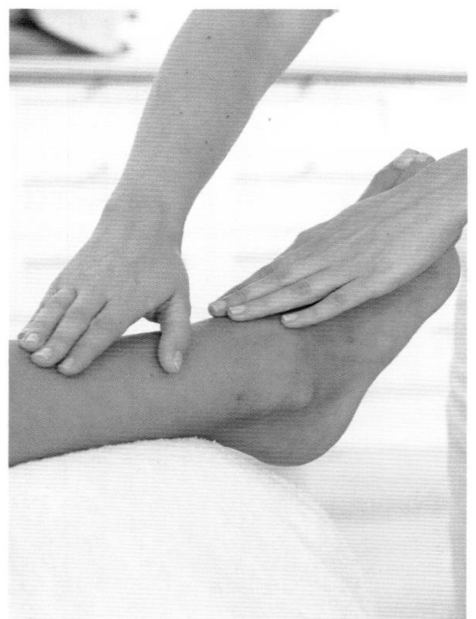

ANGEL'S TOUCH

Place both palms on the right foot and gently move the hands up the leg and then come back down again. Both hands should work together with a medium pressure. Now work on the left foot. Continue this movement for one minute on each foot.

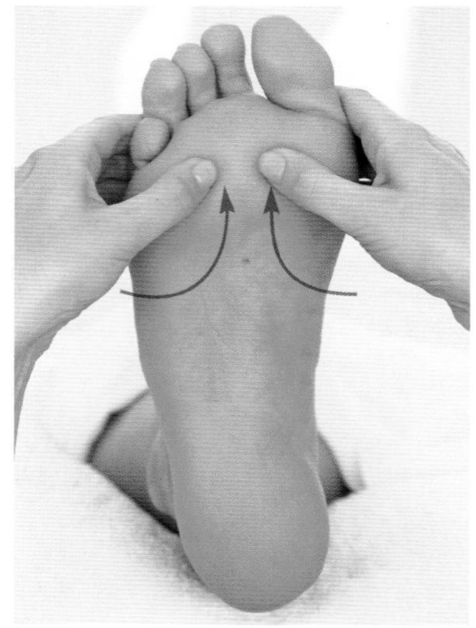

APOLLO'S BREATH

Put both hands on the right foot. Place your fingers on the dorsal aspect and your thumbs on the plantar aspect. Your thumbs should be in the lung area 2.5 cm (1 in) apart. Gently pull your fingers towards you while putting a little more pressure on the thumbs. Ask your client to visualize that, as they breathe in, their breath is reaching and healing the area of the body that needs the most help. Complete this movement five times. Now work on the left foot. Continue for 30 seconds on each foot.

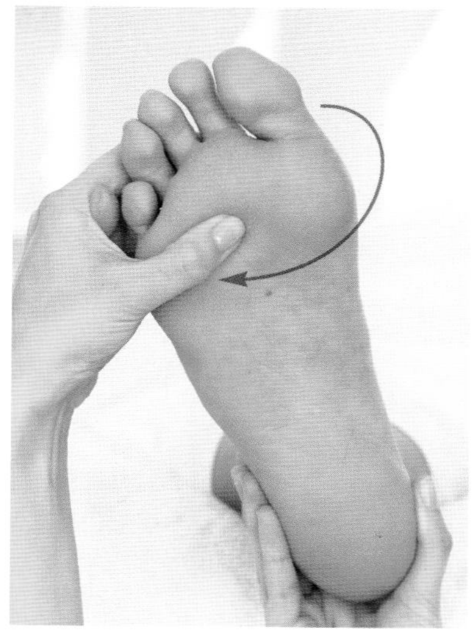

ATLAS'S ORB

Support the right foot with one hand by placing your hand under the heel. Hold the foot just under the toes with your other hand and gently rotate the foot, first clockwise and then anticlockwise, making big circles. Now work on the left foot. Continue this movement for 30 seconds on each foot.

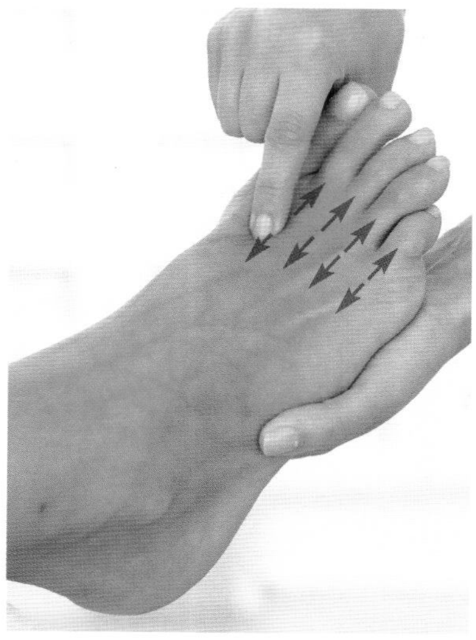

POSEIDON'S PULL

Place your index fingers on the dorsal aspect and your thumb on the plantar aspect of the right foot, in between the big toe and second toe. Rock upwards in between the toes as far as possible, within the trench between the toes. Stop when you get as far as you can. Then apply a little pressure and slide back down to the base of the big toe and second toe. Now work on the left foot. Continue this movement for 30 seconds on each foot.

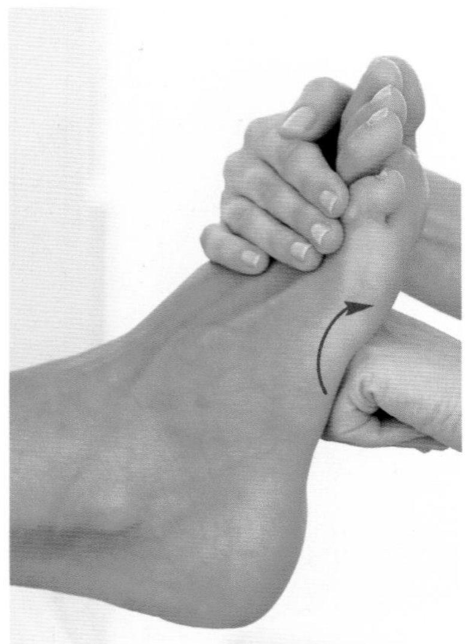

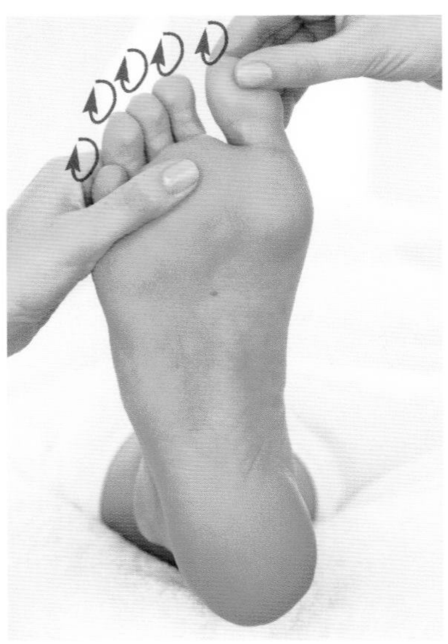

HEALING TORNADO

Support the right foot with one hand and use your other hand to make small circles halfway up the dorsal aspect of the foot. Gradually make larger circles covering the whole foot. Repeat this technique with a medium pressure five times and, as you do so, imagine healing energy building up in your hands and readying you for the treatment; you may feel your hands becoming hot. Now work on the left foot. Continue this movement for 30 seconds on each foot.

TOE ROTATION

Support the right foot and use your index finger and thumb, first on the big toe, to make small clockwise and anticlockwise circles. Repeat for the second, third, fourth and fifth toes. Now work on the left foot. Continue this movement for 30 seconds on each foot.

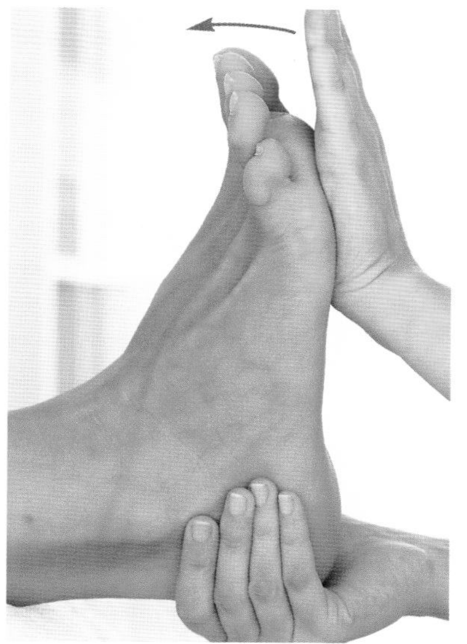

HERMES STRETCH

Support the right foot with one hand. Using your other hand, gently push the foot back and stretch the Achilles tendon. Hold for ten seconds. Now work on the left foot. Continue this movement for 30 seconds on each foot.

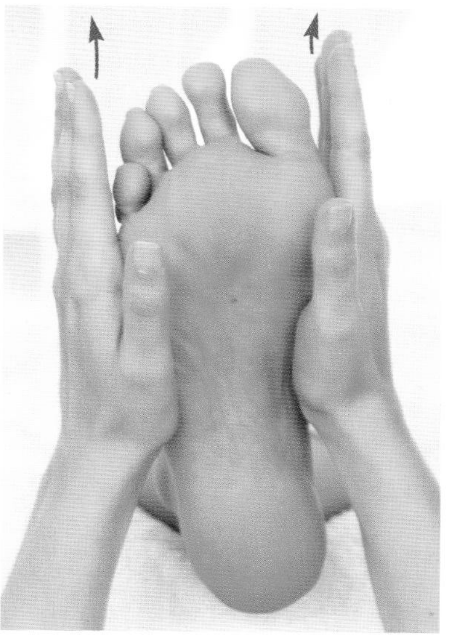

PHOENIX RISING

Place both palms on either side of the right foot. Gently roll your hands from the top of the foot down to the heel. Hold the heel and softly raise your hands back to the top of the foot. Repeat this powerful movement five times. Now work on the left foot. Continue this movement for 30 seconds on each foot.

Basic techniques

On the following pages there are four powerful reflexology techniques that will help you access the reflex points. The more you practise these techniques, the more your sequence will flow – and creating a smooth flow is important for your client's relaxation.

Giving the correct depth of pressure comes with time, and should in any case vary throughout your reflexology sequence. Generally, if someone is unwell, elderly or young, your pressure should be light, as this avoids a healing crisis reaction (see page 92). Your speed, however, should always be the same throughout the treatment.

Supporting the foot

It is important to support the foot well to ensure that it is comfortable for the client throughout the treatment. Having a calm, comforting hold on the foot will make your client feel secure and relaxed, knowing their foot is properly supported. You should use light to medium pressure.

The secret of a good supporting hold is to use one hand to apply the reflexology and the other hand to support the foot. So in effect you have one working hand and one supporting hand. Use your supporting hand on the reverse side of your working hand, thumb or finger. In this way you always make sure the client's foot is comfortable.

If you over-use your thumbs you could be at risk of repetitive strain injury or carpal tunnel syndrome. The best tip I can offer is to keep your thumb close to your hand throughout as much of the treatment as possible. If your hand or thumb does start to hurt just reduce the pressure. Some of the best treatments I have had have been given with a light touch which often deals with the cause of a symptom, and often the cause is stress.

If you use your thumb print rather than the tip of your thumb during the treatment you will find it will be a much more relaxing treatment to receive.

Learning to use the correct amount of pressure for each client comes with experience – temper the pressure to suit the situation and your client's needs.

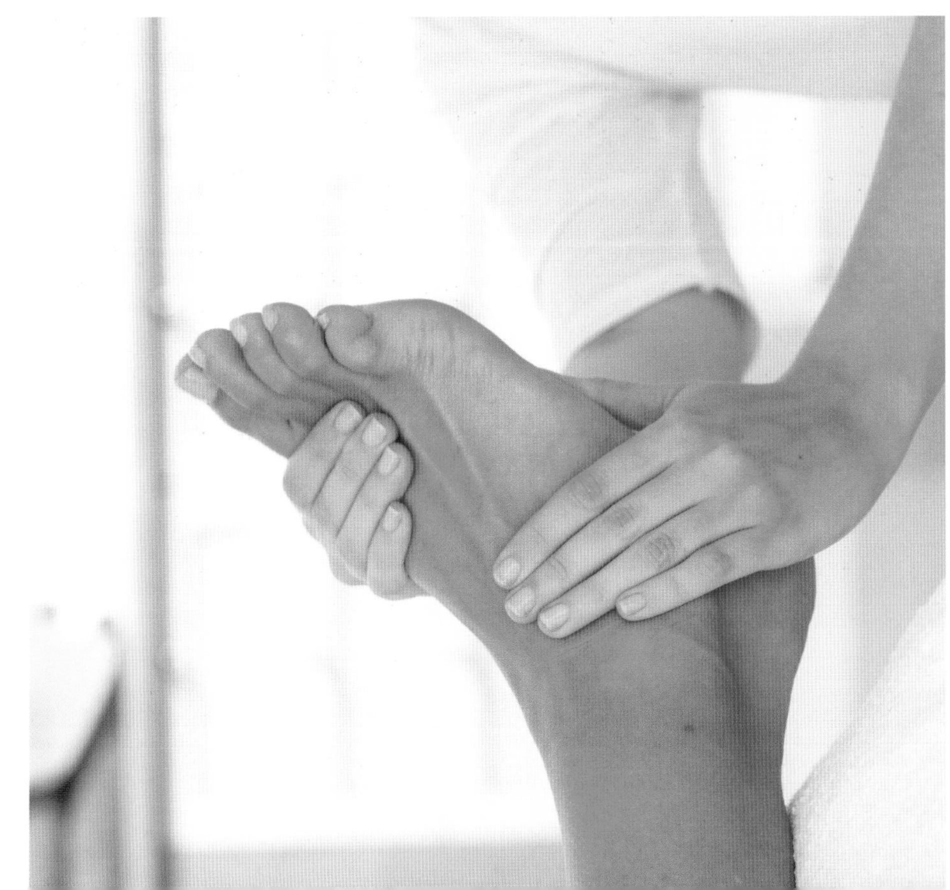

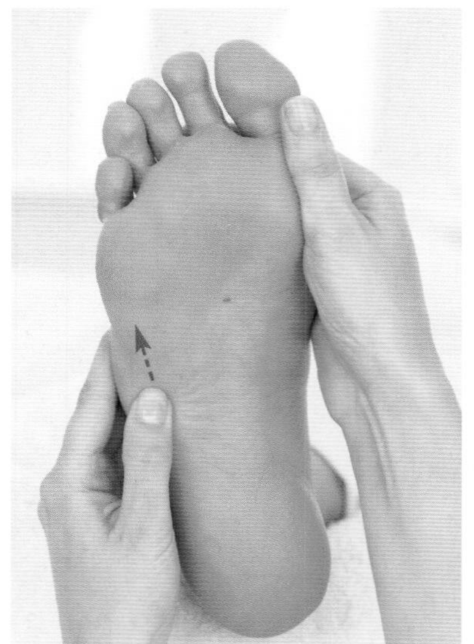

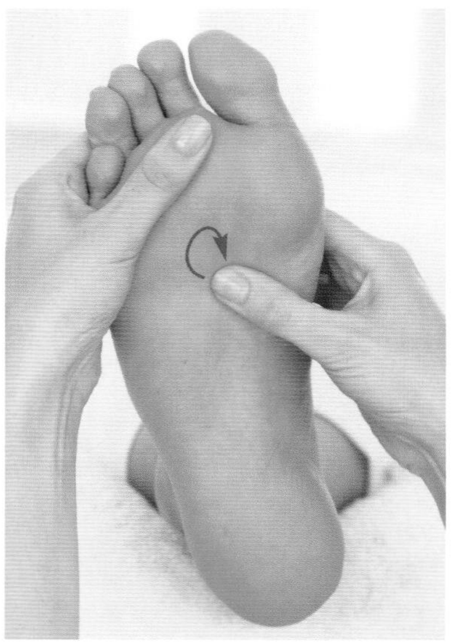

WALKING

Use your thumb or finger and simply walk it forward, taking one step at a time. The best part of the thumb to use is your thumbprint. Your thumb or finger should move across the foot in tiny steps, in the direction of your nail (never backwards). The aim is to find the crystals on a reflex area and disburse them. You should generally use medium pressure with this technique.

CIRCLES

When you work on a reflex point, use your thumb or finger to make circles. These don't just stimulate a point, but also initiate the body's self-healing mechanisms to help parts of the body work at optimum levels. When you find crystals, use circles to break them down and open up the energy pathways. You should generally use medium pressure and should stay on a point for anything from six to 20 seconds.

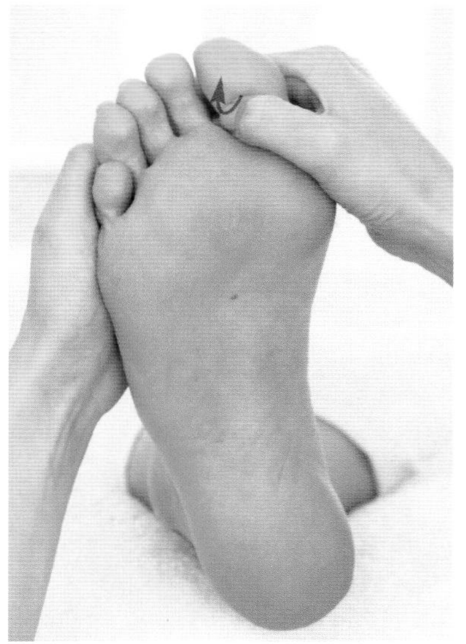

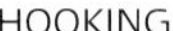

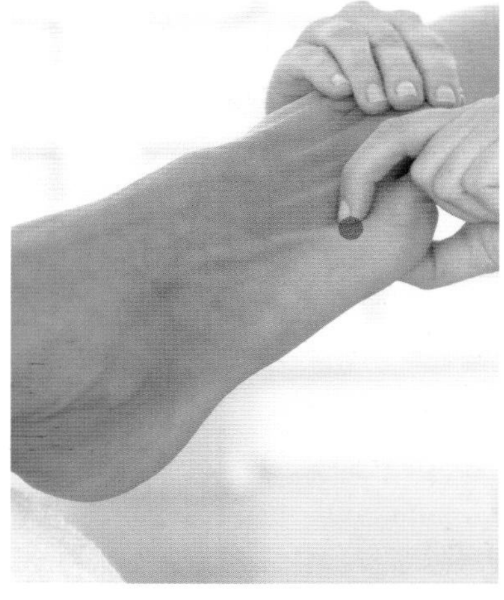

HOOKING

Use this technique to access reflex points that are hidden under tissues and muscles. Form a hook by bending the thumb, then place the thumbprint into a reflex point and use the hook to gouge into that point. Work the reflex point by gently moving your thumb to break down uric acid and calcium deposits. You should generally use medium pressure with this technique.

ROCKING

This technique helps you access a reflex point at a deep level, and saves on wear and tear of the thumb. Place your index finger on the dorsal aspect of the foot and your thumb on the plantar aspect. Use your index finger to rock up an area and to rock back and forth on a point. This technique is really useful if for some reason you cannot use your thumbs. You should generally use medium pressure and should stay on a point for anything from six to 20 seconds.

A quick reference

These pages contain some quick-reference charts that you should familiarize yourself with before you start treatment. A quick recap of these charts should make it easier for you to follow the general foot treatment (see pages 136–167). In addition, refer back to pages 40–49 to remind yourself of the various foot reflexology charts.

The zones of the body

See how easy it is to find zones one to five on each foot. Zone one starts at the big toe, and zone five ends with the fifth toe. Here is a tip that you will find useful during the treatment: zone one is the most important zone in the body, and includes the central nervous system, pituitary gland, spine, brain and reproductive organs. Generally, you will find that zone one is the most sensitive zone.

The bones of the feet

Before you start your treatment, have a quick look back to pages 54–57 to remind yourself of the bones of the feet, so that when a treatment suggests working under a specific metatarsal head, you will know exactly where is meant.

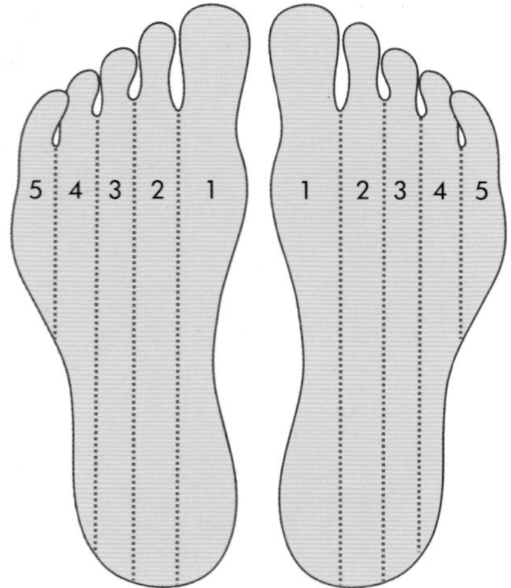

Zone 1 – big toe
Zone 2 – second toe
Zone 3 – third toe
Zone 4 – fourth toe
Zone 5 – little toe

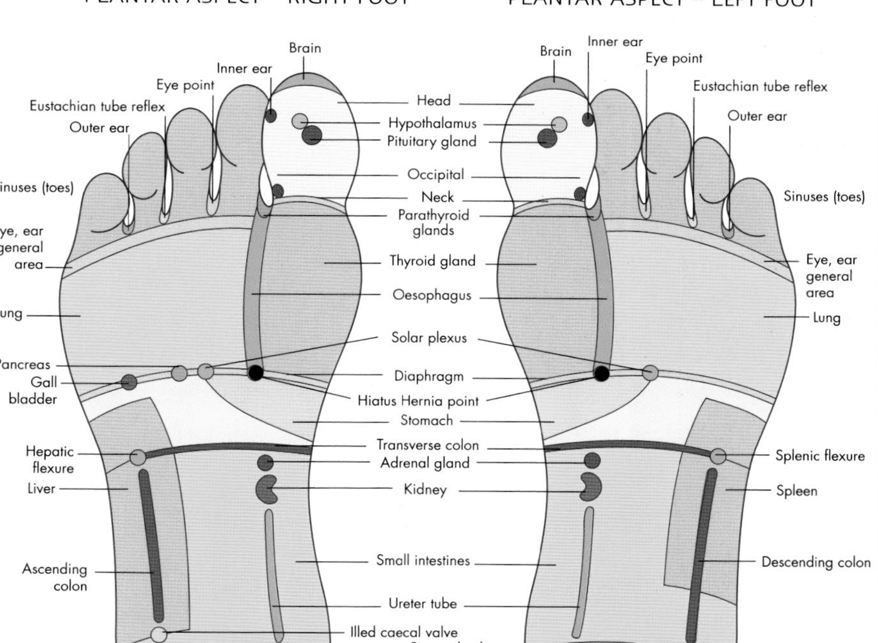
PLANTAR ASPECT – RIGHT FOOT
PLANTAR ASPECT – LEFT FOOT
Brain
Inner ear
Eye point
Eustachian tube reflex
Outer ear
Sinuses (toes)
Eye, ear general area
Lung
Pancreas
Gall bladder
Hepatic flexure
Liver
Ascending colon
Head
Hypothalamus
Pituitary gland
Occipital
Neck
Parathyroid glands
Thyroid gland
Oesophagus
Solar plexus
Diaphragm
Hiatus Hernia point
Stomach
Transverse colon
Adrenal gland
Kidney
Small intestines
Ureter tube
Illed caecal valve
Appendix
Sigmoid colon
Sciatic area
Brain
Inner ear
Eye point
Eustachian tube reflex
Outer ear
Sinuses (toes)
Eye, ear general area
Lung
Splenic flexure
Spleen
Descending colon
Sigmoid flexure

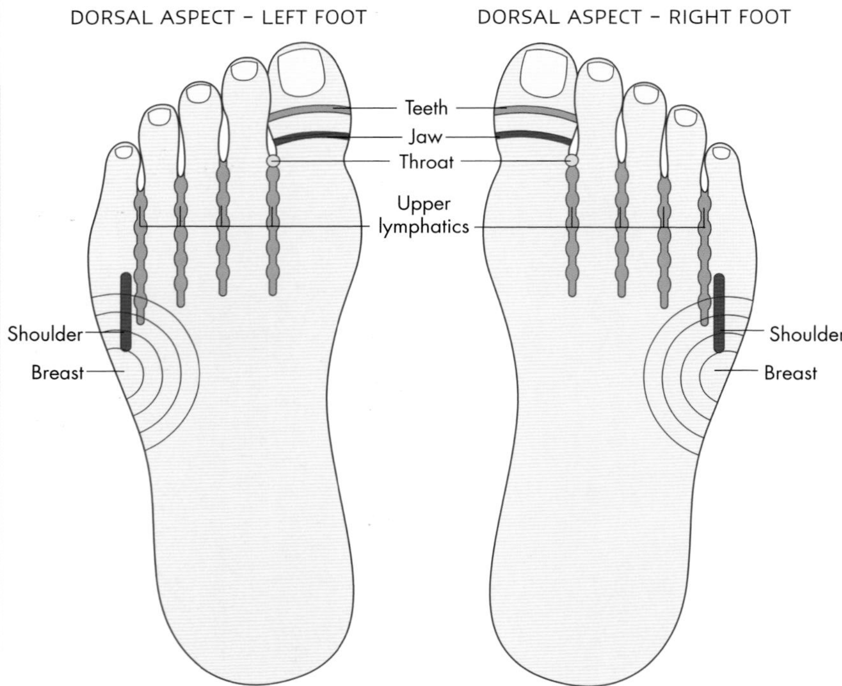

DIRECTION OF PRESSURE

In the illustrations in this book relating to reflexology treatment, the direction of pressure is shown by a dotted line. Your pressure should vary according to whom you are treating. Always use light pressure on children, the elderly and those who are ill.

MEDIAL FOOT MAP

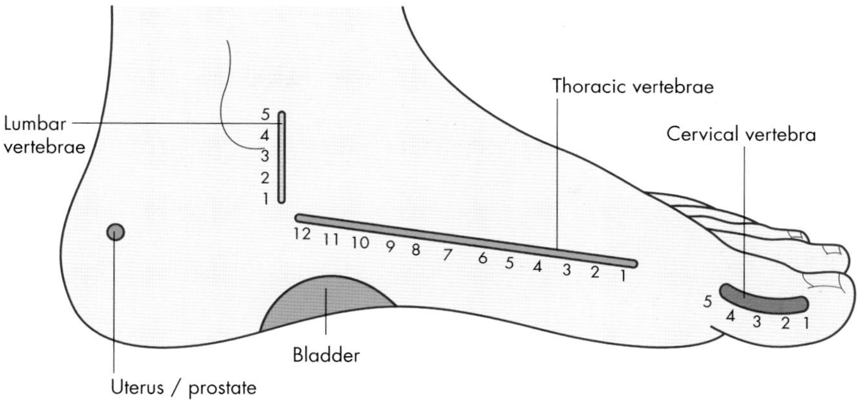

LATERAL FOOT MAP

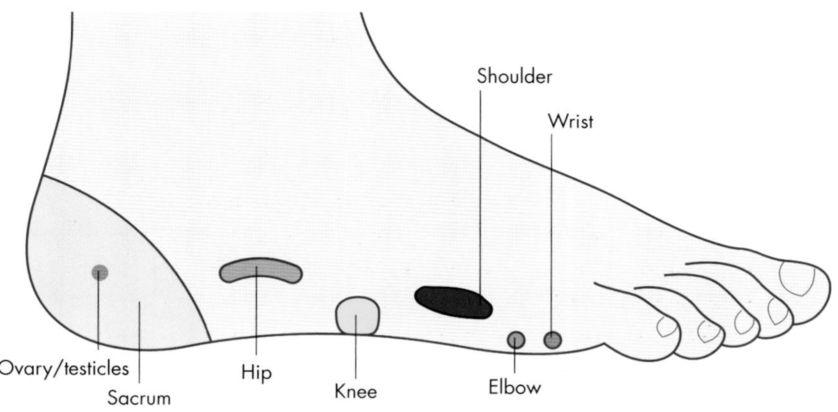

General foot treatment

Start and end your treatment with the relaxation techniques described on pages 122–127. Apply the following sequence first on the right foot and then on the left foot, using slow, confident movements. Once you have completed work on the right foot, cover it with a towel to keep it warm and comfortable while you work on the left foot.

The general foot treatment is designed to create a sense of pure relaxation, as well as ease the symptoms of most common conditions. Using this sequence once to three times a week will help to build up the body's immune system to fight infections and diseases. The whole treatment should take around 30 minutes. Use a light pressure over all the reflexes, and always take into consideration any contra-indications.

Crystals and body ecology

Remember that if you find any crystals, you need to work over them to disperse them. If your client experiences any pain, reduce the pressure to avoid causing further discomfort and work lightly over the area. Both crystals and pain indicate a reflex that is out of balance, which means that there has been, still is or could be a problem in the related body area.

Sometimes, however, you are simply dealing with body ecology, which means that something in the client's environment has altered the physiology of their body – for example, a change in diet, more or less exercise, or stress suffered during the course of the week.

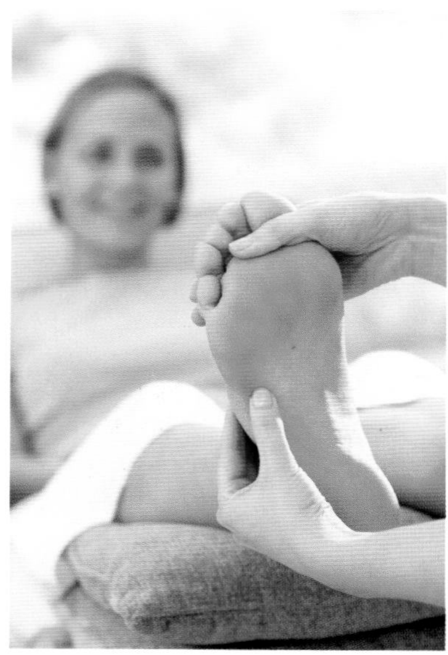

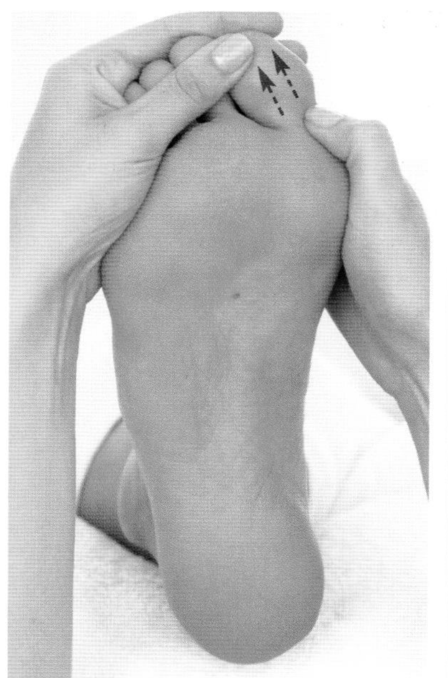

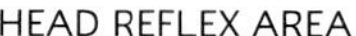

HEAD REFLEX AREA

Support the big toe with the fingers of one hand. Use your other thumb to walk up from the neckline to the top of the big toe. Repeat this several times in lines up the toe. This is a great reflex point to help with headaches or problems affecting the head.

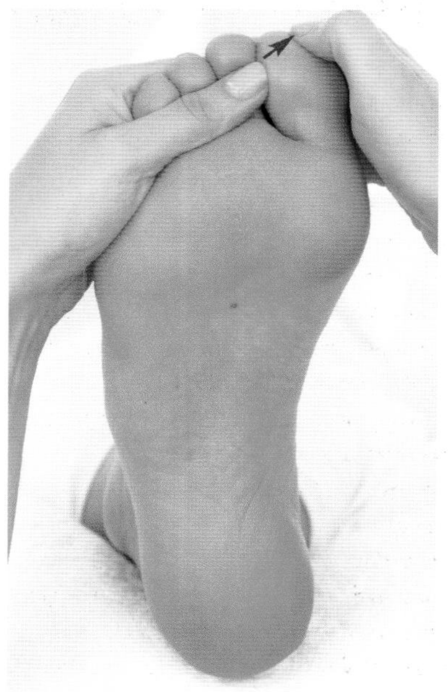

BRAIN REFLEX AREA

Support the big toe with the fingers of one hand. Use the thumb of your working hand to walk along the top of the big toe. Repeat this movement six times. This helps to give people a sense of well-being and balance, and to relieve headaches and stress. The brain reflex area can also assist in fighting depression and coping positively with life.

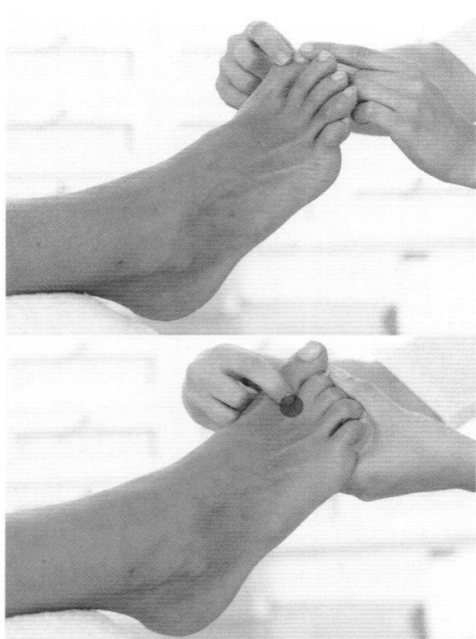

TEETH AND JAW REFLEX AREAS/THROAT REFLEX POINT

Support the foot with one hand. For the teeth, starting just below the nail, use your index finger to walk horizontally across the big toe. Repeat three times. Then, for the jaw reflex, starting just below the joint on the big toe, use your index finger to walk horizontally across the big toe. Repeat three times. Now press into the throat reflex and make small circles to work this point. Make eye contact with the client, so that you can reduce the pressure to avoid discomfort, if necessary. This reflex point helps any condition affecting the throat.

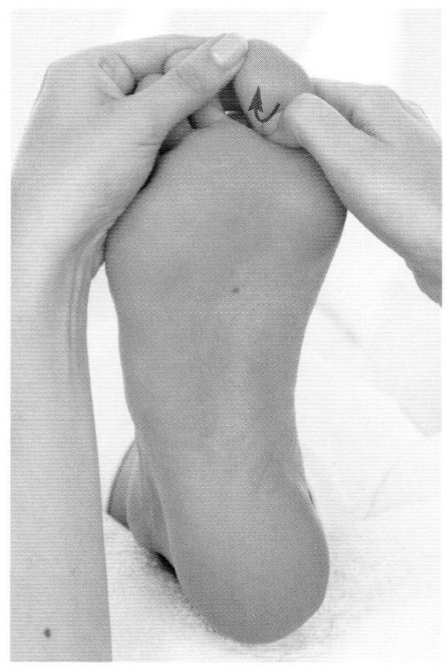

OCCIPITAL REFLEX POINT

Support the right foot, then walk along the base of the big toe with your right thumb and hook into the crease between the big toe and second toe. You will find a bone that juts out – place your thumb here and hook into the reflex point for ten seconds. This point is sensitive on most people because daily stresses affect the base of the skull.

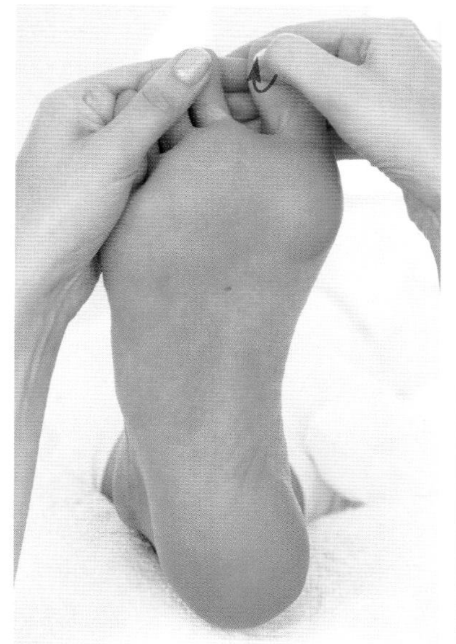

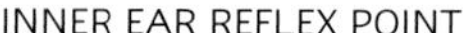

INNER EAR REFLEX POINT

Take two large steps up towards the top of the toe from the occipital reflex point. Place your thumb on the inner ear reflex and hook into the reflex point for ten seconds to work this area.

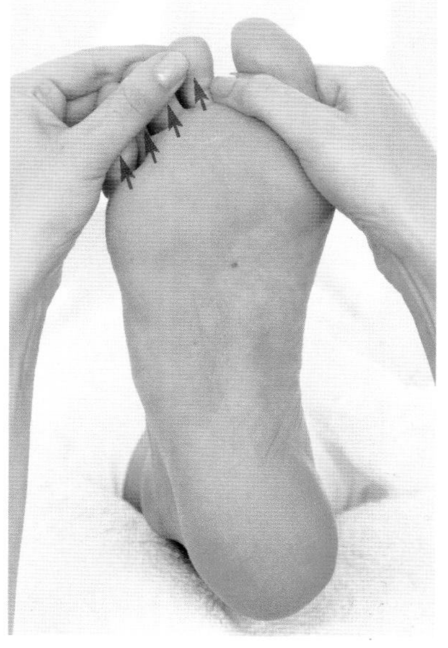

SINUS REFLEX AREA

Support the toes with one hand. Use your other thumb to walk up the medial aspect of the toes and then the lateral aspect, beginning at the second toe and working your way to the fifth toe. Use very small steps to cover as much surface area as you can. Continue in this manner through all the toes, completing the sequence twice. Working on the sinus reflexes can have amazing results in draining and strengthening the sinuses.

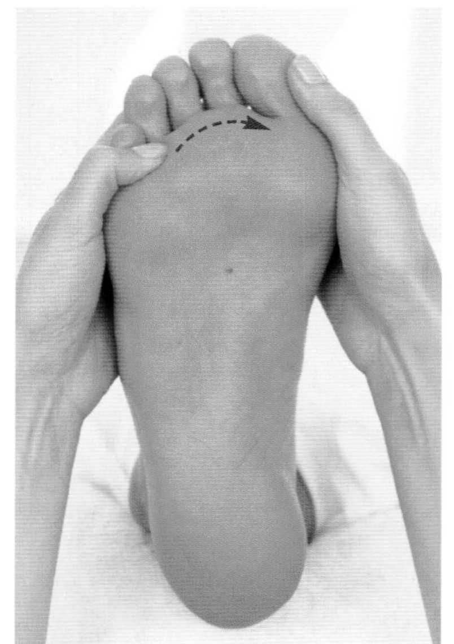

EYE/EAR GENERAL REFLEX AREA

Walk with your thumb from under the base of the second toe all the way along to the fifth toe. This whole section represents the eye/ear general area reflex. Walk across this area four times. This move helps with any problems affecting the eyes and ears.

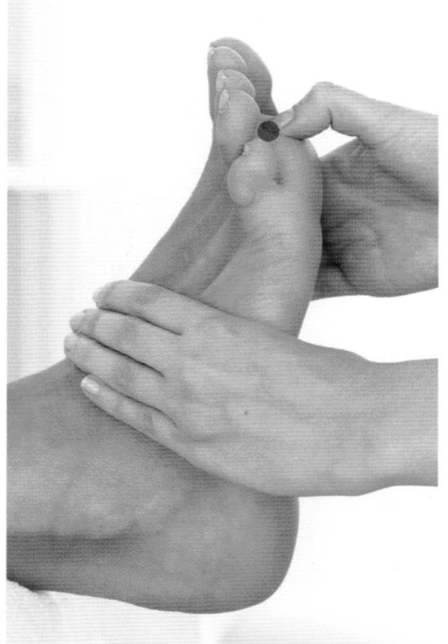

EYE REFLEX POINT

Place your thumb between the second and third toes. Press down and hook towards the big toe, working the point for six seconds. The eye reflex point on the right foot represents the right eye and that on the left foot represents the left eye. This move can help with all problems relating to the eyes.

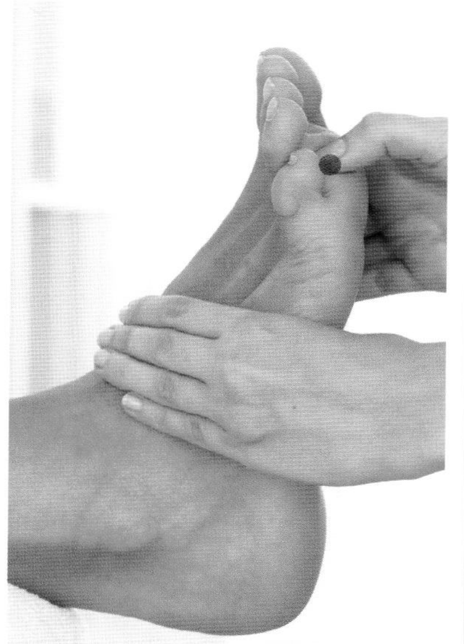

EUSTACHIAN TUBE REFLEX POINT

Place your thumb between the third and fourth toes. Press down and hook towards the big toe, working the point for six seconds. This point helps with inner ear disorders, aches and infections. It is also helps the inner ear to equalize in different altitudes – for example, when you are flying or if you need your ears to 'pop' while diving.

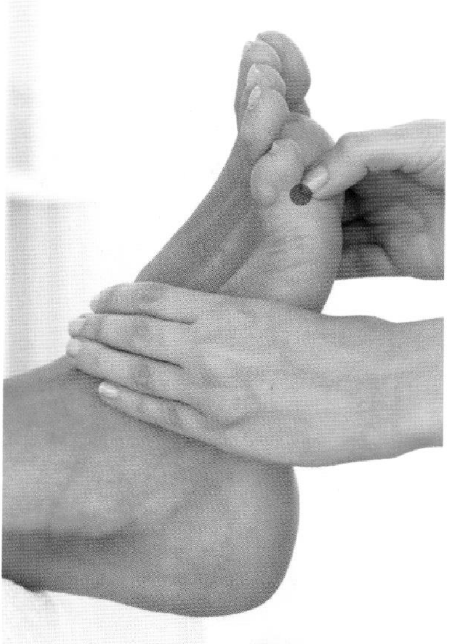

OUTER EAR REFLEX POINT

Place your thumb between the fourth and fifth toes. Press down and hook towards the big toe, working this reflex point for six seconds. You can identify conditions such as eczema on the outer ear.

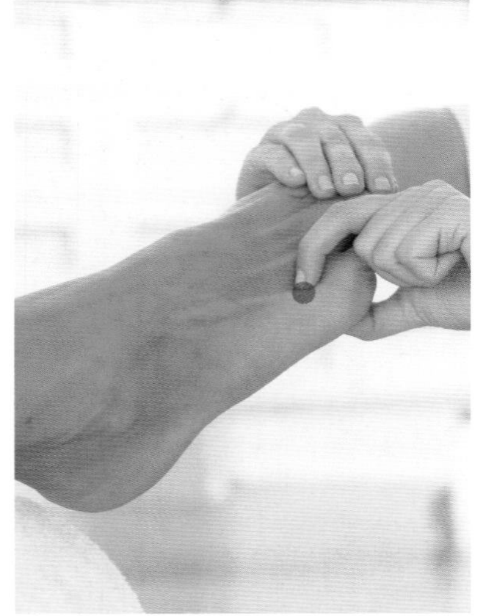

SHOULDER REFLEX POINT

This reflex point is found on the dorsal aspect of the foot, in between the fourth and fifth metatarsals. The simplest way to find it is to place your index finger and thumb at the base of the fourth and fifth toes. Slowly rock down for four steps, following the edge of the foot. When you hit the shoulder reflex point, stop and use the rocking technique for six seconds. Working this point can ease many problems that affect the shoulder, as well as relieving tension and increasing mobility in the area.

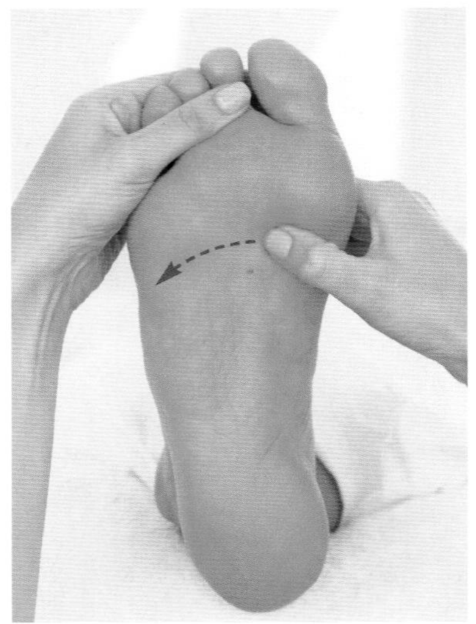

DIAPHRAGM REFLEX AREA

Support the foot with one hand, and use the thumb of your other hand to work under the metatarsal heads across the plantar aspect from medial to lateral. Use slow steps and repeat this move four times. Working the diaphragm reflex area can help with anxiety attacks, general stress and respiratory problems.

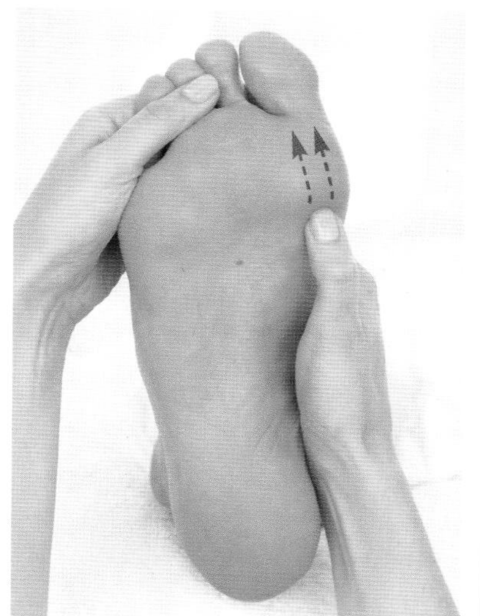

THYROID REFLEX AREA

Use one hand to pull the toes back, so that you will be able to find any crystals more easily. Use the thumb of your other hand to work the ball of the foot, from the diaphragm line all the way up to the neckline. Repeat this movement slowly six times over the area for 30 seconds. Working the thyroid reflex area can help regulate the body's energy levels, and also helps with the maintenance of body weight.

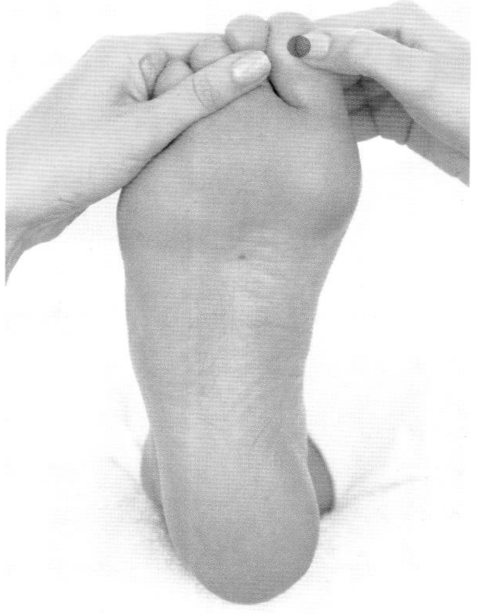

PITUITARY REFLEX POINT

This point is found in the middle of the plantar aspect of the big toe. Support the big toe with the fingers of one hand and use your other thumb to make a cross, to find the centre of the big toe. Place your thumb in the middle, then hook in with a medium pressure for ten seconds. This point helps to balance all of your hormones, by regulating and controlling their activities and many body processes. It is an important reflex point to help with female and male endocrine-system problems and complaints.

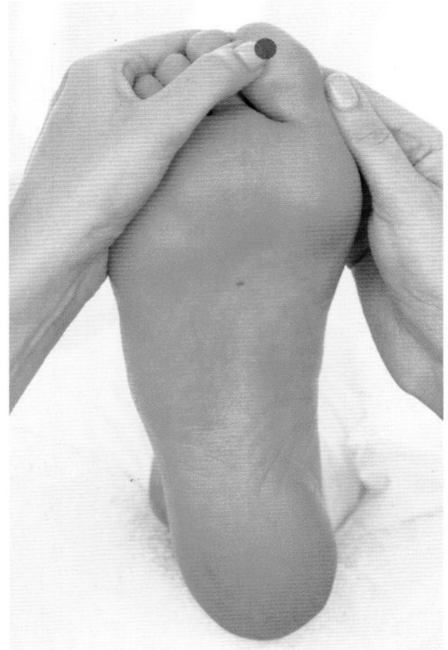

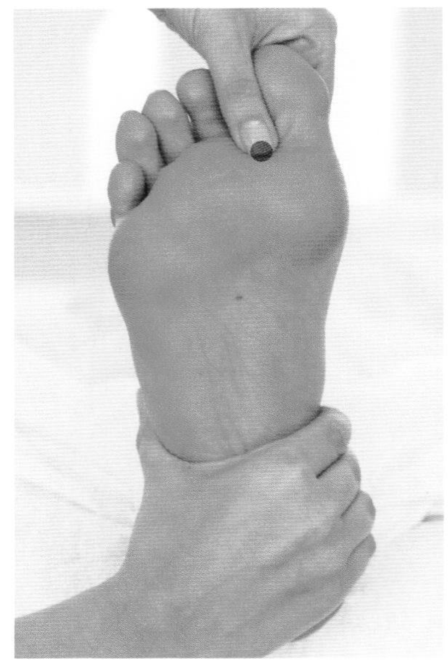

HYPOTHALAMUS REFLEX POINT

Move your thumb one step up, towards the tip of the big toe, and take a small step laterally. Hook in for ten seconds. Together with the pituitary gland, the hypothalamus regulates body temperature and sleep/wake cycles, and helps people to cope with the effects of stress.

PARATHYROID REFLEX POINT

This point is found in between the big toe and the second toe. Use your index finger and thumb to pinch the section of skin between the first and second toes. Hold the pressure and gently make circles for six seconds. This reflex point helps to control the levels of calcium in the blood, which can regulate muscle and bone density and nerve function, as well as helping with disorders relating to the parathyroid glands.

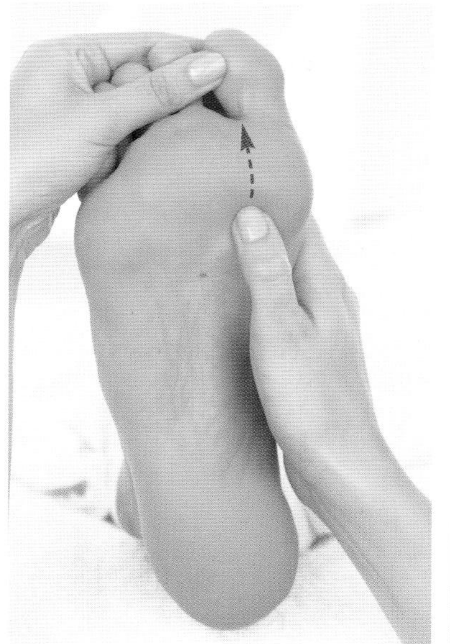

OESOPHAGUS REFLEX AREA

Support the foot with one hand, and place the thumb of your other hand at the diaphragm line in between zones one and two. Work your thumb up in between the metatarsals, from the diaphragm line to the eye/ear general reflex area (see page 140). Repeat this process four times. Working this area can ease disorders of the oesophagus, bad breath, trouble in swallowing and heartburn.

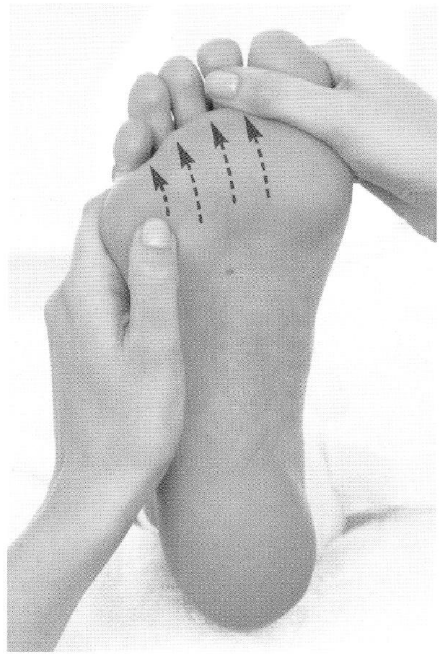

LUNG REFLEX AREA

Support the foot with one hand, and use the thumb of your other hand to work up from the diaphragm line to the eye/ear general reflex area (see page 140). You should be working in between the metatarsals to properly stimulate the lung. Repeat this process twice, making sure that you have worked in between all the metatarsals. Working this area can ease disorders of the lungs, as well as helping to strengthen their functions.

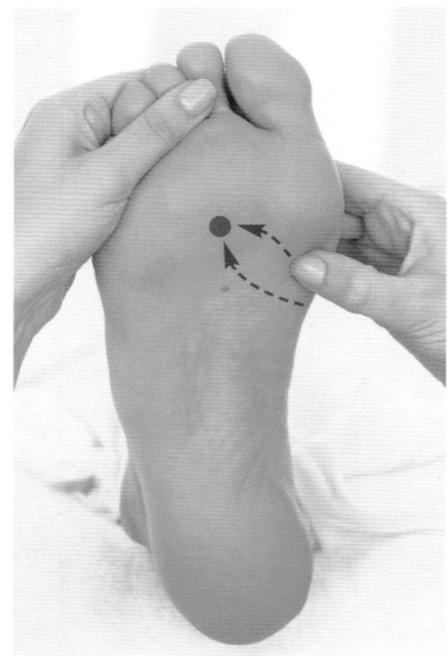

STOMACH REFLEX AREA

This reflex area is located just under the ball of the foot. Support the foot with one hand, and place your other thumb just below the thyroid reflex area (see page 143). Gently work up towards the solar plexus three to four times. People with stomach disorders may find this area sensitive, or you may feel crystals here. Work this area to help ease stomach complaints, such as ulcers, and help with the production of digestive juices.

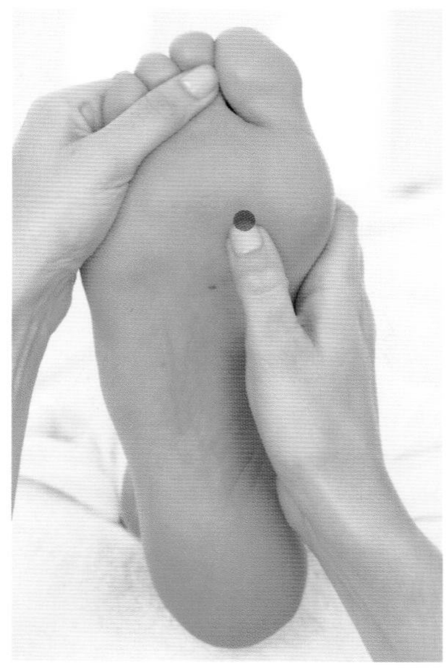

HIATUS HERNIA REFLEX POINT

This point is located along the diaphragm line, in between zones one and two. Flex the foot back with one hand, and place the thumb of your other hand on the hiatus hernia point. Stay on this point making circles for 12 seconds. A hiatus hernia is a common condition – a protrusion of part of the stomach through a weak area in the diaphragm. By working this reflex you can help with the associated symptoms, including acid reflux, heartburn and pain.

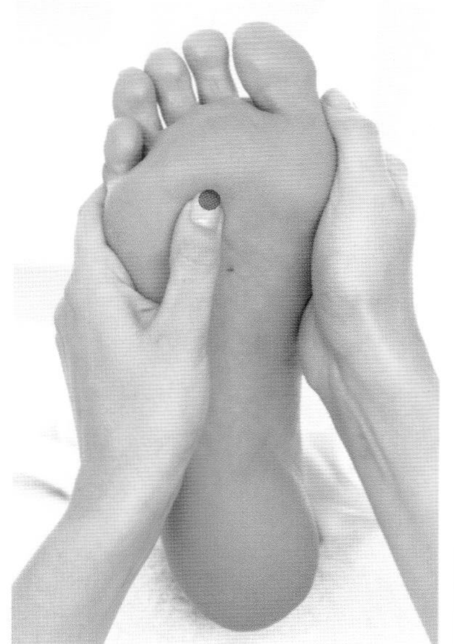

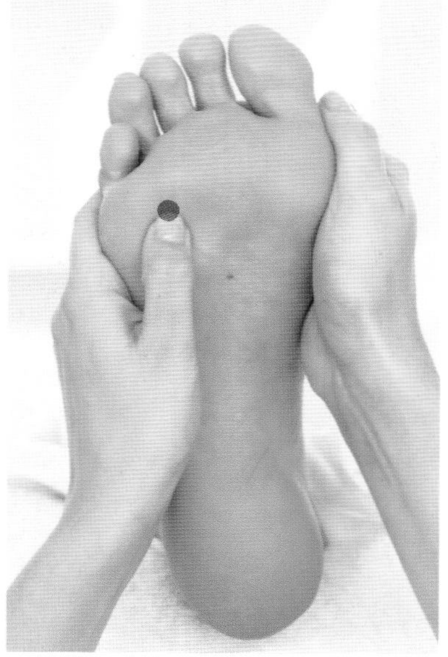

PANCREAS REFLEX POINT

This reflex point is only found on the right foot. Place your thumb on the third toe, tracing a line down to below the diaphragm line. Push up into the joint and hook up for six seconds. Working the pancreas reflex point can help with good digestion, by secreting digestive enzymes to break down fats and by helping to balance blood-sugar levels with the production of insulin.

GALL BLADDER REFLEX POINT

This reflex point is only found on the right foot. Place your thumb on the fourth toe and trace a line down to below the diaphragm line. Push up into the joint and hook up for six seconds. The gall bladder is the body's own dishwashing-liquid bottle and squeezes out bile, which has a detergent-like effect on the fats we eat. Working this point can help with gall bladder problems.

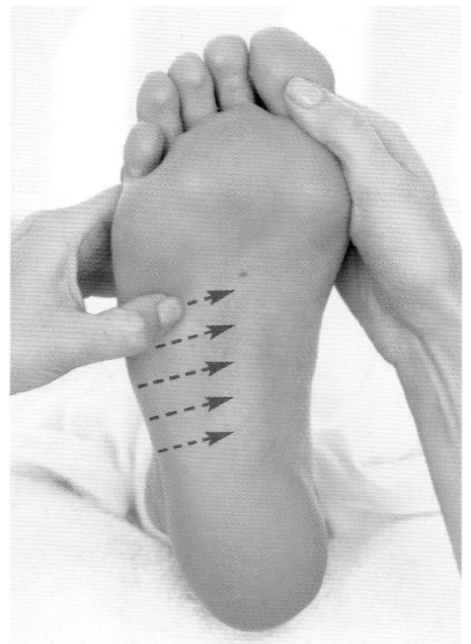

LIVER REFLEX AREA

This reflex area is only found on the right foot. Support the foot with your right hand, and place your left thumb just underneath the diaphragm line. Work slowly and precisely, horizontally across the foot, from zone five to zone three. Proceed in one direction. Continue in this manner until you get just above the redness of the heel. Complete the process twice. This can help regulate levels of the many chemicals and glucose in the blood, dispose of used hormones and in clearing the blood of drugs and toxins.

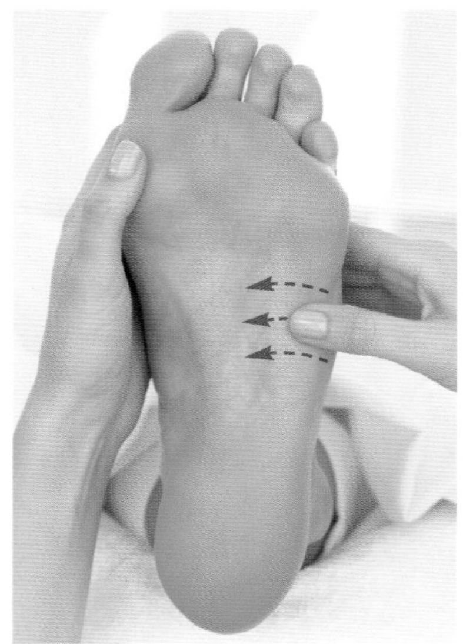

SPLEEN REFLEX AREA

This reflex area is only found on the left foot. Support the foot with your left hand, and place your right thumb just underneath the diaphragm line. Work slowly and precisely, horizontally across the foot, into zones five and four and just into zone three. Proceed in one direction. Continue in this manner for four horizontal lines. Complete the spleen reflex twice. Working this reflex will help to fight infection in the body as well as destroy old blood cells.

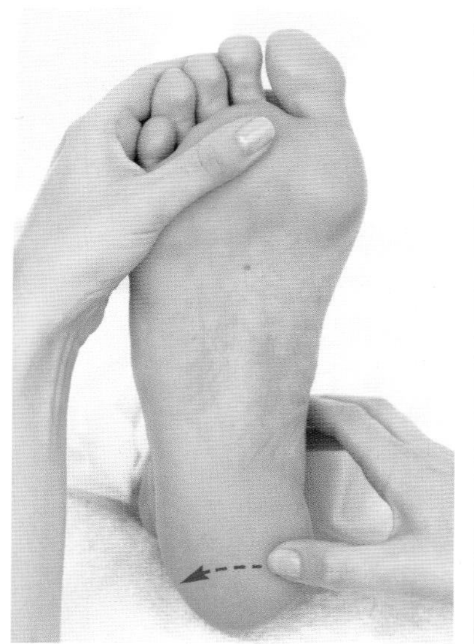

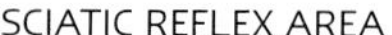

SCIATIC REFLEX AREA

This area runs horizontally across the redness of the heel. Support the foot with one hand, and place your other thumb halfway up the redness of the heel. Walk across the plantar aspect from medial to lateral, then swap hands and walk back again. By working this reflex area you can help with sciatica, especially with pain that radiates along the sciatic nerve and may extend down through the legs to the feet. Repeat this move five times.

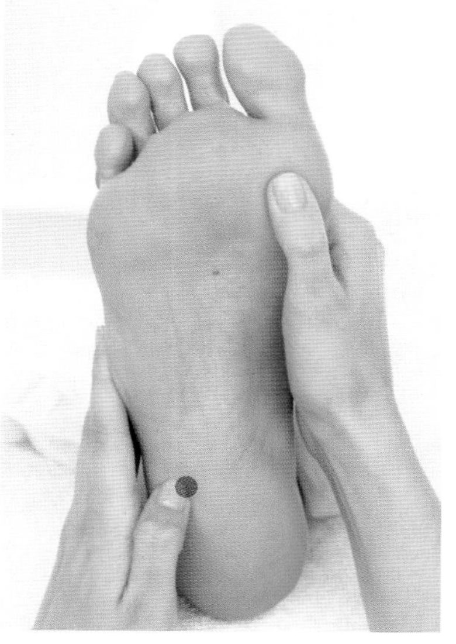

APPENDIX REFLEX POINT

This reflex point is only found on the right foot. Place your left thumb on the fourth toe and slide all the way down to the redness of the heel. Push in and make circles for six seconds. Because the appendix contains a large amount of lymphoid tissue, by working this reflex point you can help boost the body's immune system against local infection here.

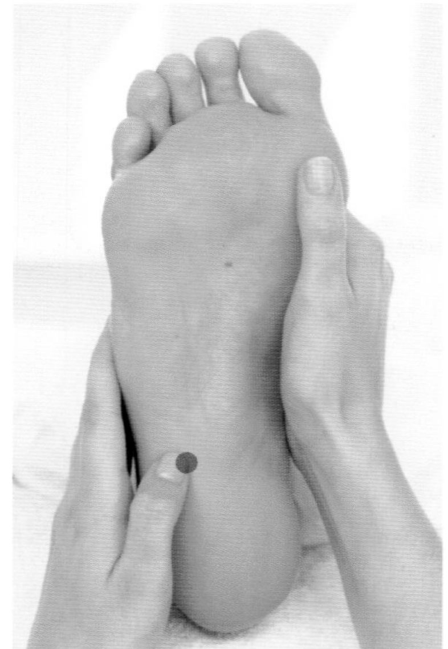

ILEOCAECAL VALVE REFLEX POINT

This reflex point is only found on the right foot. Place your left thumb on the appendix reflex point (see page 149), and take half a thumbprint up towards the fourth toe. Push in and make circles for six seconds. This valve prevents the backflow of waste matter from the large to the small intestine and assists in good digestion and mucus balance in the body.

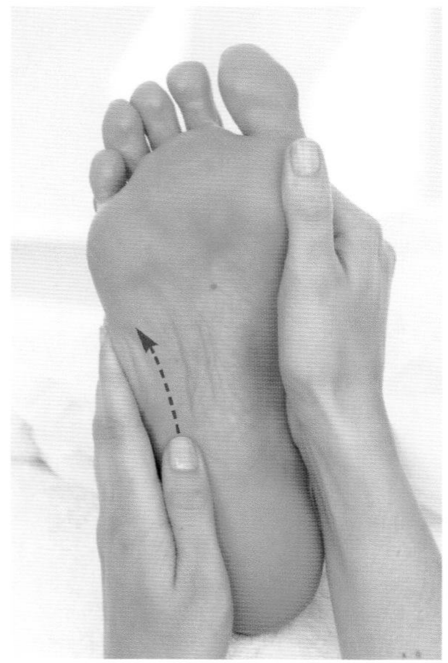

ASCENDING COLON REFLEX AREA

This reflex area is only found on the right foot. Use your left thumb to walk up zone four from the ileocaecal valve point (see left) to work this first part of the colon. Continue in this manner until you get to the hepatic flexure point (see opposite), which is halfway up the foot. Work the ascending colon reflex area twice and with slow movements, to help stimulate the peristaltic muscular action of the colon.

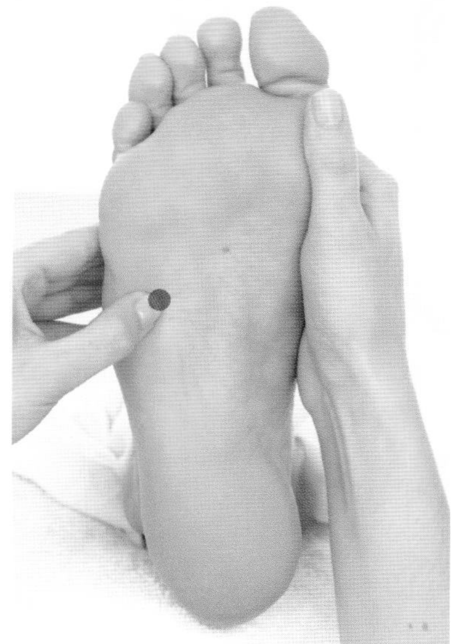

HEPATIC FLEXURE POINT

This reflex point is only found on the right foot. Continuing up from the ascending colon, stop halfway up the foot at the hepatic flexure point. Hook in for six seconds. By working this reflex point you can help with the correct functioning of the colon, which in turn encourages the liver to work better.

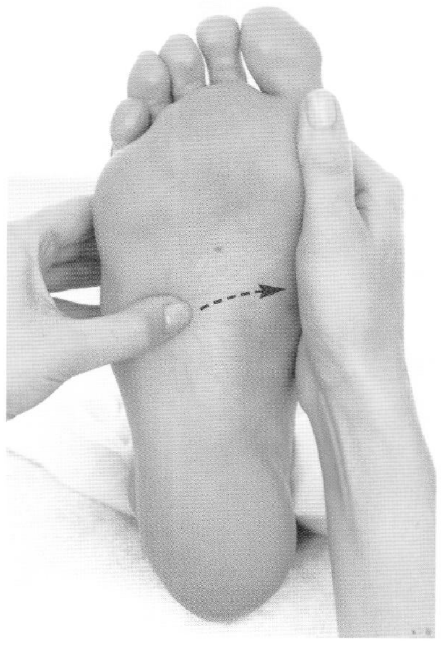

TRANSVERSE COLON REFLEX AREA

This reflex area is found horizontally across the plantar aspect of the foot, from lateral to medial. Work across from the hepatic flexure point, ending up just underneath the stomach reflex (see page 146). Work the transverse colon twice to help with good bowel movements.

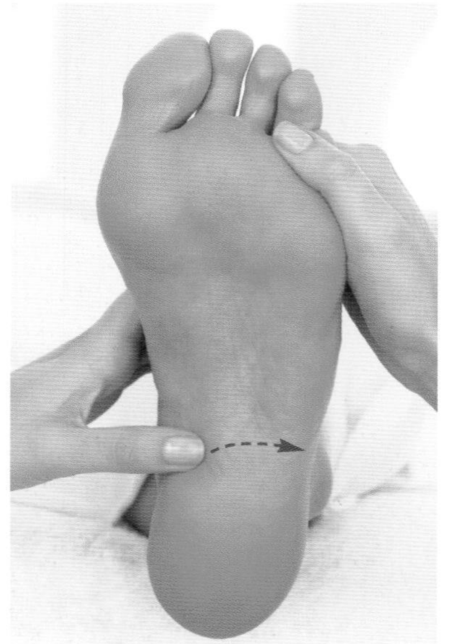

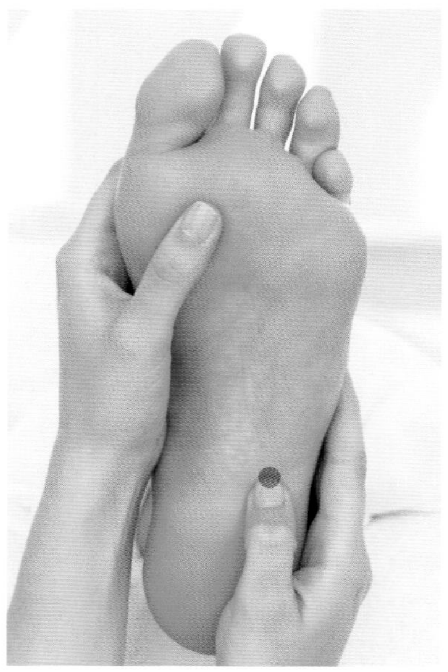

SIGMOID COLON REFLEX AREA

This reflex area is only found on the left foot. Place your left thumb at the medial aspect of the foot and just above the redness of the heel. Walk across the redness of the heel to zone four. The sigmoid colon has the specialized job of contracting vigorously to maintain high pressure and regulate the movement of stools into the rectum. Working this reflex area can help with constipation, haemorrhoids and diverticulitis.

SIGMOID FLEXURE REFLEX POINT

This reflex point is only found on the left foot. Swap thumbs in zone four, placing your right thumb on the sigmoid flexure reflex point. Push in and hook the point for six seconds. This can help the colon to function more efficiently.

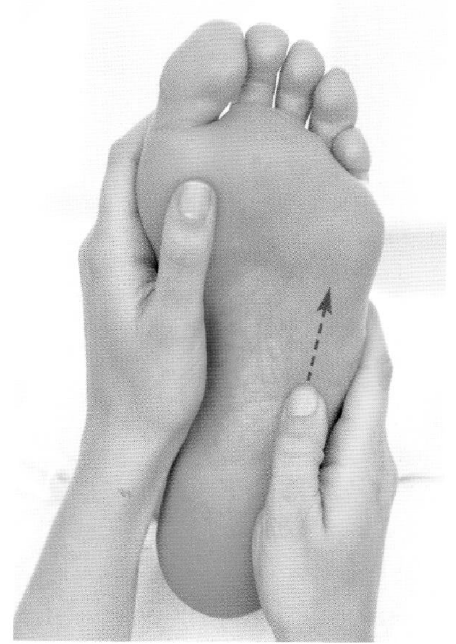

DESCENDING COLON REFLEX AREA

This reflex area is only found on the left foot. Use your right thumb to walk up zone four from the sigmoid flexure reflex point, to work this part of the colon. Continue in this manner until you get halfway up the foot. Work the descending colon reflex area twice. By working it you can promote adequate enzyme activity in the colon, which is necessary throughout the whole of the gastro-intestinal tract.

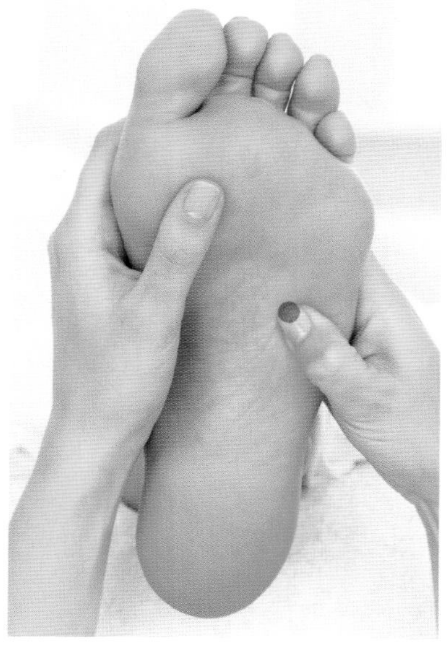

SPLENIC FLEXURE REFLEX POINT

This reflex point is only found on the left foot. Continuing up from the descending colon reflex area, stop halfway up the foot for the splenic flexure point. Hook in for six seconds. By working this point you can help with splenic flexure syndrome, which is the trapping of gas at the splenic flexure (a bend in the colon), causing distension and bloating.

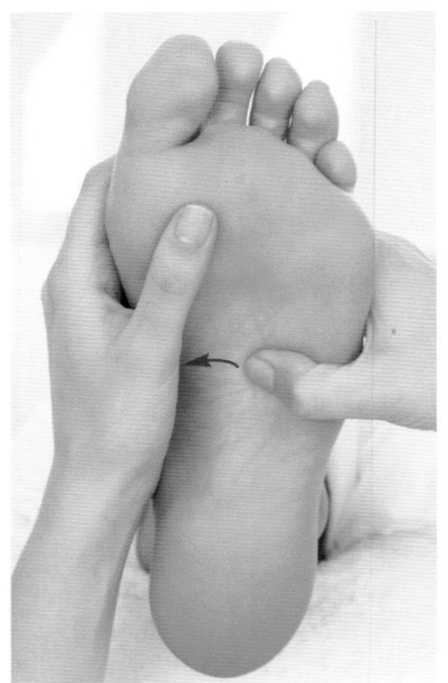

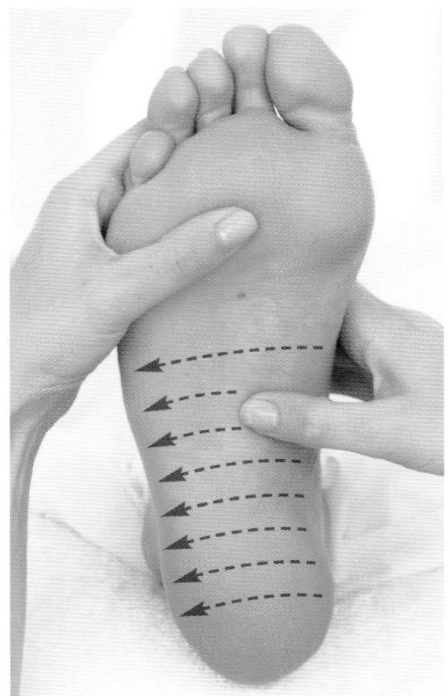

TRANSVERSE COLON REFLEX AREA

This reflex area is found horizontally across the plantar aspect of the foot from lateral to medial. Work across from the splenic flexure reflex point, ending up just underneath the stomach reflex (see page 146). Work the transverse colon twice to help with good bowel movements. Working this area on both feet during the sequence ensures better results.

SMALL INTESTINE REFLEX AREA

Walk across the foot horizontally with either thumb. Start just below the transverse colon reflex area (see left) and continue in this manner down to the base of the heel. The small intestine is where the most extensive part of digestion occurs. Most food products are absorbed there, so working this area can help with the absorption of essential vitamins.

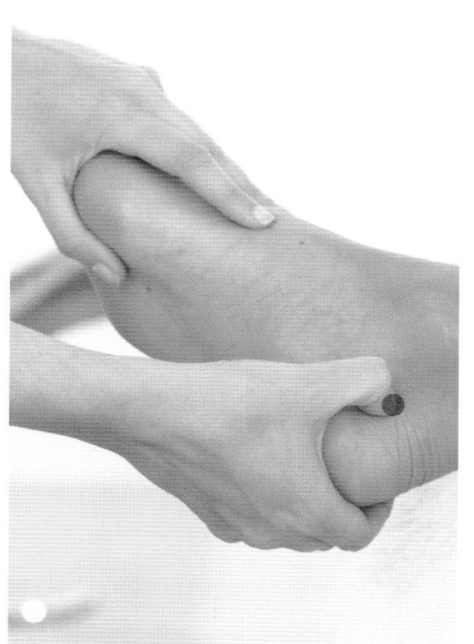

UTERUS/PROSTATE REFLEX POINT

Work on the medial side of the foot. Place your index finger approximately halfway between the back of the heel and the ankle bone. Push in gently and make circles for ten seconds. By working the uterus and prostate reflex points you can help with good general reproductive health.

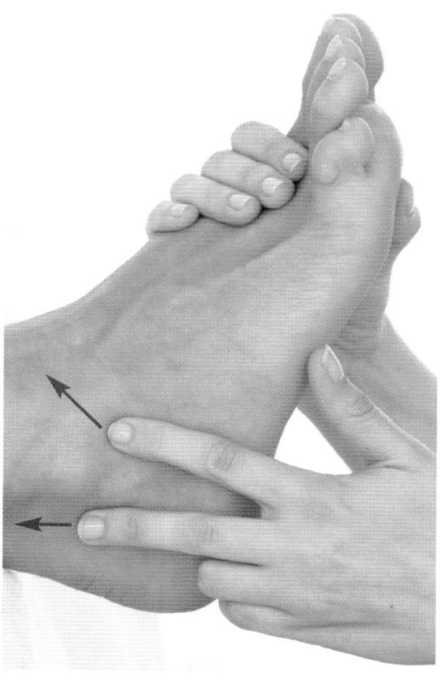

LYMPHATICS OF THE GROIN REFLEX AREA

This area is found on either side of the ankle bone. Use your index finger to rock up on either side of the ankle bone slowly for ten seconds. Working this reflex area helps to increase the body's defences against infection and cancer in the lower part of the body; it could also be sensitive if the client is menstruating.

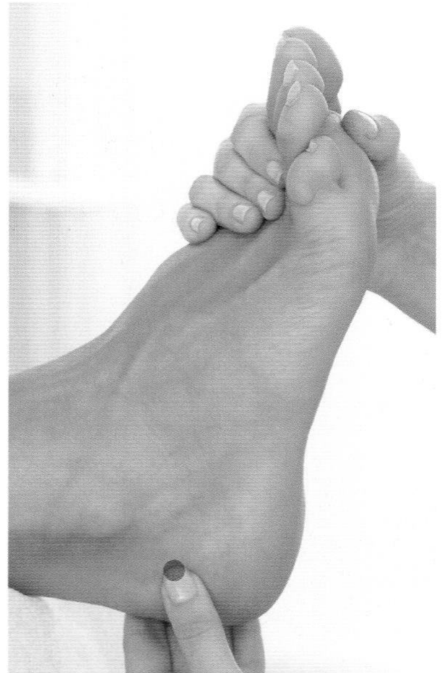

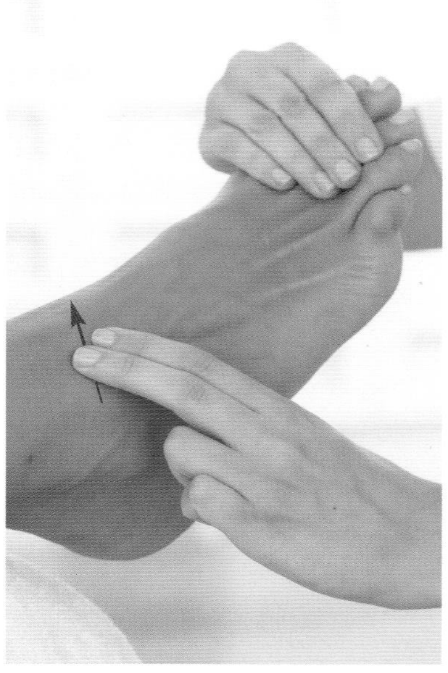

OVARY/TESTICLE REFLEX POINT

Work on the lateral side of foot. Place your index finger approximately halfway between the back of the heel and the ankle bone. Push in gently and make circles for ten seconds. By working the ovary and testicle reflex points you can help with the production of sex hormones, as well as regulating ovulation and healthy sperm production.

FALLOPIAN TUBE/VAS DEFERENS REFLEX AREA

This reflex area is located across the top of the foot. Use your index and middle fingers to walk from the lateral to the medial aspect of the foot, connecting ankle bone to ankle bone and back again. Continue in this manner for six seconds. This is a good area to work on to help fertility issues.

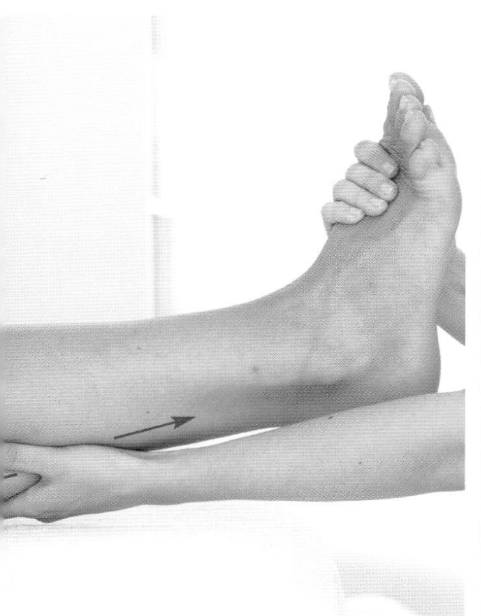

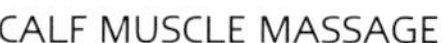

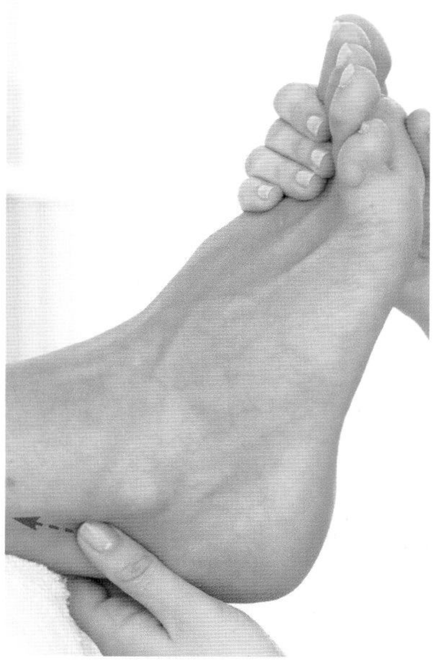

CALF MUSCLE MASSAGE

Using both hands, massage the calf muscle behind the leg and work up towards the knee. Continue this movement gently for ten seconds. This can help with the circulation of the blood and lymph back up to the heart, to be reoxygenated and to take away waste products.

RECTUM/ANUS REFLEX AREA

Use your thumb and index finger to gently squeeze behind the entire Achilles tendon, down to the heel. Working this reflex area can help with defecation and the pain associated with inflammation in the rectum. Continue for 10 seconds.

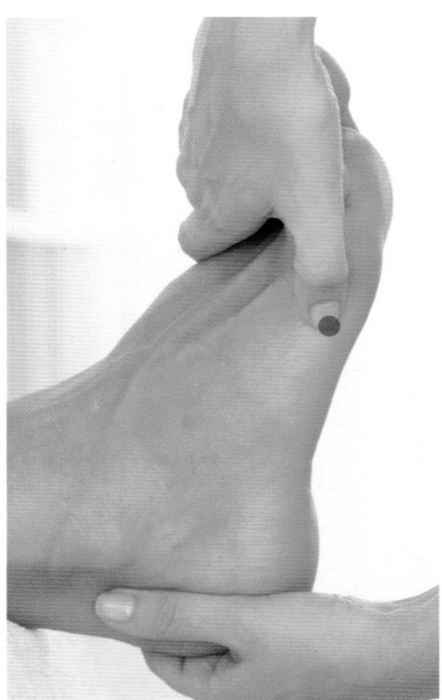

WRIST REFLEX POINT

Use your thumb to walk one step down the lateral aspect of the foot from the fifth toe. Push in to rock the wrist reflex point, and then make circles for six seconds. This is a good reflex point to work to help with conditions such as carpal tunnel syndrome and repetitive strain injury.

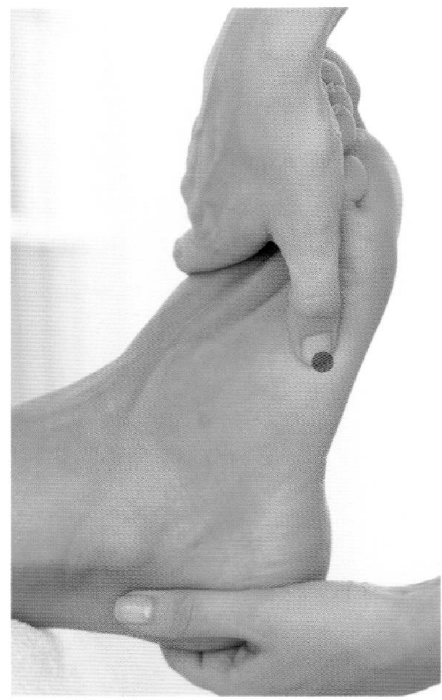

ELBOW REFLEX POINT

From the wrist reflex point take one step for the elbow reflex point. Push in to work the elbow reflex point, and rock on the point for six seconds. This reflex point helps with nerve problems in the arm, arthritis affecting the elbow, golfer's or tennis elbow and speeding up the healing of fractures in this area.

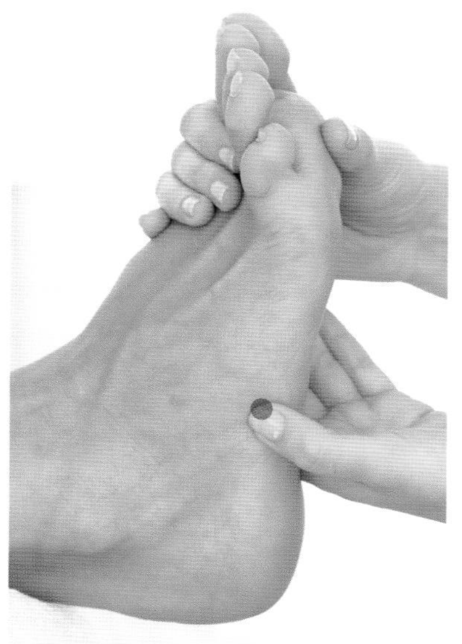

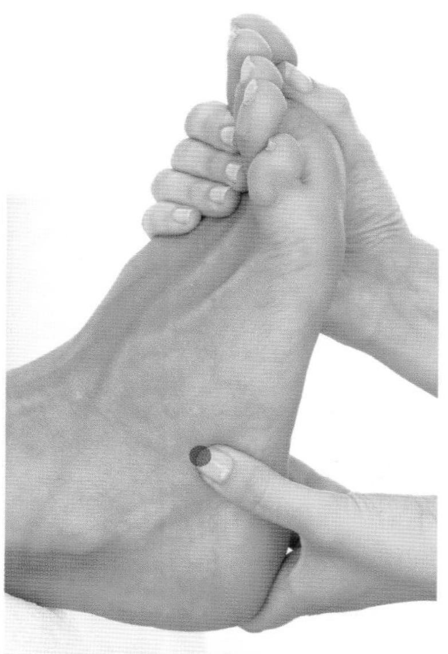

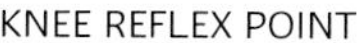

KNEE REFLEX POINT

Use your thumb to take two steps from the elbow reflex point to the knee reflex point. You can feel this point as a small bony protrusion on the side of the foot. Push in to hook on it for six seconds. This reflex point helps to reduce the pain associated with ligament sprains and arthritis and strengthens the knee joint for optimum sports performance.

HIP REFLEX POINT

Using your thumb, take two diagonal steps from the knee reflex point to the ankle bone. Rock the point to help stimulate this area. Work this point for six seconds. By working the hip reflex point you can ease hip disorders such as arthritis, help to heal fractures, recovery from hip surgery and pain in the hip.

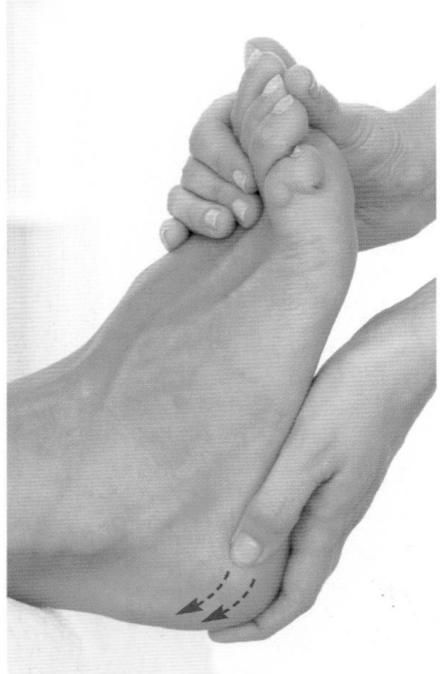

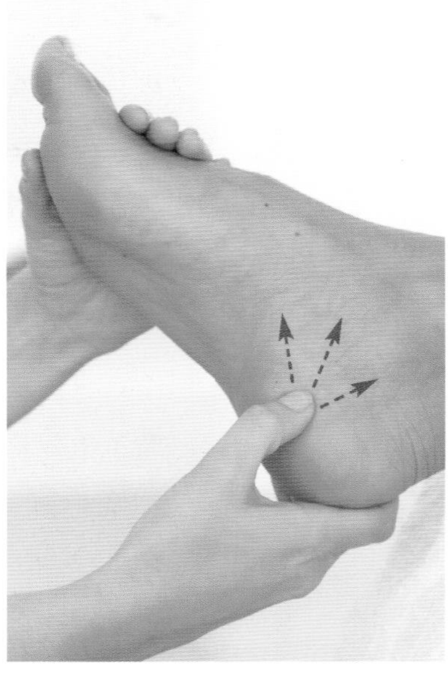

LOWER BACK/SACRUM REFLEX AREA

Use your finger in a rocking technique to work from the knee reflex point (see page 159) to the back quadrant of the heel, working with slow, precise movements for ten seconds. Continue this method, covering the last section of the heel and always keeping low to avoid going over the ovary or testicle reflex point (see page 156). Working this area helps to ease the pain of lower backache.

BLADDER REFLEX AREA

Use your thumb to fan out (like the spokes of a bicycle wheel) over the soft area on the medial aspect of the foot until you reach the spinal reflex, always returning to the place you started from. Work on this area six times. Don't be surprised to find crystals here if your client has cystitis; just keep working to disperse the crystals.

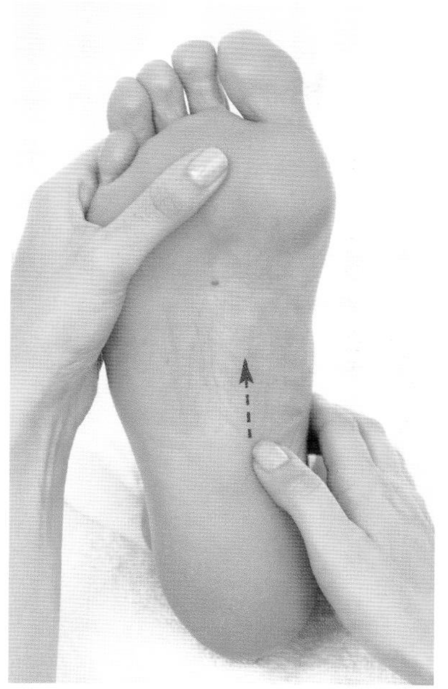

URETER TUBE REFLEX AREA

Flex the foot back a little and walk slowly up the tendon that you will find one-third of the way into the foot. Repeat this movement four times. Most people don't drink enough water for their body's needs, and this can show up as crystals in the ureter tube reflex area.

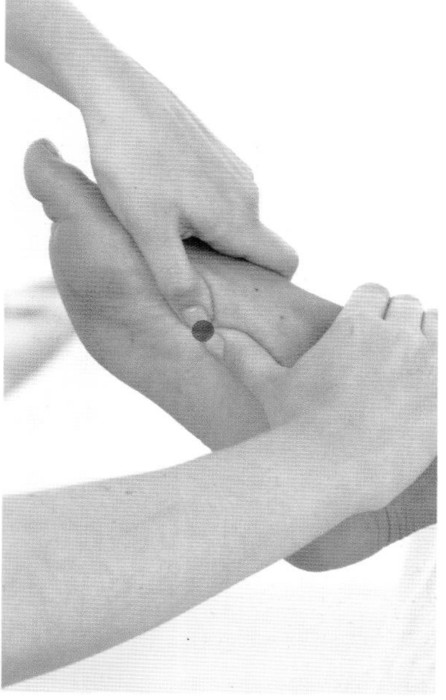

KIDNEY/ADRENAL REFLEX POINTS

The adrenal glands lie on the kidney, and you can find these reflexes on the top of the ureter tube reflex area. When you have reached the top of the ureter tube reflex, place your two thumbs together and gently pull-apart to tear into the kidney and adrenal reflexes, increasing and reducing your pressure. Work in this manner for ten seconds. These are naturally sensitive reflexes, and working them can assist in reducing pain in the body, as well as helping the body to cope with stress.

WORKING THE SPINE

The spinal reflexes are arranged so that each move your thumb or finger takes represents a specific vertebra, so if you work carefully you can accurately identify which vertebra is causing a problem. Work underneath or against the bone to access the spine, and apply gentle pressure. Frequent, light treatments can offer pain relief. You can use any of the movements given on pages 164–165, depending on the client's needs.

The groupings of vertebrae are as follows:

- The seven cervical vertebrae support the neck and head.
- The 12 thoracic vertebrae anchor the ribs.
- The five lumbar vertebrae towards the bottom of the spine are strong weight-bearing regions and provide a centre of gravity during movement.
- The five sacral vertebrae and the four coccygeal vertebrae are fused.

When you use reflexology on the spinal reflexes you are working on a number of different levels:

1 Helping with problems like backache and with spinal injuries and disorders. When you work the spine, certain areas will appear sensitive; these are the specific vertebrae that may be causing the problem. Working on them gently over time can help reduce the pain/tension/muscle spasm and strengthen the area.

2 Assisting with emotional issues, because the central nervous system is composed of the brain and spinal cord, which is protected by the spinal column. By working the spine, you are helping to turn off the body's 'fight-or-flight' response and turn on the parasympathetic nervous system, which promotes a state of balance and well-being.

3 Working the whole body, through the spinal nerve roots that connect the spinal cord to all parts of the body.

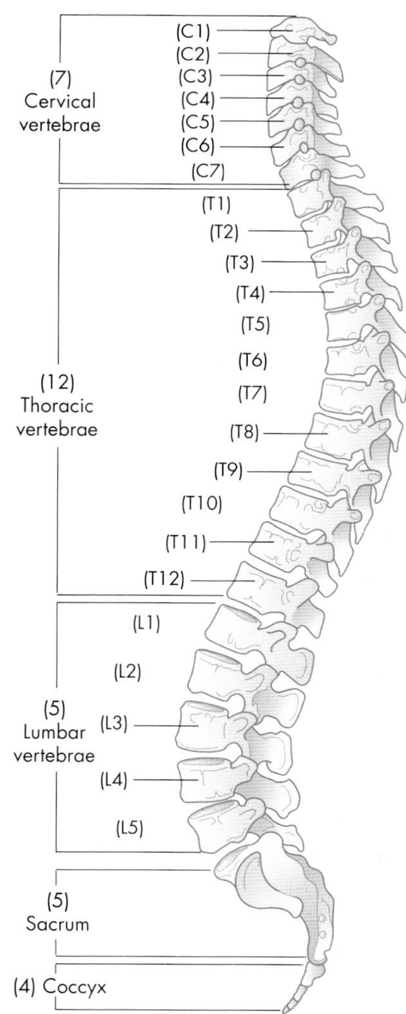

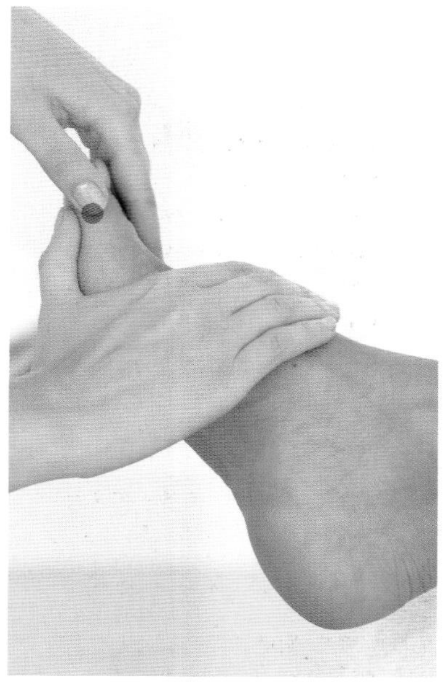

CERVICAL VERTEBRAE REFLEX AREA

This lies on the medial aspect of the big toe and in between the joints (but you do not work on the joints because of many different factors that could affect them). Support the big toe with one hand. Use the thumb of the other hand to make seven small steps, remembering that each step represents a specific vertebra. Walk towards the foot. Repeat the movement five times.

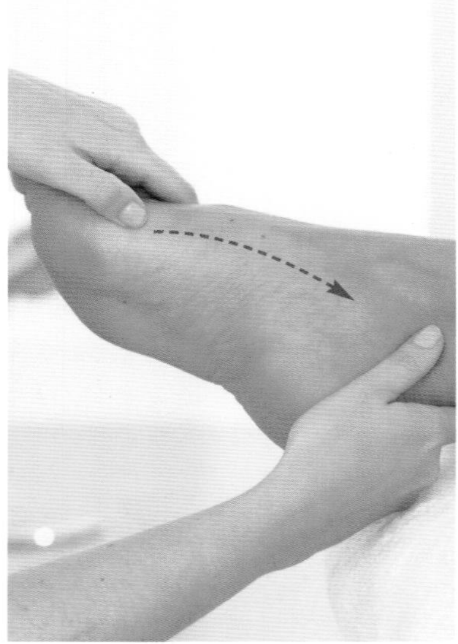

THORACIC VERTEBRAE REFLEX AREA

Take 12 steps from the base of the joint of the big toe to work the thoracic vertebrae reflex area. You should end up on a bone called the navicular, which feels like a knuckle and is halfway between the bladder reflex area (see page 160) and the ankle. The key to working on the spine is light pressure to avoid a healing crisis reaction (see page 92) and increased frequency of treatments – such as three to four times a week.

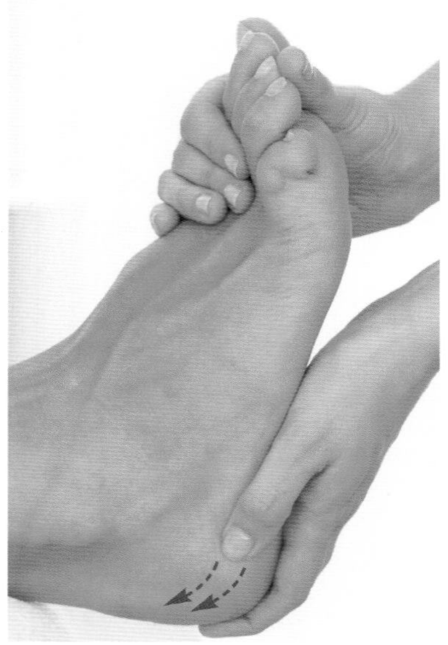

LOWER BACK/SACRUM REFLEX AREA

Use your finger in a rocking technique to work from the knee reflex point (see page 159) to the back quadrant of the heel, working with slow, precise movements for ten seconds. Continue this method, covering the last section of the heel and always keeping low to avoid going over the ovary or testicle reflex point (see page 156). Working this area twice in the sequence ensures better results.

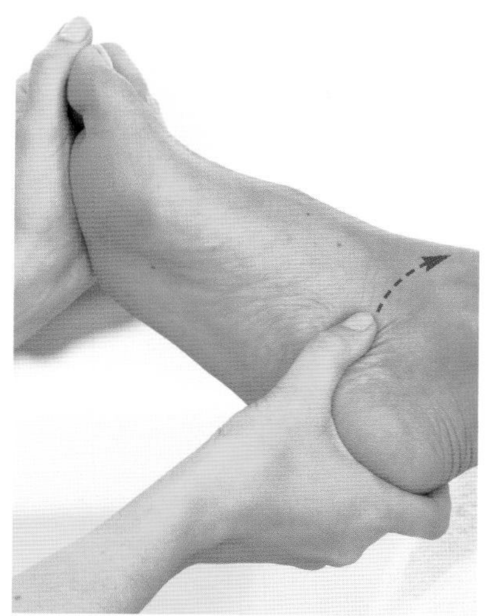

LUMBAR VERTEBRAE REFLEX AREA

Walk around the navicular bone, which represents lumbar one; take five steps up to the dip in front of the ankle bone, which represents lumbar five. Push into lumbar five and make small circles for six seconds. Repeat the movement twice.

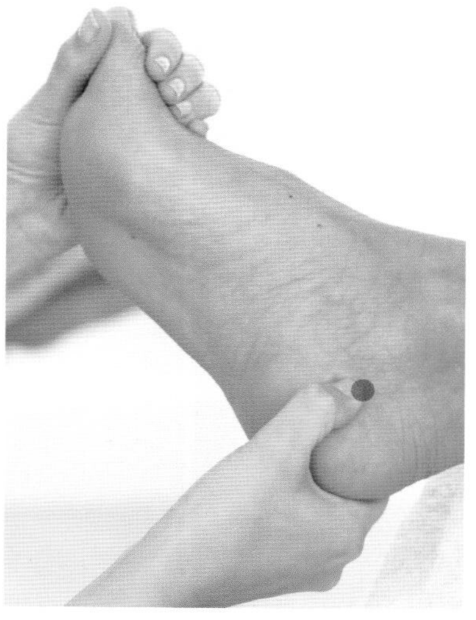

COCCYX REFLEX POINT

Place your thumb on the bladder reflex area (see page 160) and take two large steps along the medial aspect of the heel. Push in and make large circles.

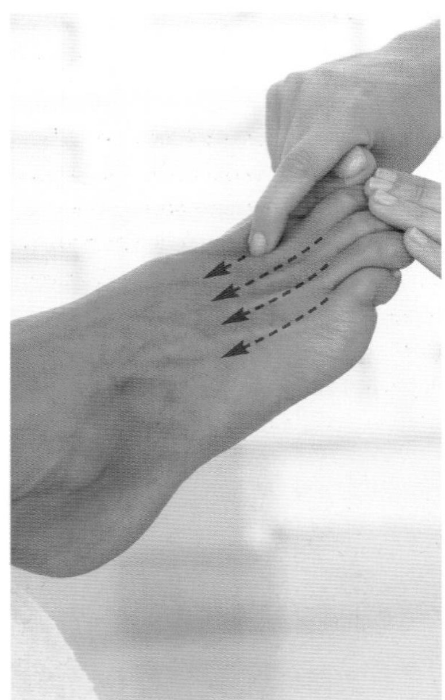

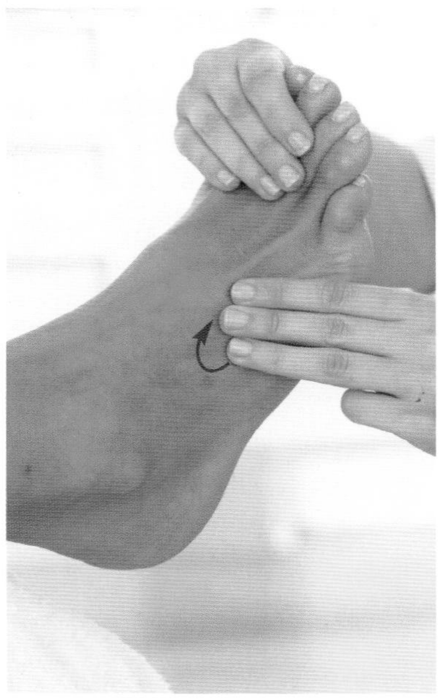

UPPER LYMPHATIC REFLEX AREA

Use the rocking technique on the dorsal aspect, working from the base of the toes towards the ankle in between the metatarsals. Work with a medium pressure up as far as you can, then slide back to make circles lightly between the clefts of the toes. Repeat this method twice to strengthen the body's immune system.

BREAST REFLEX AREA

This reflex area is located halfway down the dorsal aspect of the foot. Support the foot with one hand, and place three fingers of the other hand halfway up the foot in between zones four and five. Make large, gentle circles to work this area. By working this reflex you can help with disorders of the breast, including infection, benign tumours and the breast tenderness associated with menstruation.

Closing the treatment

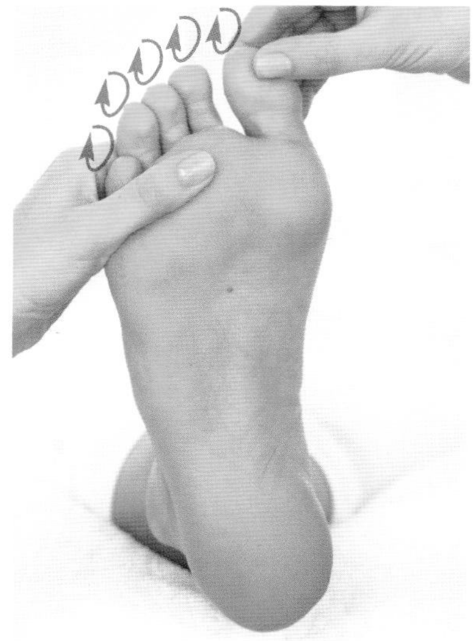

TOE ROTATION

Hold the base of the toes with the fingers of one hand, and rotate them with the fingers of your other hand to energize your client. When you have finished the right foot, move on to the left foot. Once you have completed both feet, use the techniques for relaxing the feet (see pages 122–127), ending up with inner energy breathing to close the treatment.

Aftercare

Now that your treatment is complete, the first question you should ask is how is your client feeling? Once they have answered that question, cover their feet with a towel and go and wash your hands. When you come back to your client, offer them a glass of water. This will help to flush away any toxins that have been released during the reflexology session.

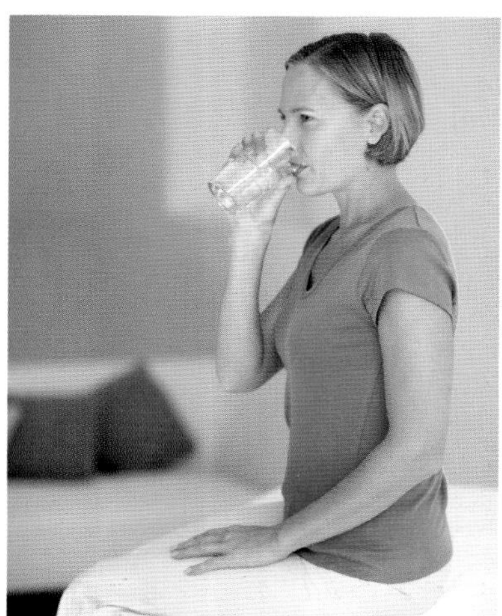

Drinking hot or cold water after a treatment helps flush out toxins from the system.

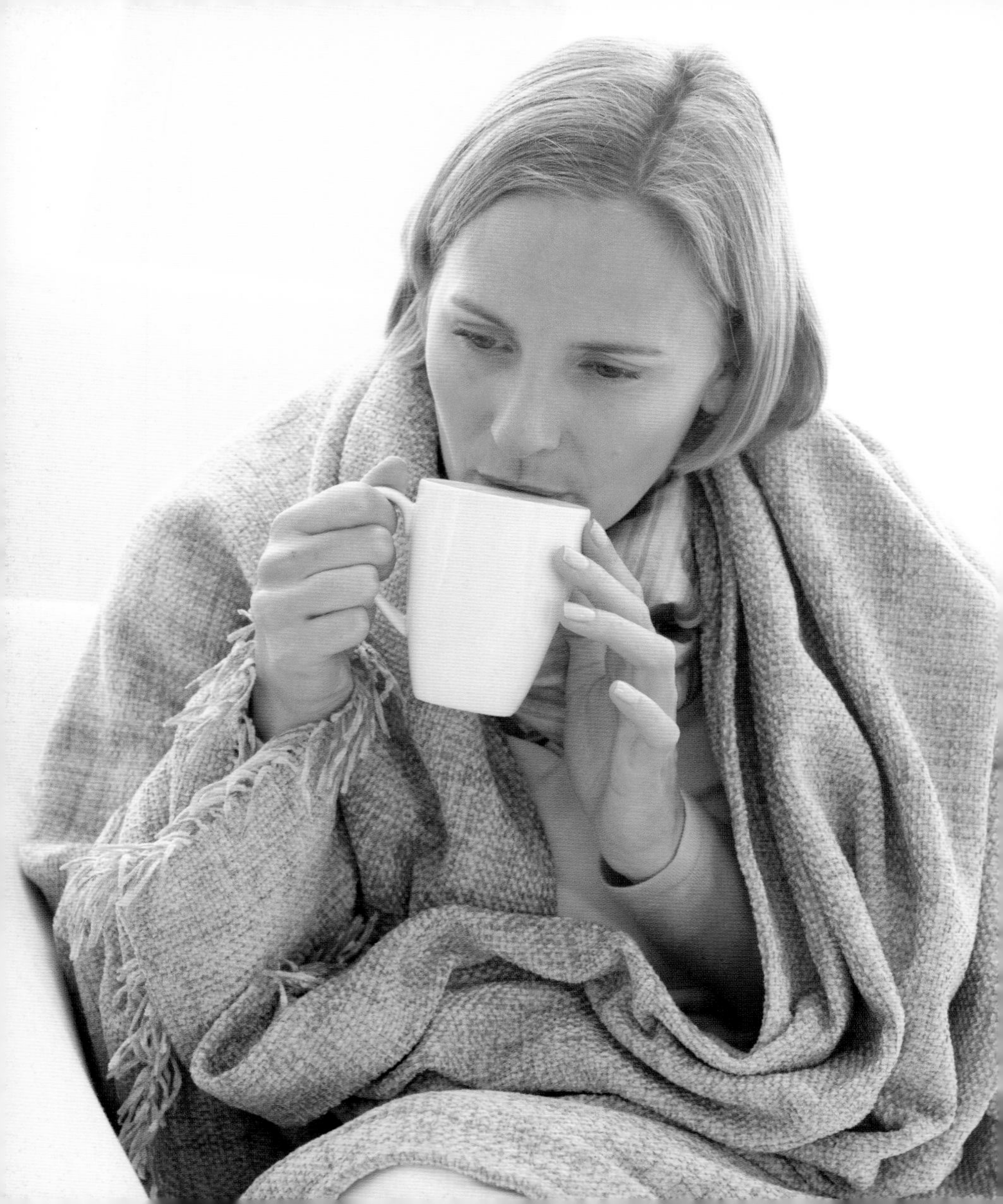

PART 5

Reflexology for common ailments

How to use this part

In this part of the book there are simple, effective reflexology sequences to help you treat common ailments, ranging from acne and asthma to psoriasis and a sore throat. They are grouped by body system (see below), so that all the circulatory and respiratory conditions, for example, come together in one section.

I have devised a new form of reflexology called 'power reflexology', which focuses directly on a particular condition and can be applied within ten minutes. For these unique sequences you should spend five minutes on the right foot and five minutes on the left foot.

Because power reflexology is based upon short sequences it is a slightly firmer treatment. However, if you are treating someone as often as twice a day, ensure you use a lighter pressure. For this type of reflexology, oil is a more appropriate massage media than powder, as it will allow you to apply a firmer pressure (see page 111).

When you are applying a firmer treatment, bear in mind to keep your fingers close to the working thumb.This will reduce the risk of injuring your hand due to the firmer pressure. Try strengthening your hands using the techniques on pages 362–363 and your will notice the difference during and after the treatment.

First, find somewhere to carry out your treatment and organize a comfortable place for your client to relax in, as described in Part 3 (see pages 100–103). Always start and end your treatment with two relaxation techniques (see pages 122–127); I also suggest that you include inner energy breathing (see page 123) because it is beneficial for all these common ailments. Use the basic techniques described in Part 4 (see pages 128–131) and refer to the quick reference charts (see pages 132–135) as necessary to remind yourself of the position of the reflex areas, points and zones.

Where advice on food is given in this chapter, always consult a qualified nutritional therapist, especially concerning vitamin and herbal supplements. Most local health food stores employ a nutritional therapist who will offer you free advice.

Inner energy breathing is a wonderful way to start and end any treatment session. Focus your energies and breathe deeply.

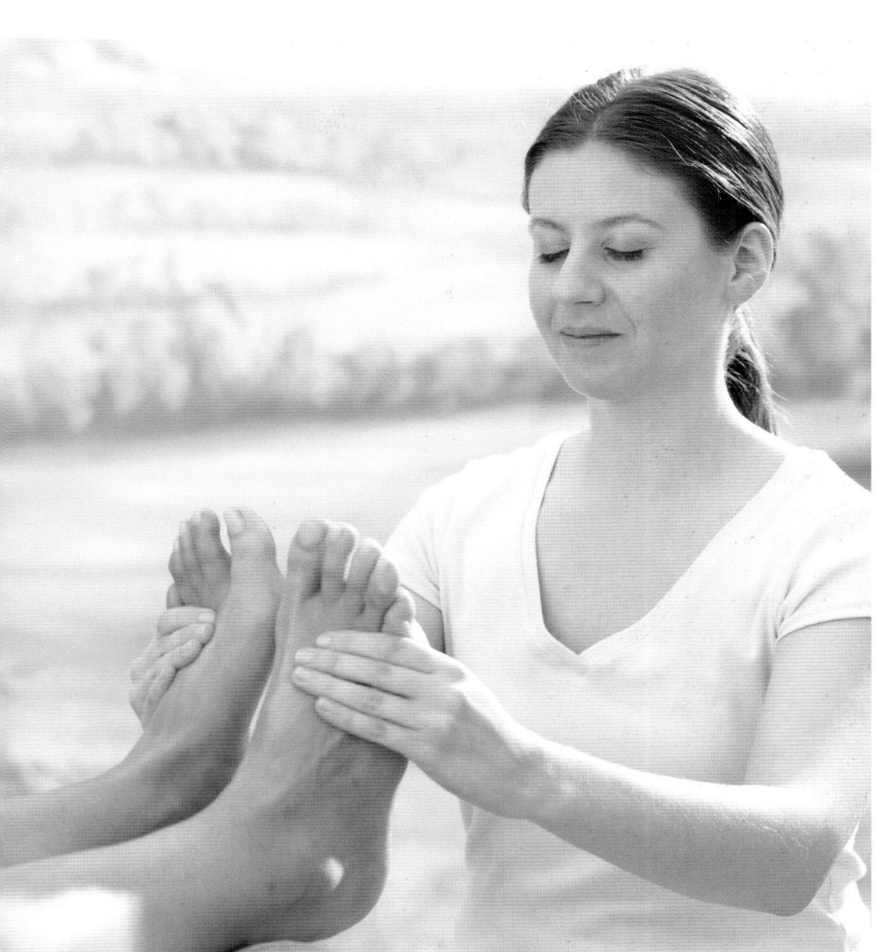

Asthma

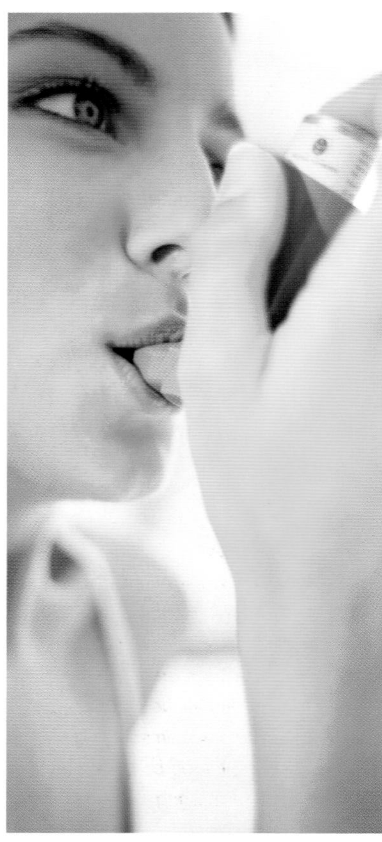

An attack of asthma can be triggered by dust, animal dander, different types of pollen or by airborne pollutants.

This is a lung disease characterized by recurrent episodes of breathlessness caused by constricted airways, although in some forms of the disease there is no known cause. During an asthma attack the muscle walls within the lungs constrict, and there is an increase of mucus and inflammation, making it very hard to breathe normally. Typical symptoms during an attack are coughing, wheezing, a feeling of tightness in the chest and difficulty in breathing. A predisposition to asthma may be hereditary. Stress and anxiety can bring on an attack.

REFLEX AREAS/POINTS TO WORK

- Pituitary
- Lungs
- Diaphragm
- Adrenals
- Thoracic vertebrae
- Solar plexus

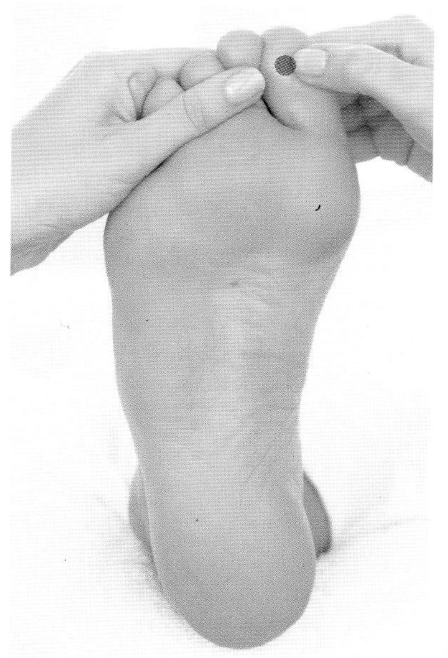

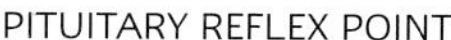

PITUITARY REFLEX POINT

Support the big toe with the fingers of one hand, and use your other thumb to make a cross to find the centre of the big toe. Place your thumb into the centre, push in and make circles for 15 seconds.

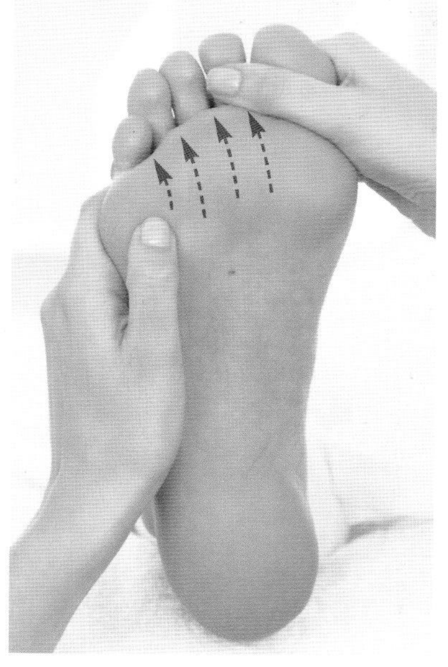

LUNG REFLEX AREA

Flex the foot back with one hand to create skin tension. Use the thumb of your other hand to work up from the diaphragm line to the eye/ear general area. You should be working in between the metatarsals. Repeat this process five times, making sure you have worked in between all the metatarsals, dispersing crystals as you proceed.

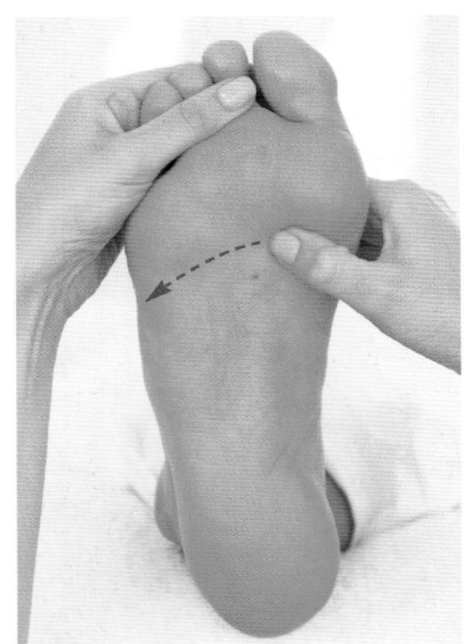

DIAPHRAGM REFLEX AREA

Flex the foot back with one hand to create skin tension. Use the thumb of your other hand to work under the metatarsal heads, across from the lateral aspect to the medial aspect of the foot. Use slow steps and repeat this movement six times.

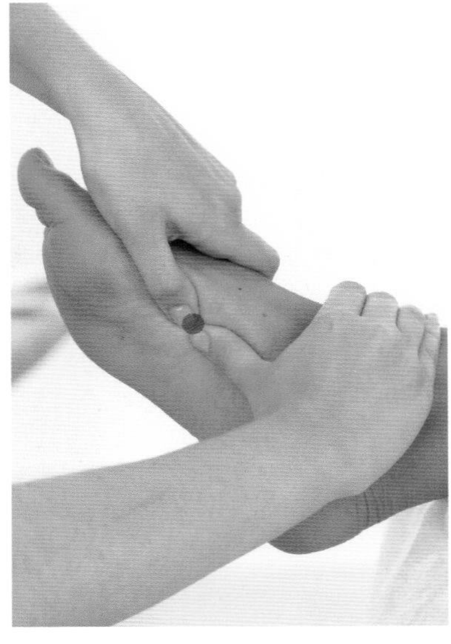

ADRENAL REFLEX POINT

You can find the adrenal reflexes in zone one, three steps down from the ball of the foot. Place both thumbs together and gently push into the adrenal reflexes, making small circles. Work in this manner for 15 seconds.

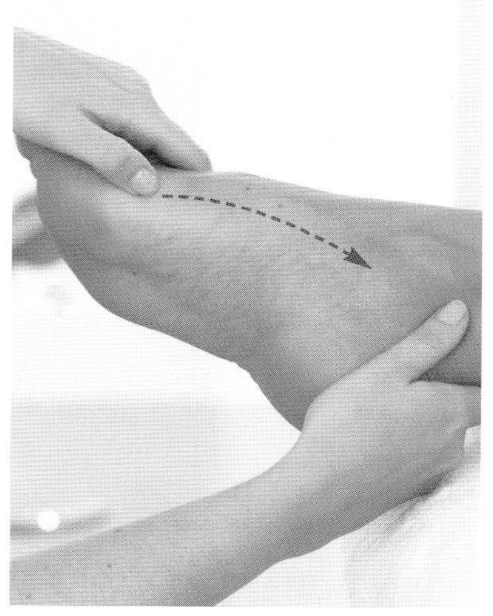

THORACIC VERTEBRAE REFLEX AREA

Support the foot and take 12 steps from the base of the joint of the big toe to work the thoracic vertebrae. You should end up on a bone called the navicular, which feels like a knuckle and is halfway between the bladder point and the ankle. Each step represents a specific vertebra and should be slow, with light to medium pressure. Repeat this movement five times to access spinal nerve roots for the lungs.

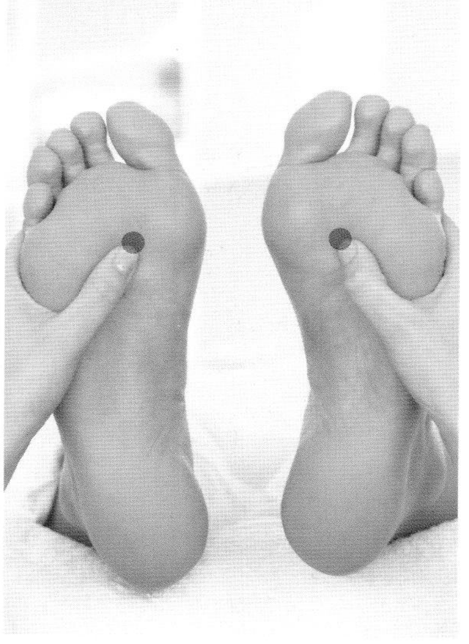

SOLAR PLEXUS REFLEX POINT

Place your left thumb on the solar plexus reflex point on the right foot, and your right thumb on the solar plexus reflex point on the left foot. Ask your client to take a deep breath in for five seconds, while you make small circles on the solar plexus point. Ask them to hold their breath for five seconds as you continue to work on this point. Ask them to breathe out for five seconds, and reduce the pressure on the solar plexus reflex point. Repeat this movement six times.

Influenza

Influenza affects the upper respiratory tract, is commonly known as 'flu' and is highly contagious because it is spread by coughing or sneezing. The symptoms of flu begin like those of a common cold and include headaches, body aches and pains, and feeling tired; as it progresses it is often accompanied by a fever one moment and chills the next. Sufferers frequently have a dry throat and cough. Influenza is only dangerous for the weak, frail and those over 65. It can make someone more susceptible to pneumonia, sinus problems and ear infections.

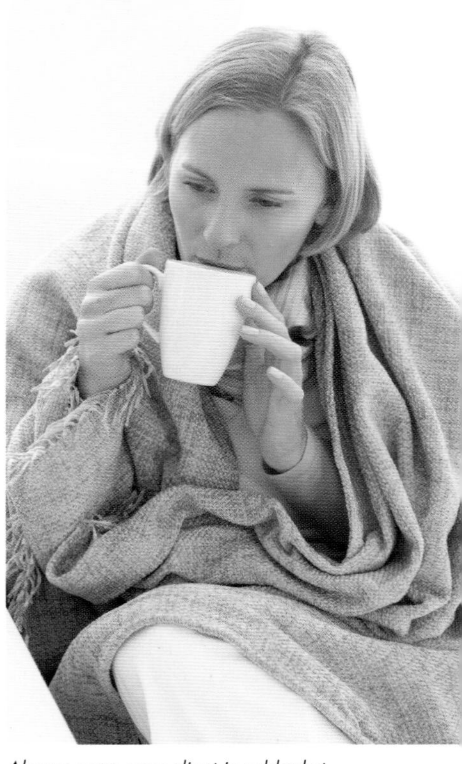

Always wrap your client in a blanket before you start the treatment. This is especially important if suffering with flu.

REFLEX AREAS/POINTS TO WORK

- Head
- Upper lymphatics
- Lungs
- Thyroid
- Spleen
- Thoracic vertebrae

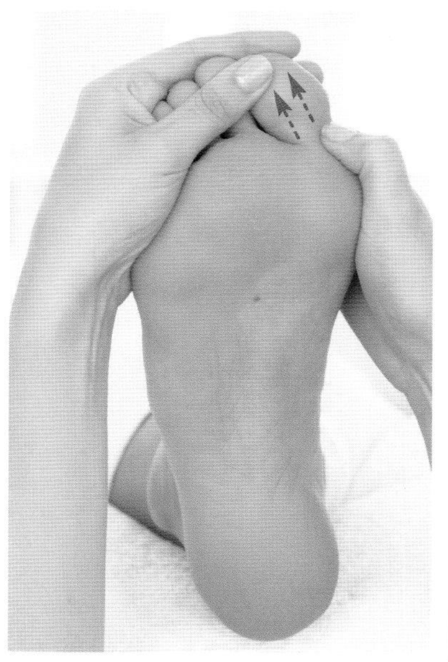

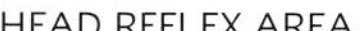

HEAD REFLEX AREA

Support the big toe with the fingers of one hand. Use your other thumb to walk up from the neckline to the top of the big toe. Repeat this several times in lines up the toe. This is a great reflex to help with headaches or problems affecting the head, associated with influenza.

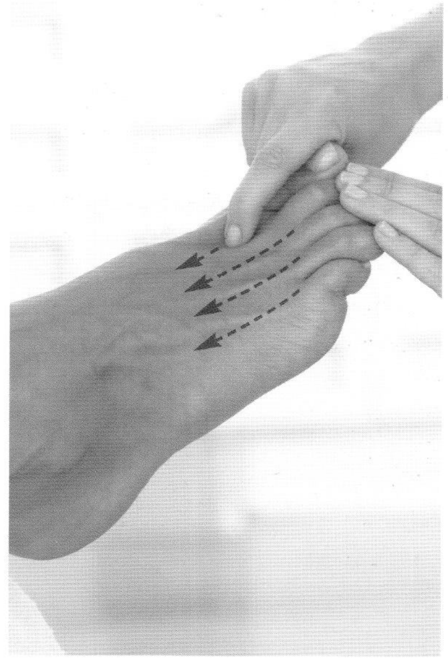

UPPER LYMPHATIC REFLEX AREA

Work on the dorsal aspect of the foot, using your index finger and thumb to walk up from the base of the toes towards the ankle in between the metatarsals. Work with a medium pressure up as far as you can, then slide back to make circles lightly between the clefts of the toes. Repeat this movement six times to strengthen the body's immune system.

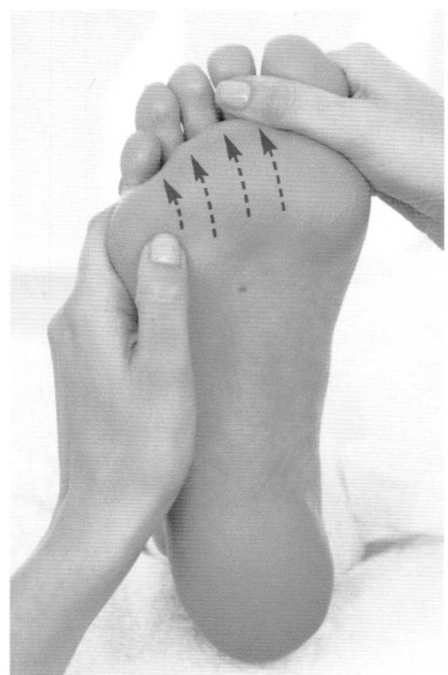

LUNG REFLEX AREA

Flex the foot back with one hand to create skin tension. Use the thumb of your other hand to work up from the diaphragm line to the eye/ear general area. You should be working in between the metatarsals. Repeat this process seven times, making sure you have worked in between all the metatarsals.

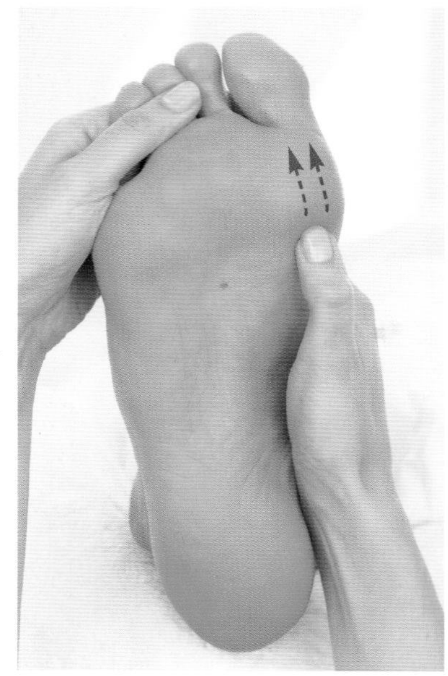

THYROID REFLEX AREA

Use one hand to pull the toes back so that you will be able to find any crystals more easily. Use the thumb of your other hand to work the ball of the foot from the diaphragm line all the way up to the neckline. Repeat this movement slowly seven times over the reflex area. Working the thyroid reflex can help regulate the body's energy levels.

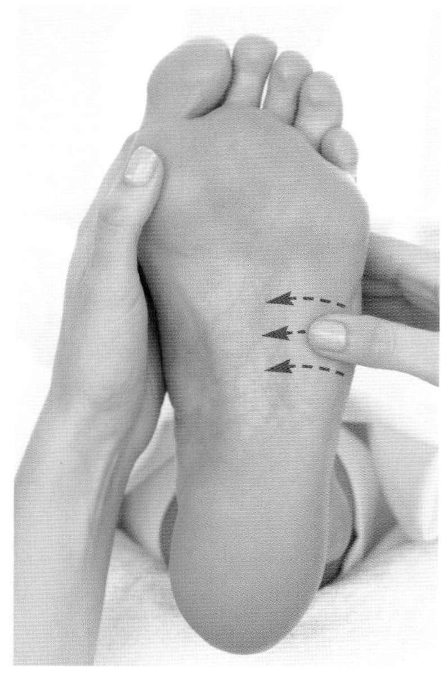

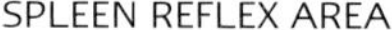

SPLEEN REFLEX AREA

This reflex area is only found on the left foot. Support the foot with your left hand, and place your right thumb just underneath the diaphragm line. Work slowly and precisely, horizontally across the foot, into zones five and four and just into zone three. Proceed in one direction. Continue in this manner for four horizontal lines. Complete the spleen reflex five times.

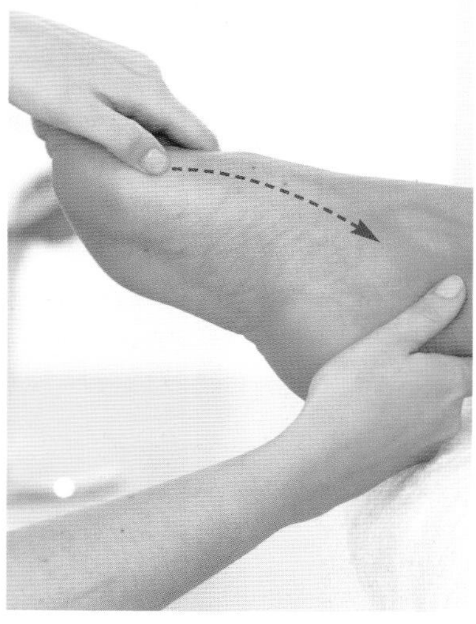

THORACIC VERTEBRAE REFLEX AREA

Support the foot and take 12 steps from the base of the joint of the big toe to work the thoracic vertebrae. You should end up on a bone called the navicular, which feels like a knuckle and is halfway between the bladder point and the ankle. Each step represents a specific vertebra and should be slow, with light to medium pressure. Repeat the movement six times.

Sore throat

This is a very common viral or bacterial infection and can be the first symptom of a cold, influenza or an upper respiratory tract infection. A sore throat can be caused by something that irritates the back of the throat, including: tooth and gum infections, chronic coughing, dust, extremely hot drinks or food, some air pollutants and smoke. A sore throat affects the front of the neck and the passage that runs down the back of the mouth and nose to the upper part of the oesophagus, and causes pain and tenderness. There will probably be pain or discomfort when swallowing. Gargling with salt water every few hours can help to relieve a sore throat.

REFLEX AREAS/POINTS TO WORK

- Head
- Cervical vertebrae
- Oesophagus
- Spleen
- Adrenals
- Upper lymphatics

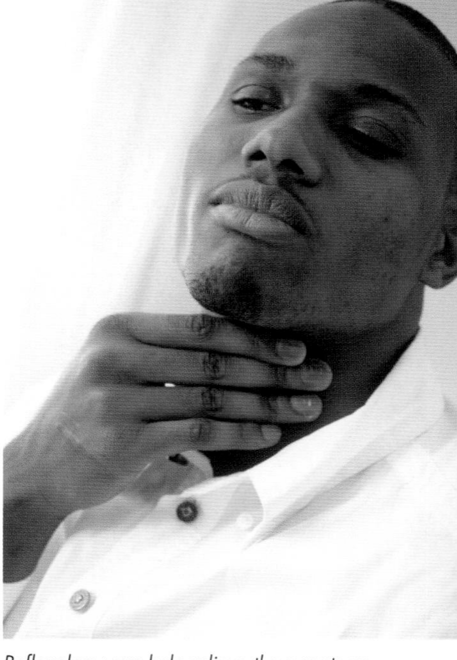

Reflexology can help relieve the symptoms associated with a sore throat. Try gargling with salt water to ease soreness.

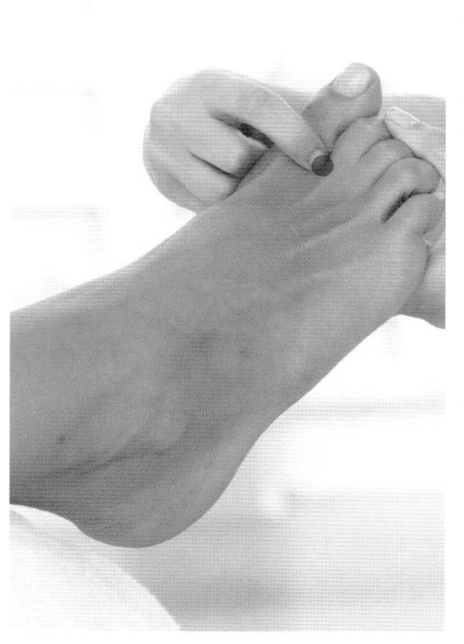

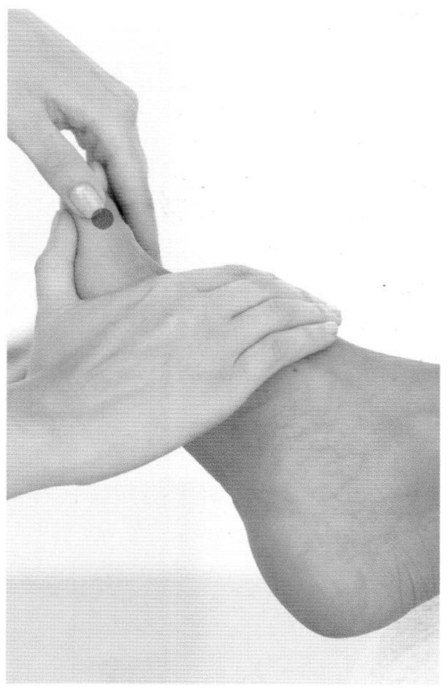

THROAT REFLEX POINT

Start just below the joint of the big toe; using your index finger, walk horizontallty across the big toe and press into the throat reflex and make circles for seven seconds.

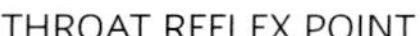

CERVICAL VERTEBRAE REFLEX AREA

This reflex area lies on the medial aspect of the big toe and in between the joints (you do not actually work on the joints because many different factors could affect them). Support the big toe with one hand. Use the thumb of the other hand to make seven small steps, remembering that each step represents a specific vertebra. Walk towards the foot. Repeat the movement six times.

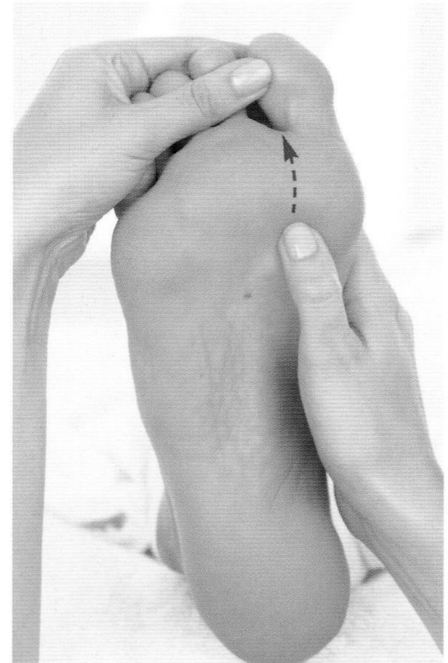

OESOPHAGUS REFLEX AREA

Flex the foot back with one hand to create skin tension. Place the thumb of your other hand at the diaphragm line in between zones one and two. Work up in between the metatarsals from the diaphragm line to the eye/ear general area. Continue in this manner six times. Working this area can help with disorders of the oesophagus, bad breath, trouble in swallowing and heartburn and symptoms of a sore throat.

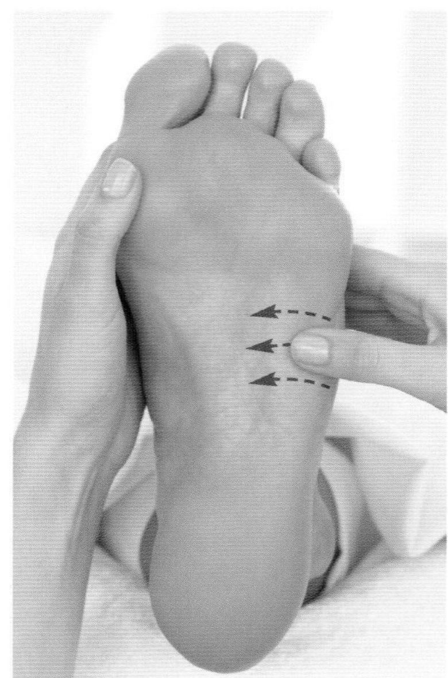

SPLEEN REFLEX AREA

This reflex area is only found on the left foot. Support the foot with your left hand and place your right thumb just underneath the diaphragm line. Work slowly and precisely, horizontally across the foot, into zones five and four and just into zone three. Proceed in one direction. Continue in this manner for four horizontal lines. Complete the spleen reflex five times.

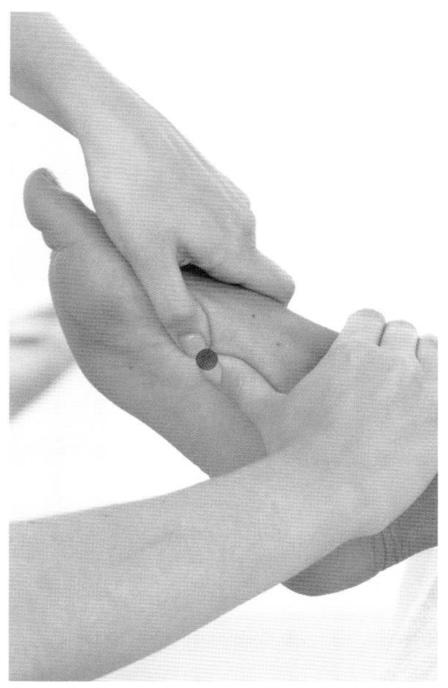

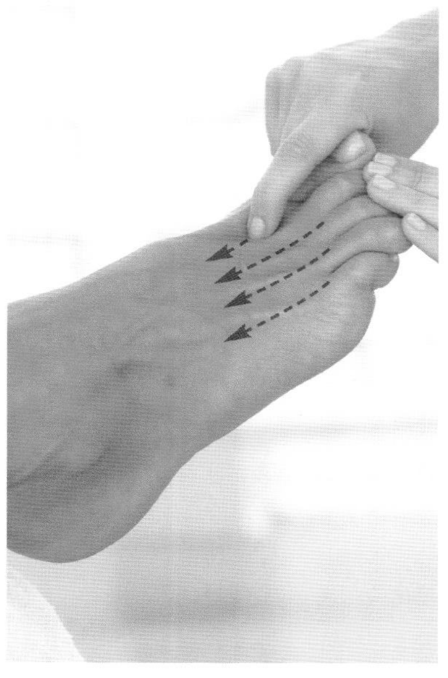

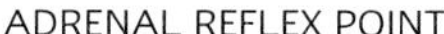

ADRENAL REFLEX POINT

You can find the adrenal reflexes in zone one, three steps down from the ball of the foot. Place your two thumbs together and gently push into the adrenal reflexes, making small circles. Work in this manner for 15 seconds.

UPPER LYMPHATIC REFLEX AREA

Work on the dorsal aspect of the foot, using your index finger and thumb to walk up from the base of the toes towards the ankle in between the metatarsals. Work with a medium pressure up as far as you can, then slide back to make circles lightly between the clefts of the toes. Repeat this movement six times to strengthen the body's immune system.

Common cold

There are more than 200 viruses that cause the common cold, which is experienced as an infection of the upper respiratory tract. Typical symptoms include a sore throat, sneezing, watery eyes, head congestion, headaches, fever and aches and pains. Most colds clear up in around eight days, but occasionally – if someone has a weak or immature immune system – a cold can lead to more serious infections, such as bronchitis, pneumonia or flu. Avoid sugar if you are susceptible to a cold, because all sugars can reduce the body's ability to fight infection by 50 per cent.

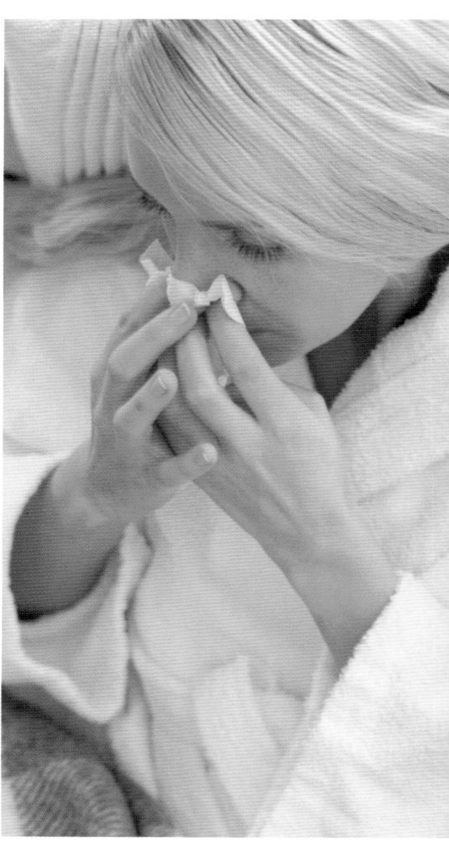

Never reuse tissues as this will reinfect you and prolong the cold. Blow gently from one nostril at a time.

REFLEX AREAS/POINTS TO WORK

- Head
- Pituitary
- Eye/ear general area
- Cervical vertebrae
- Thoracic vertebrae
- Upper lymphatics

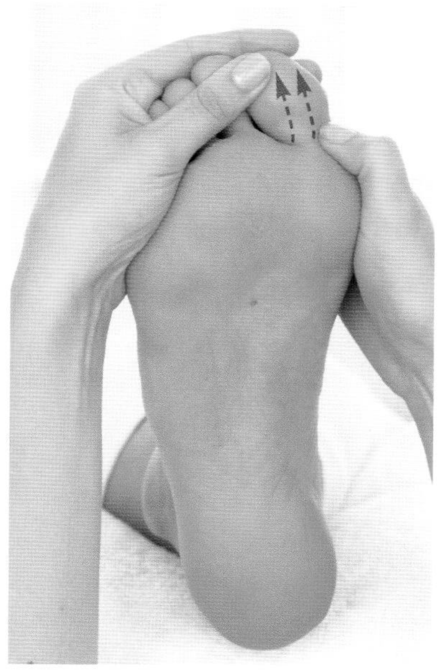

HEAD REFLEX AREA

Support the big toe with the fingers of one hand. Use your thumb to walk up from the neckline to the top of the big toe. Repeat this several times in lines up the toe. This should help with headaches or problems affecting the head.

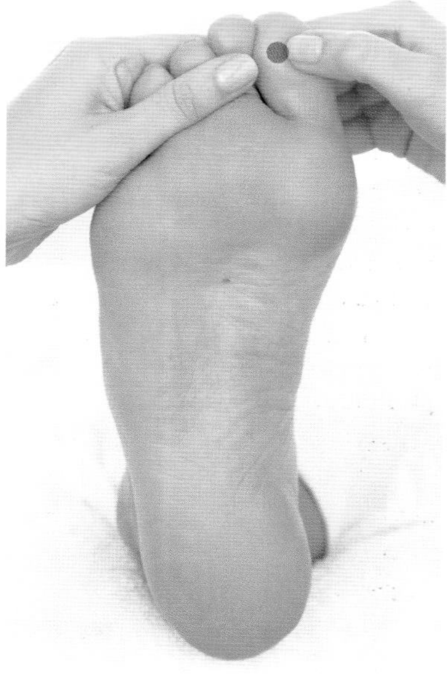

PITUITARY REFLEX POINT

Support the big toe with the fingers of one hand, and use your other thumb to make a cross to find the centre of the big toe. Place your thumb into the centre, push in and make circles for ten seconds.

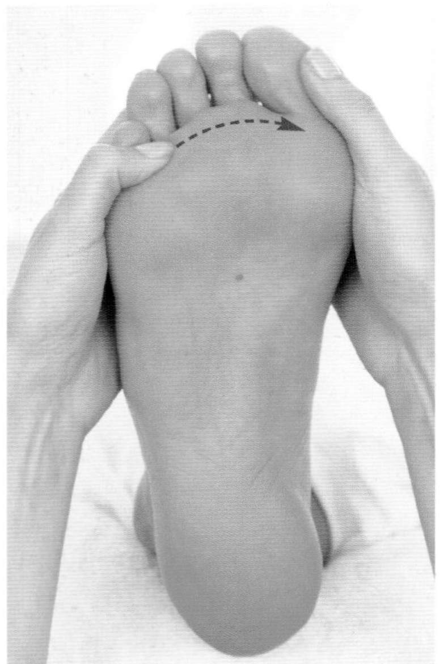

EYE/EAR GENERAL REFLEX AREA

Flex the toes back with one hand to create skin tension and make it easier for you to feel any crystals. Walk with your thumb from under the base of the second toe all the way along to the fifth toe. Repeat this move six times.

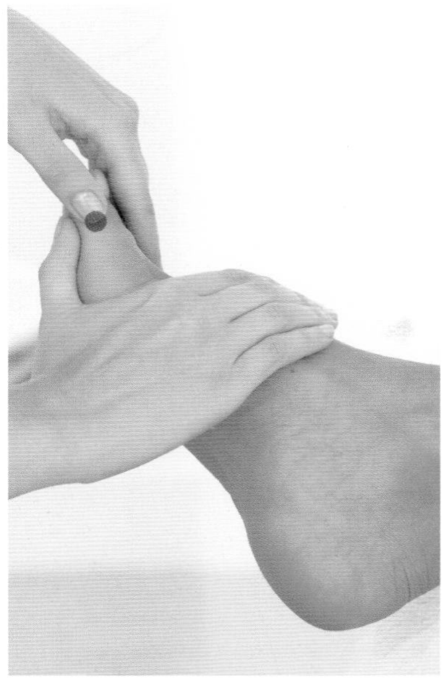

CERVICAL VERTEBRAE REFLEX AREA

This reflex area lies on the medial aspect of the big toe and in between the joints (you do not actually work on the joints, because many different factors could affect them). Support the big toe with one hand. Use the thumb of your other hand to make seven small steps, remembering that each step represents a specific vertebra. Walk towards the foot. Repeat the movement five times.

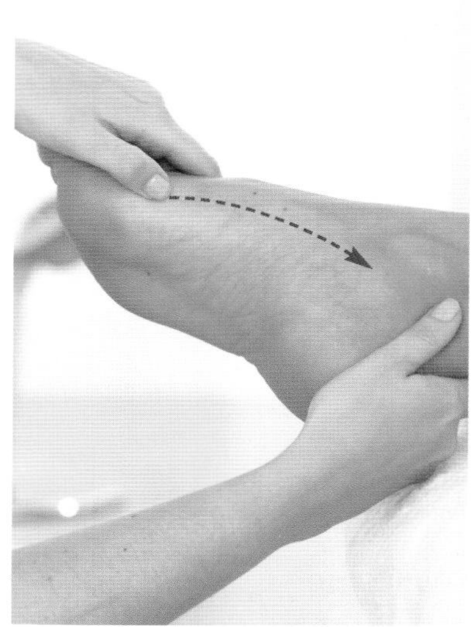

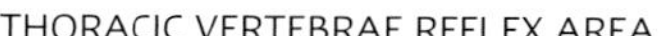

THORACIC VERTEBRAE REFLEX AREA

Support the foot and take 12 steps from the base of the joint of the big toe to work the thoracic vertebrae. You should end up on a bone called the navicular, which feels like a knuckle and is halfway between the bladder point and the ankle. Each step represents a specific vertebra and should be slow, with light to medium pressure. Repeat the movement three times to access spinal nerve roots.

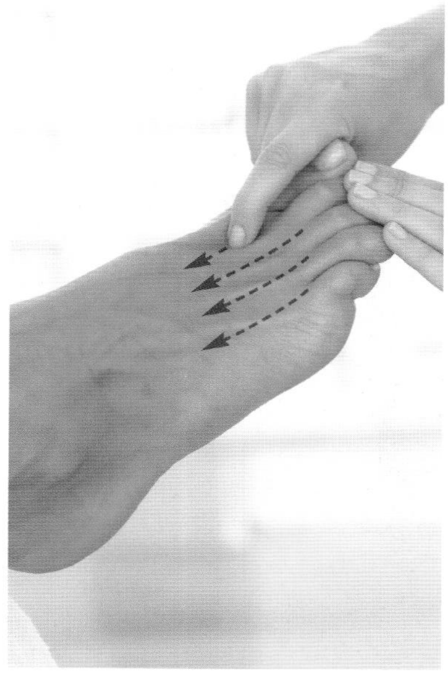

UPPER LYMPHATIC REFLEX AREA

Work on the dorsal aspect of the foot, using your index finger and thumb to walk up from the base of the toes towards the ankle in between the metatarsals. Work with a medium pressure up as far as you can, then slide back to make circles lightly between the clefts of the toes. Repeat this movement six times to strengthen the body's immune system.

Irritable bowel syndrome

It is estimated that one in five adults is affected by this syndrome, which is twice as common in women as it is in men. Irritable bowel syndrome (IBS) is a chronic or long-term condition affecting the small or large bowel. It causes pain or discomfort and an altered bowel habit, and affects the rate at which the contents of the bowel move. The symptoms affect the digestive tract, causing irregular bowel movements, diarrhoea, constipation, bloating, abdominal pain, nausea and flatulence. The stools are the shape of rabbit droppings and often contain an accumulation of mucus. Headaches and tiredness are also associated with the condition.

REFLEX AREAS/POINTS TO WORK

- Ascending colon
- Transverse colon
- Sigmoid colon
- Descending colon
- Pituitary
- Adrenals

IBS can be triggered by stress, food intolerances and an imbalance of good bacteria in the bowel.

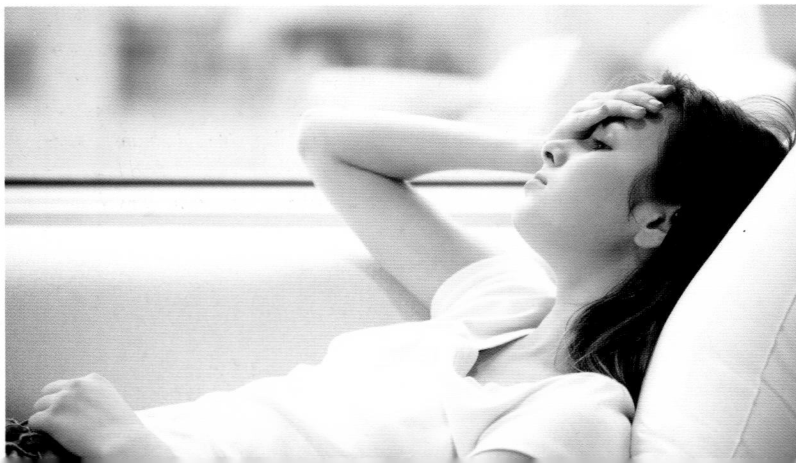

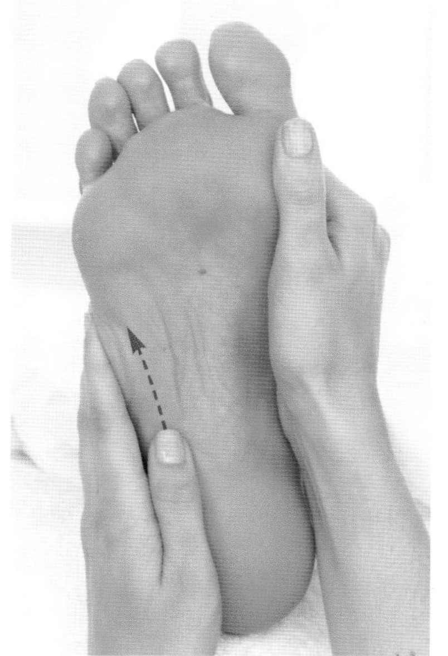

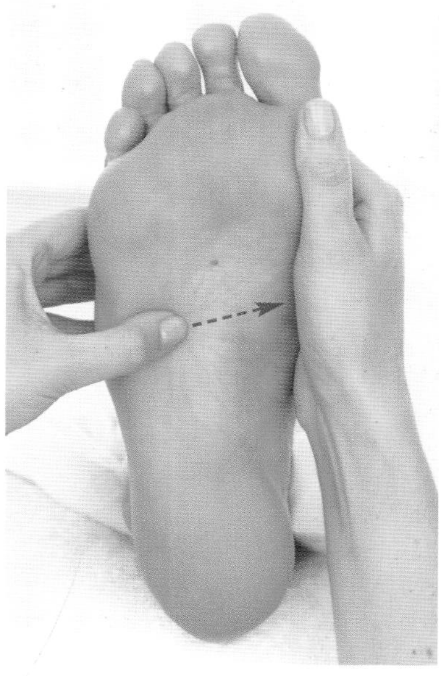

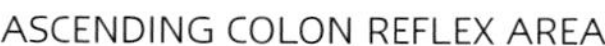

ASCENDING COLON REFLEX AREA

This reflex area is only found on the right foot. Use your left thumb to walk up zone four from the redness of the heel, to work this first part of the colon. Continue in this manner until you get halfway up the foot. Work the ascending colon reflex area six times and in slow movements.

TRANSVERSE COLON REFLEX AREA

This reflex area is found horizontally across the foot, from the lateral aspect to the medial. Work across from the top of the ascending colon to just underneath the stomach reflex. Work the transverse colon six times to encourage good bowel movements and calm the bowel.

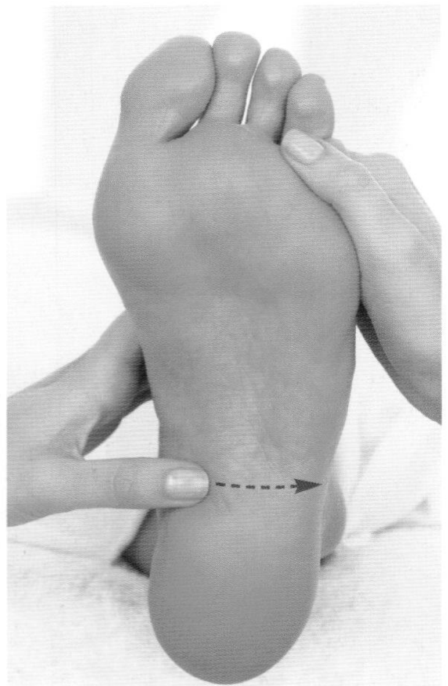

SIGMOID COLON REFLEX AREA

This reflex area is only found on the left foot. Place your left thumb on the medial aspect of the foot and just above the redness of the heel. Use slow movements to walk across the sigmoid colon all the way to zone four. Work this reflex area six times and in slow movements.

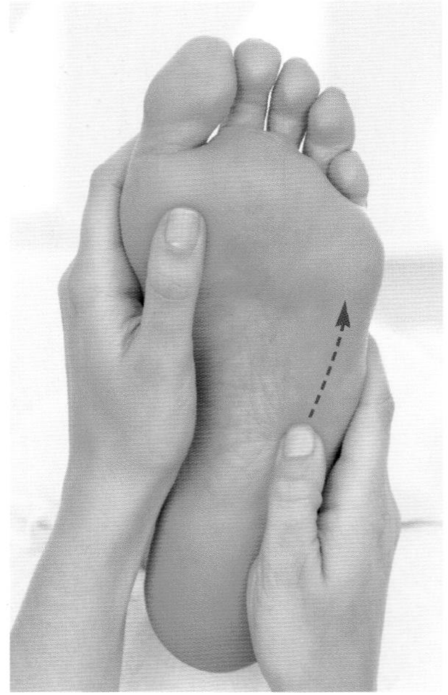

DESCENDING COLON REFLEX AREA

This reflex area is only found on the left foot. Use your right thumb to walk up zone four to work the descending colon. Continue in this manner until you get halfway up the foot. Work the descending colon reflex area six times and in slow movements, making circles as you proceed up the foot.

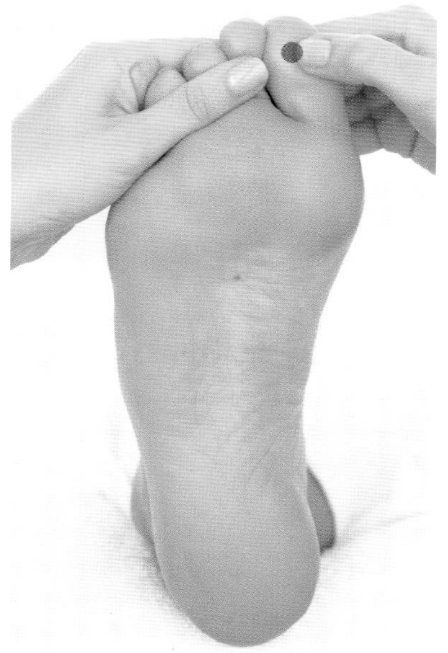

PITUITARY REFLEX POINT

Support the big toe with the fingers of one hand, and use your other thumb to make a cross to find the centre of the big toe. Place your thumb into the centre, push in and make circles for ten seconds.

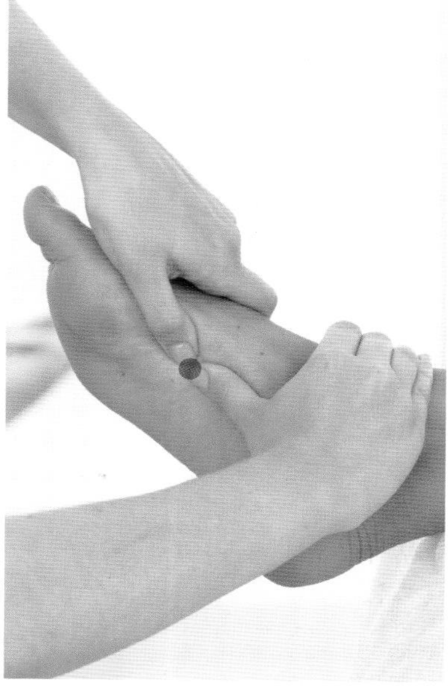

ADRENAL REFLEX POINT

You can find the adrenal reflexes in zone one, three steps down from the ball of the foot. Place your two thumbs together and gently push into the adrenal reflexes, making small circles. Work in this manner for 15 seconds.

Constipation

This condition occurs when waste material moves too slowly through the large bowel, resulting in infrequent and painful elimination and hard, dry faeces. Constipation can give rise to a number of different ailments, including bad breath, depression, fatigue, flatulence, bloating, headaches, haemorrhoids (piles) and insomnia. It is important to move the bowels on a daily basis because harmful toxins can form after this period. In many cases constipation may arise from insufficient amounts of fibre and fluids in the diet. Other causes could be advanced age, medication, insufficient exercise and bowel disorders.

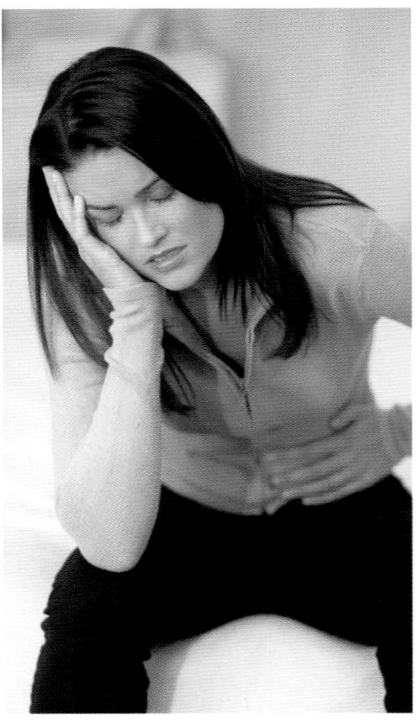

Papaya, pineapple and apples can all help relieve the symptoms of constipation. Ensure that you drink sufficient amounts of water throughout the day.

REFLEX AREAS/POINTS TO WORK

- Ascending colon
- Sigmoid colon
- Descending colon
- Thyroid
- Kidneys/adrenals
- Lumbar vertebrae

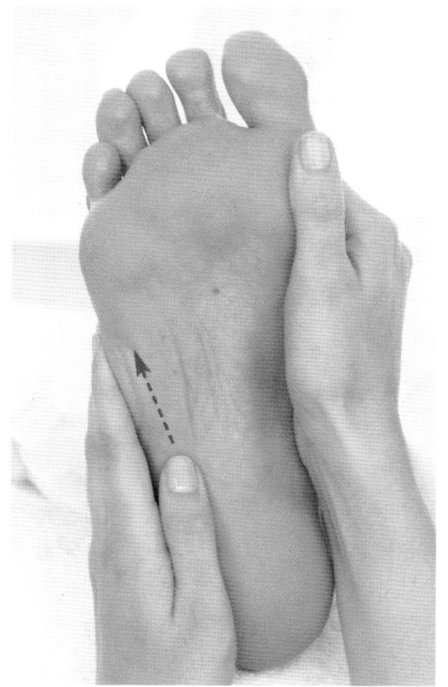

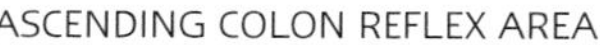

ASCENDING COLON REFLEX AREA

This reflex area is only found on the right foot. Use your left thumb to walk up zone four from the redness of the heel, to work this first part of the colon. Continue in this manner until you arrive halfway up the foot. Work this reflex area six times and in slow movements to help stimulate the peristaltic muscular action of the colon.

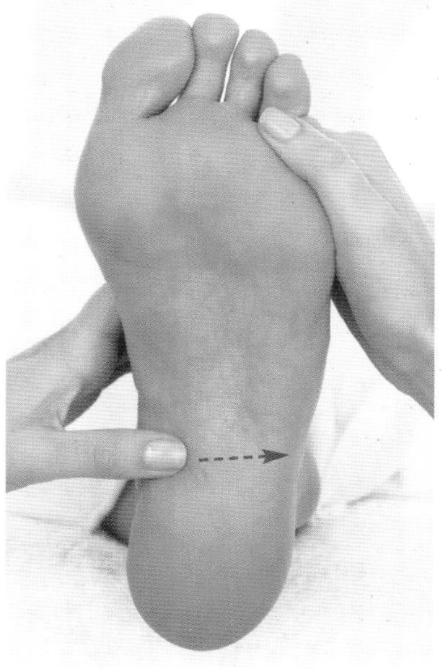

SIGMOID COLON REFLEX AREA

This reflex area is only found on the left foot. Place your left thumb at the medial aspect of the foot and just above the redness of the heel. Use slow movements to walk across the sigmoid colon all the way to zone four. Repeat this movement six times.

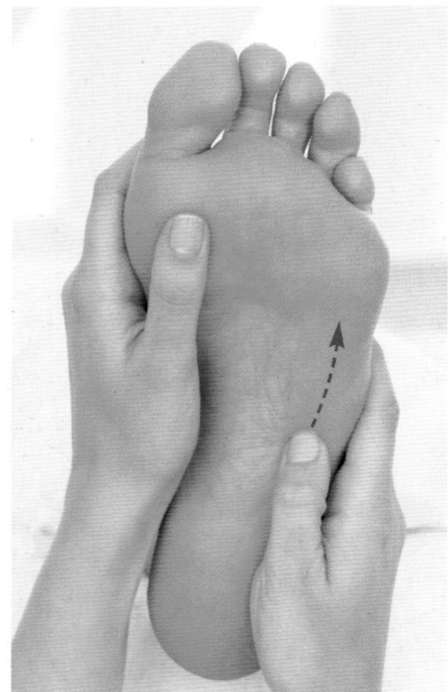

DESCENDING COLON REFLEX AREA

This reflex area is only found on the left foot. Use your right thumb to walk up zone four from the redness of the heel, to work this part of the colon. Continue in this manner until you arrive halfway up the foot. Work this reflex area six times and in slow movements to help stimulate the peristaltic muscular action of the colon.

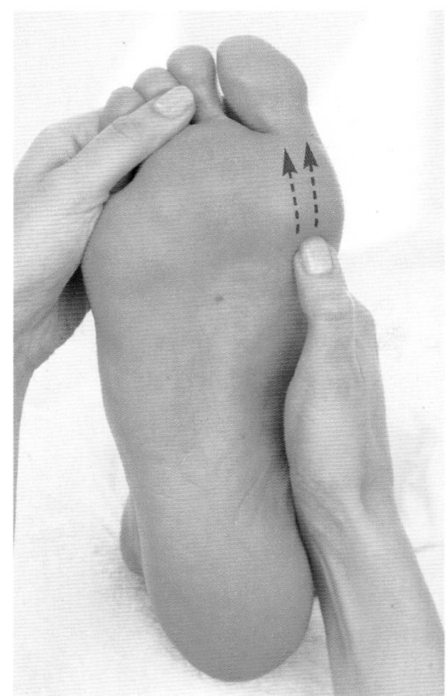

THYROID REFLEX AREA

Use one hand to pull the toes back so that you can find any crystals more easily. Use the thumb of your other hand to work the ball of the foot, from the diaphragm line all the way up to the neckline. Repeat this movement slowly seven times over the area. Working the thyroid reflex area can help to regulate the body's energy levels.

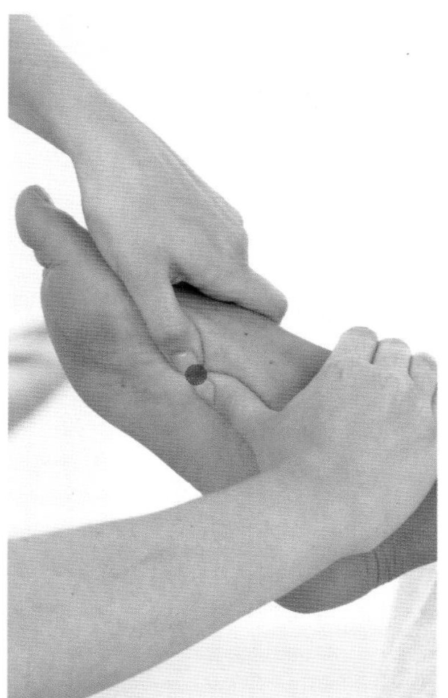

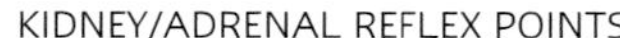

KIDNEY/ADRENAL REFLEX POINTS

You can find these reflexes in zone one, three steps down from the ball of the foot. Place your two thumbs together and gently push into the kidney/adrenal reflexes, making small circles. Work in this manner for 15 seconds.

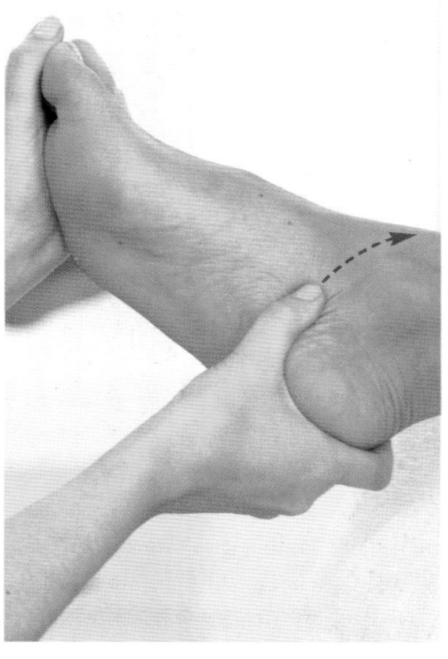

LUMBAR VERTEBRAE REFLEX AREA

Support the foot with one hand, and use the other thumb to walk around the navicular bone, which represents lumbar one, taking five steps up to the dip in front of the ankle bone, which represents lumbar five. Push into lumbar five and make small circles for six seconds. Repeat the movement six times.

Heartburn

Heartburn is experienced as a burning pain that travels up from the centre of the chest to the throat. It can occur when the muscular sphincter (a type of valve found between the stomach and the oesophagus) relaxes, allowing food and digestive juices in the stomach to travel back up the oesophagus. Having a full stomach makes this more likely to happen as it puts extra pressure on the valve. Heartburn is often made worse by lying down or bending over during an attack. Chewing food thoroughly is the first step towards good digestion. Overeating, eating too quickly or eating too many rich, fatty or spicy foods, or drinking too much alcohol, often causes heartburn, while stress can exacerbate it. Milk creates an acid environment in the stomach and should be avoided by those suffering from heartburn.

REFLEX AREAS/POINTS TO WORK

- Diaphragm
- Oesophagus
- Pancreas
- Stomach
- Lungs
- Thoracic vertebrae

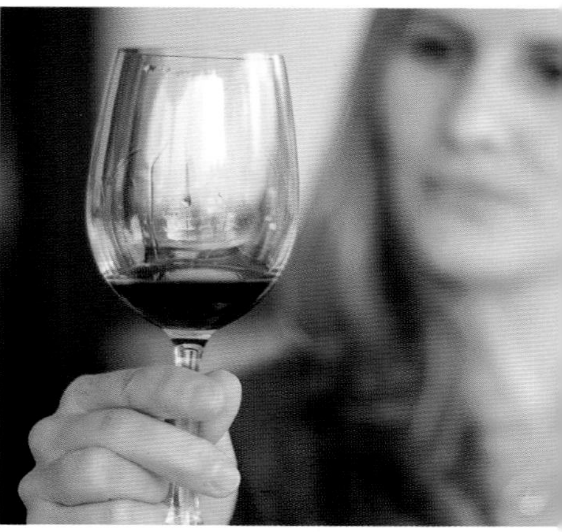

Wine can be a trigger for heartburn as can fatty foods. Overeating and not chewing your food properly can also lead to heartburn.

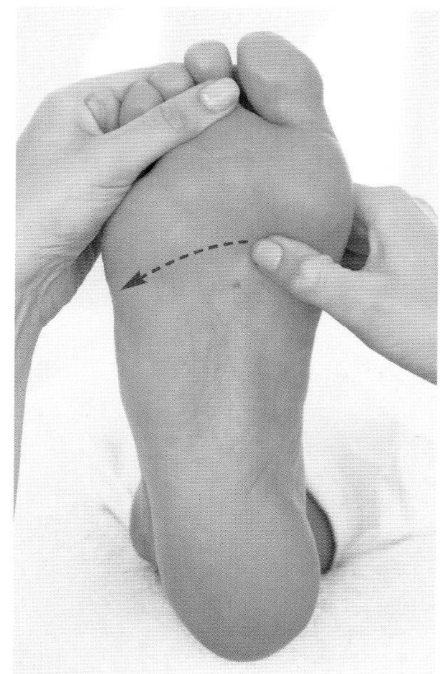

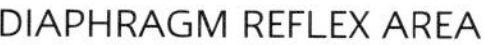

DIAPHRAGM REFLEX AREA

Flex the foot back with one hand to create skin tension. Use the thumb of your other hand to work under the metatarsal heads, across from the lateral aspect to the medial aspect of the foot. Use slow steps and repeat this movement eight times.

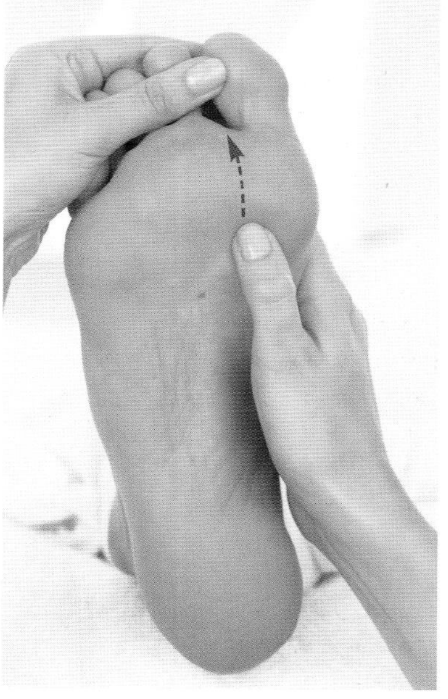

OESOPHAGUS REFLEX AREA

Flex the foot back with one hand to create skin tension. Place the thumb of your other hand at the diaphragm line in between zones one and two. Work up in between the metatarsals from the diaphragm line to the eye/ear general area. Continue in this manner six times.

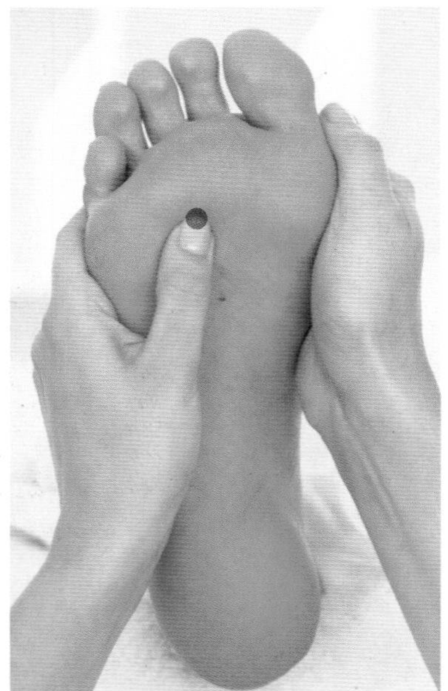

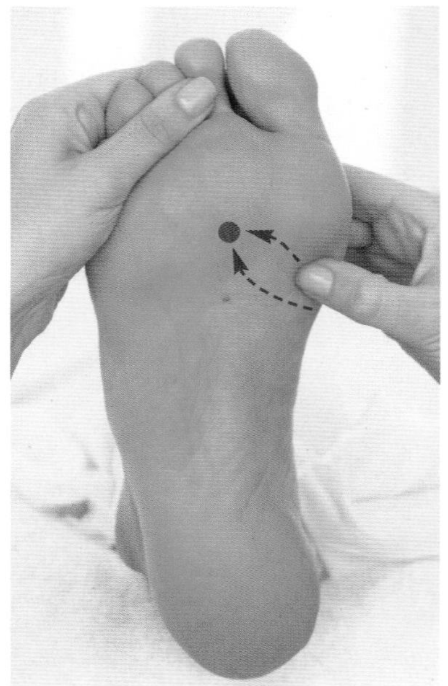

PANCREAS REFLEX POINT

This reflex point is only found on the right foot. Place your thumb on the third toe and trace a line down to below the diaphragm line. Push up into the joint and make small circles for ten seconds. Working this point can help to neutralize the adverse affects of stomach acid.

STOMACH REFLEX AREA

You will find this reflex area just under the ball of the foot. Support the foot with one hand, and place your other thumb just below the thyroid reflex area. Gently work up laterally to the solar plexus reflex, stopping there to stimulate it with circles for four seconds. Repeat this movement eight times, using slow circles as you walk.

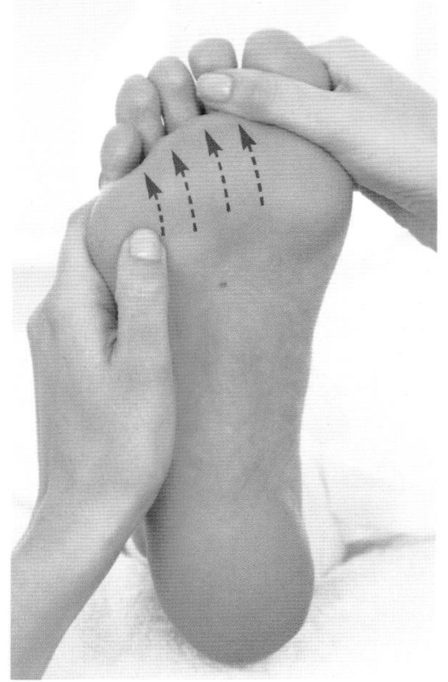

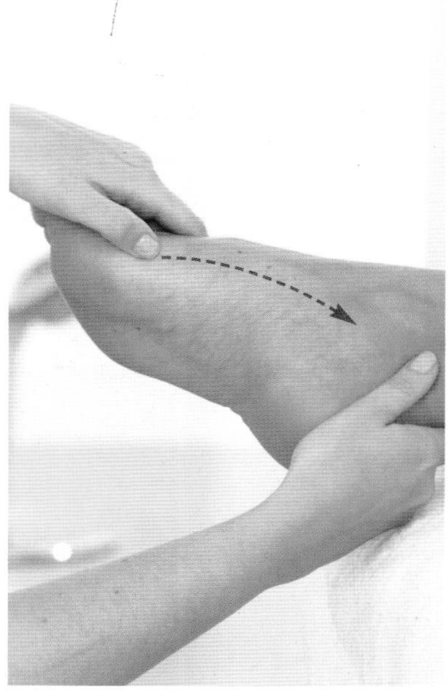

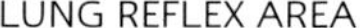

LUNG REFLEX AREA

Flex the foot back with one hand to create skin tension. Use the thumb of your other hand to work up from the diaphragm line to the eye/ear general area. You should be working in between the metatarsals. Repeat this process five times, making sure that you have worked in between all the metatarsals.

THORACIC VERTEBRAE REFLEX AREA

Support the foot and take 12 steps from the base of the joint of the big toe to work the thoracic vertebrae. You should end up on a bone called the navicular, which feels like a knuckle and is halfway between the bladder point and the ankle. Each step represents a specific vertebra and should be slow, with light to medium pressure. Repeat the movement three times to access spinal nerve roots.

Hiatus hernia

This is an abnormal protrusion of part of the stomach, which passes up through the wall of the diaphragm and causes pain and discomfort. The diaphragm is the muscular sheet that separates the lungs and chest from the abdomen. Hiatus hernia affects us more as we get older. Doctors are not sure what causes it, but people are more likely to get it if they are aged over 50, smokers, overweight or pregnant. A hiatus hernia often causes no symptoms, but may cause pain and heartburn (a feeling of warmth or burning in the chest). It is not usually a serious condition and often needs no treatment. Any symptoms can usually be treated with drugs or (if severe) an operation. It is advisable to eat small, frequent meals.

REFLEX AREAS/POINTS TO WORK

- Diaphragm
- Hiatus hernia
- Stomach
- Pituitary
- Adrenals
- Thoracic vertebrae

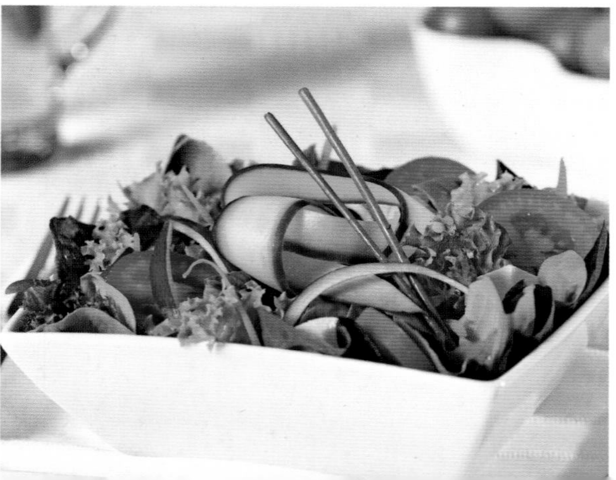

Good, fresh food is the foundation of good digestive health.

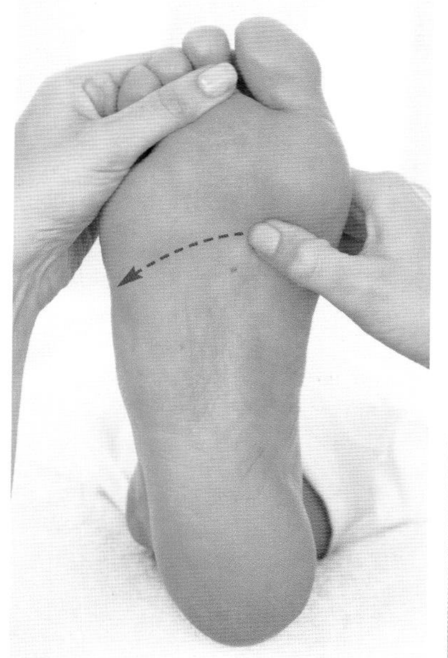

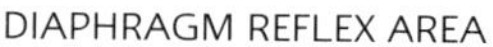

DIAPHRAGM REFLEX AREA

Flex the foot back with one hand to create skin tension. Use the thumb of your other hand to work under the metatarsal heads, across from the lateral aspect to the medial aspect of the foot. Use slow steps and repeat this movement eight times.

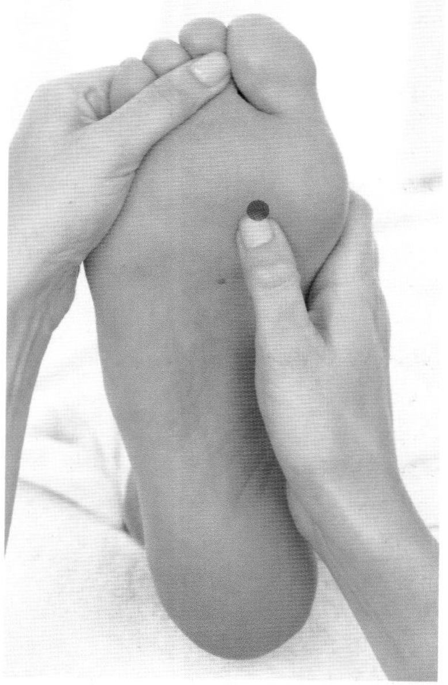

HIATUS HERNIA REFLEX POINT

Flex the foot back with one hand, and place the thumb of your other hand on the hiatus hernia point, which you can find along the diaphragm line and in between zones one and two. Stay on this point, making circles for 12 seconds.

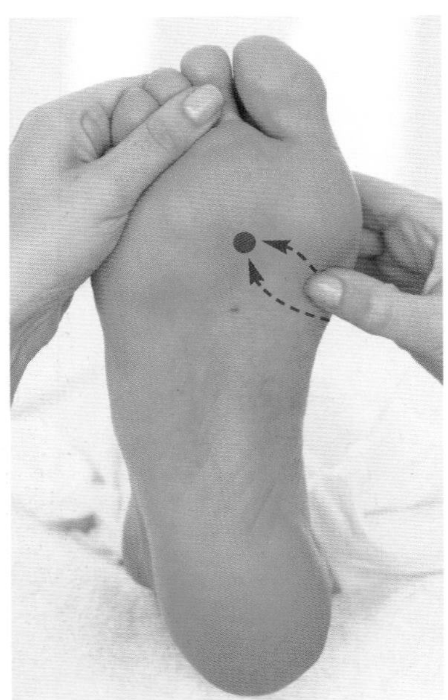

STOMACH REFLEX AREA

You will find this reflex area just under the ball of the foot. Support the foot with one hand, and place your other thumb just below the thyroid reflex area. Gently work up laterally to the solar plexus reflex, stopping there to stimulate it with circles for four seconds. Repeat this movement eight times.

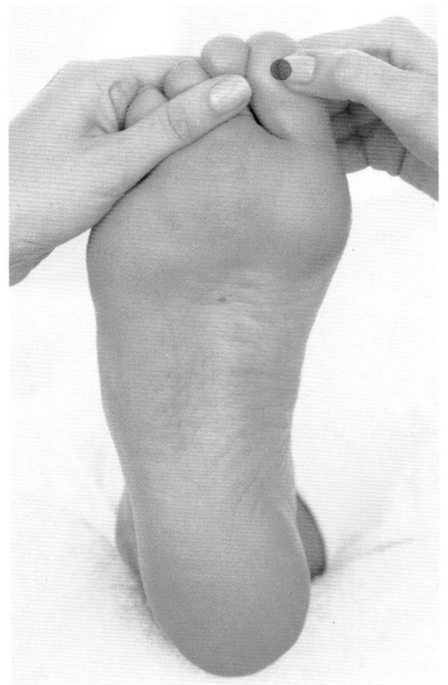

PITUITARY REFLEX POINT

Support the big toe with the fingers of one hand, and use your other thumb to make a cross to find the centre of the big toe. Place your thumb into the centre, push in and make circles for 15 seconds.

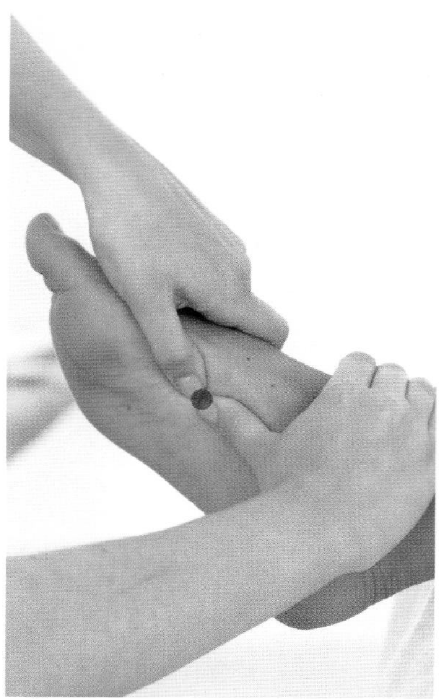

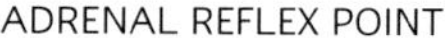

ADRENAL REFLEX POINT

You can find the adrenal reflexes in zone one, three steps down from the ball of the foot. Place your two thumbs together and gently push into the adrenal reflexes, making small circles. Work in this manner for 15 seconds.

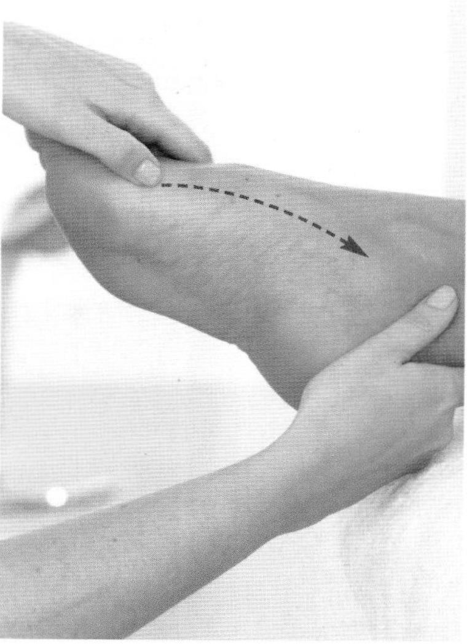

THORACIC VERTEBRAE REFLEX AREA

Support the foot and take 12 steps from the base of the joint of the big toe to work the thoracic vertebrae. You should end up on a bone called the navicular, which feels like a knuckle and is halfway between the bladder point and the ankle. Each step represents a specific vertebra and should be slow, with a light to medium pressure. Repeat the movement three times.

Osteoporosis

This condition causes the bones to weaken, making broken bones more likely. Osteoporosis is sometimes called the 'silent disease', because most people who are affected are unaware that their bones are thinning until they break one. Bones affected by osteoporosis are less dense than normal and are porous. The bones that are most at risk are the ribs, wrist, spine and hips, which are more likely to break as the result of a minor bump or fall, or even without injury (for example, a sneeze may break a rib). You are more likely to get osteoporosis if you are aged over 60 years, and the risk continues to rise as you get older.

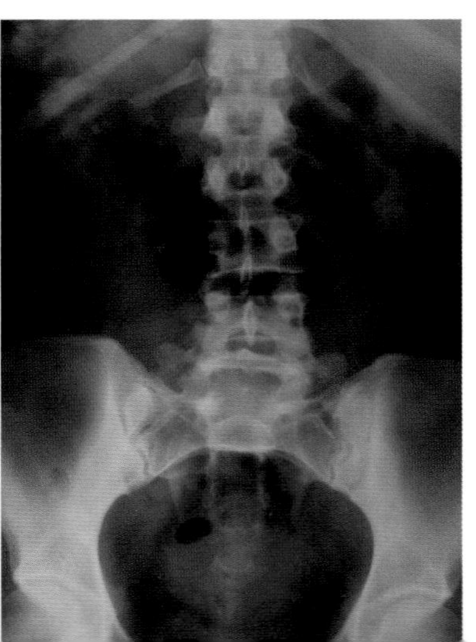

REFLEX AREAS/POINTS TO WORK

- Thyroid
- Pituitary
- Parathyroid
- Kidneys/adrenals
- Hip
- Entire spine

The condition is around four times more common in women than in men and is most common in women who have been through the menopause, because their production of oestrogen falls dramatically (and oestrogen helps to retain calcium in the bones). Long-term immobility, anorexia, inflammatory bowel disease and a family history can all increase the risk of developing osteoporosis.

Bone mineral density can be reduced to 35 per cent in osteoporosis which may result in fractures as you get older.

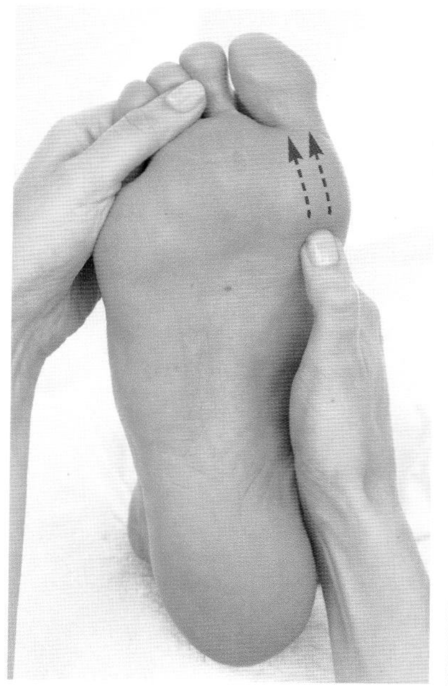

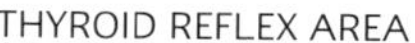

THYROID REFLEX AREA

Use the thumb of one hand to work the ball of the foot, from the diaphragm line all the way up to the neckline. Repeat this movement slowly four times over the area for one minute. This reflex area helps to control the levels of calcium in the blood.

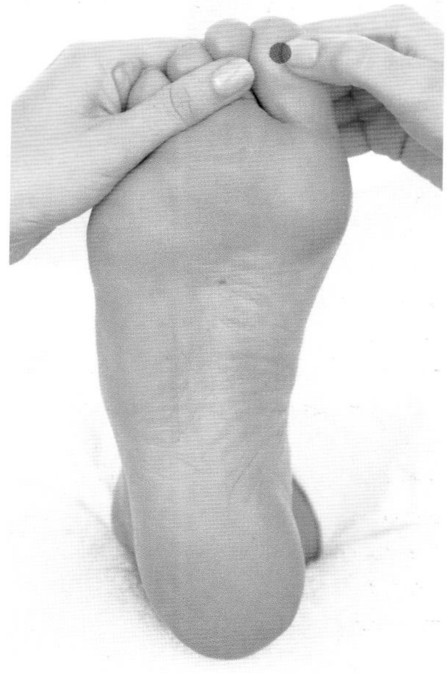

PITUITARY REFLEX POINT

Support the big toe with the fingers of one hand, and use your other thumb to make a cross to find the centre of the big toe. Place your thumb into the centre, push in and make circles for 15 seconds.

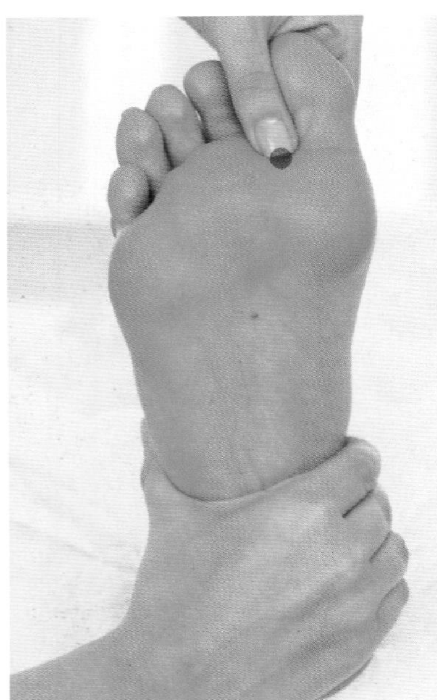

PARATHYROID REFLEX POINT

You can find this point in between the big toe and the second toe. Use your index finger and thumb to pinch the section of skin between the first and second toes. Hold the pressure and gently make circles for 15 seconds. This reflex point helps to control the levels of calcium in the blood, which can help regulate muscle and nerve function as well as easing disorders relating to the parathyroid glands.

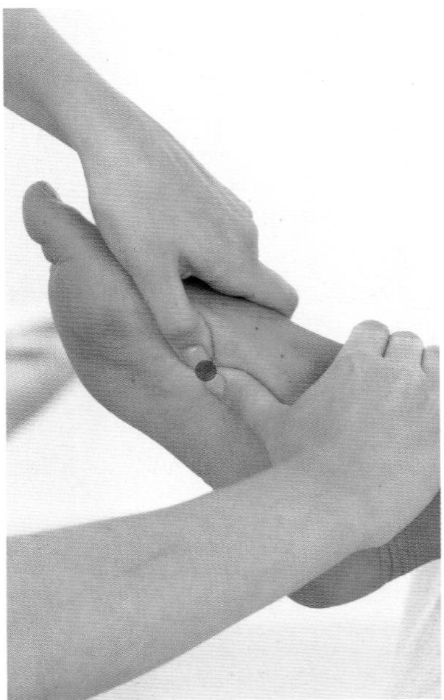

KIDNEY/ADRENAL REFLEX POINTS

You can find these reflexes in zone one, three steps down from the ball of the foot. Place your two thumbs together and gently push into the kidney/adrenal reflexes, making small circles. Work in this manner for 15 seconds.

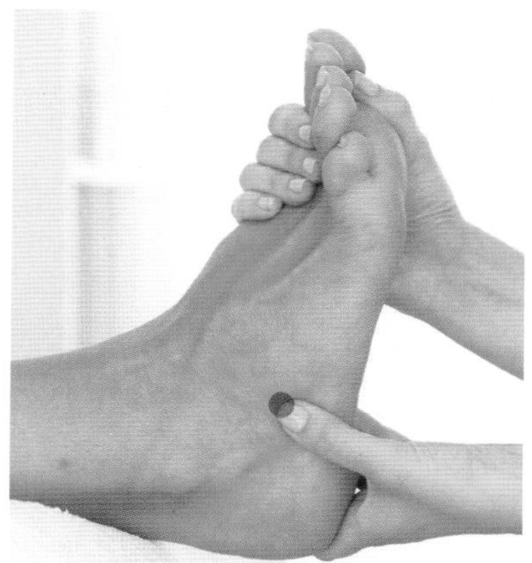

HIP REFLEX POINT

Place your thumb approximately two steps down from the ankle bone and take one step towards the fifth toe. Push in and make very big circles to help stimulate the hip reflex point. Work this point gently for 15 seconds.

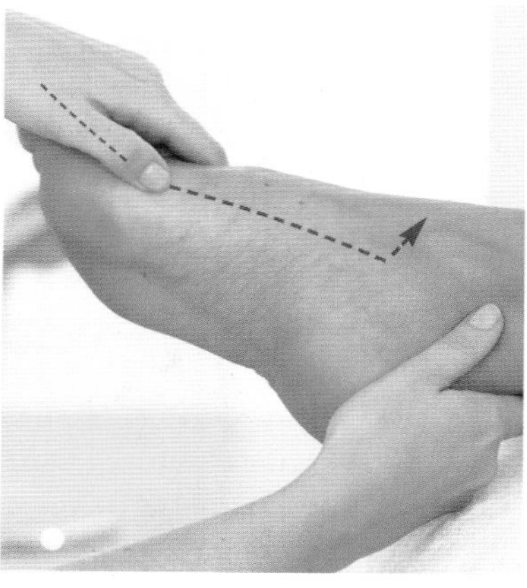

ENTIRE SPINE

Work on the medial aspect of the foot. Support the foot with one hand, and use your other thumb to make seven small steps in between the joints of the big toe, remembering that each step represents a specific vertebra. Walk towards the foot. Then take 12 gentle steps from the base of the joint of the big toe to work the thoracic vertebrae. You should end up on a bone called the navicular, which feels like a knuckle and is halfway between the bladder point and the ankle. Walk around the navicular bone, which represents lumbar one, taking five steps up to the dip in front of the ankle bone, which represents lumbar five. Repeat this movement three times.

Carpal tunnel syndrome

This syndrome can affect one or both hands. It is a fairly common condition that occurs when there is too much pressure on a nerve in the wrist. The median nerve carries sensory messages from the thumb and some fingers, and also conducts movements of the hand. Sometimes carpal tunnel syndrome can be triggered by your job, but it may be prevented by stopping or reducing the activity that stresses your fingers, hand or wrist, or by changing the way in which activities are done. It tends to be worse at night or first thing in the morning and can be made worse by strenuous wrist movements.

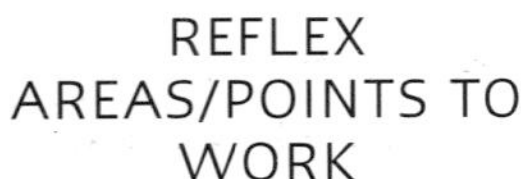

REFLEX AREAS/POINTS TO WORK

- Shoulder
- Wrist
- Elbow
- Thyroid
- Kidneys/adrenals
- Cervical vertebrae
- Thoracic vertebrae

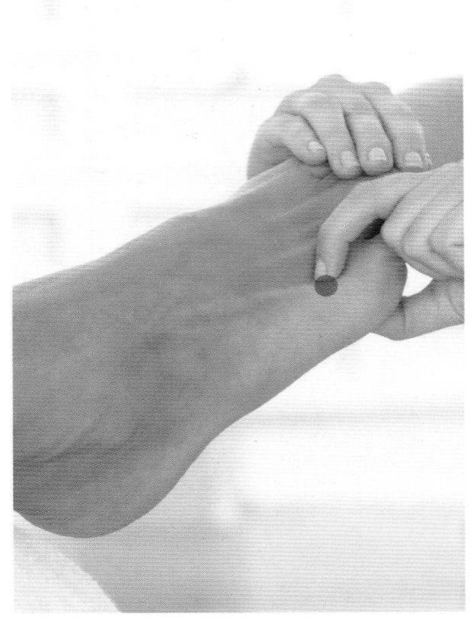

SHOULDER REFLEX POINT

You will find this reflex point on the dorsal aspect of the foot, in between the fourth and fifth metatarsals. The simplest way to find it is to place your index finger and thumb at the base of the fourth and fifth toes. Slowly walk down four steps, following the edge of the foot in a pinching movement. When you hit this sensitive reflex, stop and push in, gently making small circles for 15 seconds.

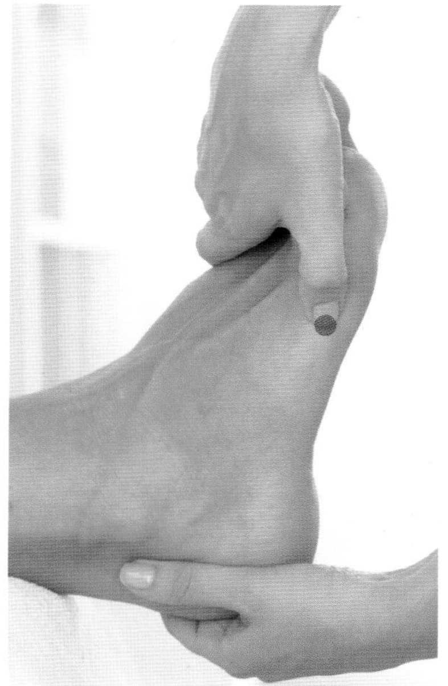

WRIST REFLEX POINT

Use your thumb to walk two steps down the lateral aspect of the foot from the fifth toe. Push in to work the wrist reflex point, making circles for 15 seconds.

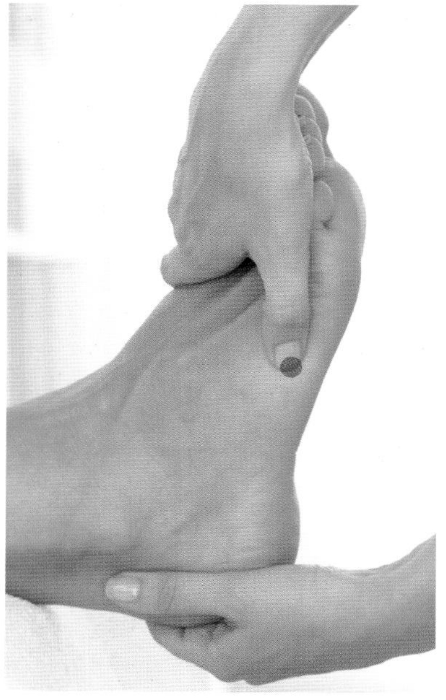

ELBOW REFLEX POINT

Use your thumb to take one large step from the wrist reflex point to the elbow reflex point. Push in to work this point, making circles for 15 seconds.

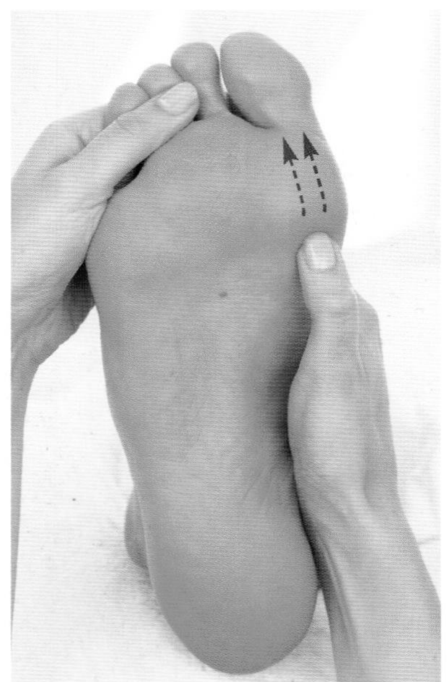

THYROID REFLEX AREA

Use one hand to pull the toes back so that you will be able to find any crystals more easily. Use the thumb of your other hand to work the ball of the foot, from the diaphragm line all the way up to the neckline. Repeat this movement slowly four times over the area, dispersing crystals as you find them.

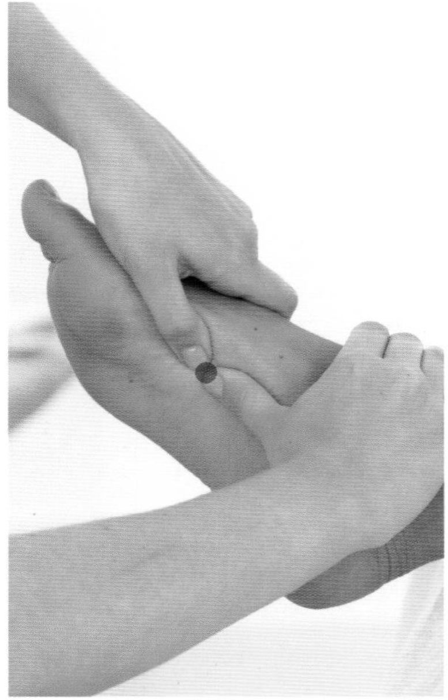

KIDNEY/ADRENAL REFLEX POINTS

You can find these reflexes in zone one, three steps down from the ball of the foot. Place your two thumbs together and gently push into the kidney/adrenal reflexes, making small circles. Work in this manner for 15 seconds.

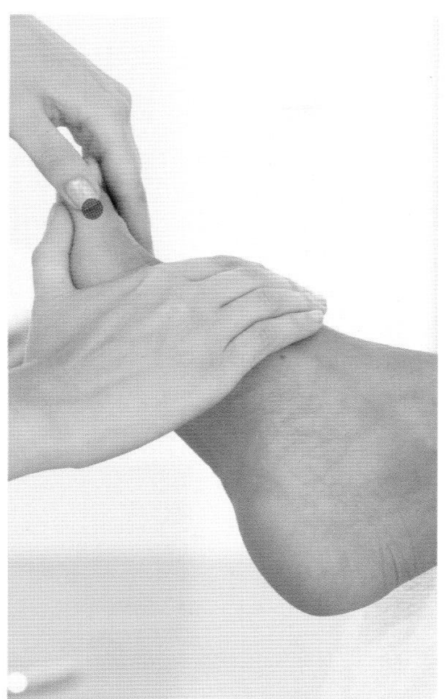

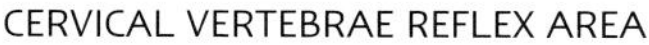

CERVICAL VERTEBRAE REFLEX AREA

This reflex area lies on the medial aspect of the big toe and in between the joints (you do not actually work on the joints, because many different factors could affect them). Support the big toe with one hand. Use the thumb of your other hand to make seven small steps, remembering that each step represents a specific vertebra. Walk towards the foot. Repeat the movement five times.

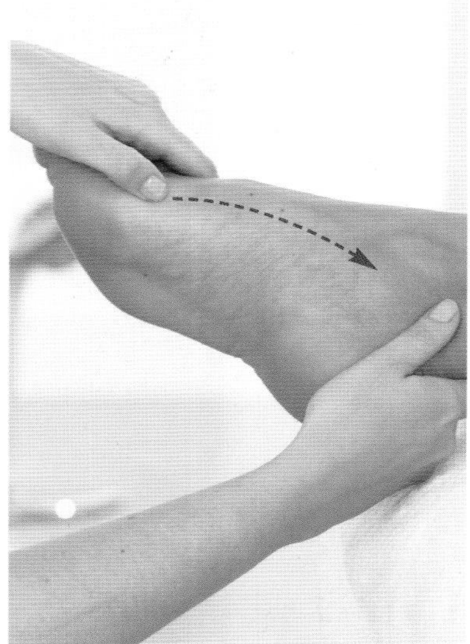

THORACIC VERTEBRAE REFLEX AREA

Support the foot and take 12 steps from the base of the joint of the big toe to work the thoracic vertebrae. You should end up on a bone called the navicular, which feels like a knuckle and is halfway between the bladder point and the ankle. Each step represents a specific vertebra and should be slow, with light to medium pressure. Repeat the movement five times.

Osteoarthritis

Osteoarthritis affects three times as many women as it does men, and is characterized by inflammation of some joints, causing creaking, stiffness, swelling and loss of joint function, deformity and pain. It is aggravated by mechanical stress, which can wear down the protective cartilage that lines the joints in the body. Osteoarthritis occurs in almost all people over 60, although not everyone has symptoms. Weakness and shrinkage of the surrounding muscles may occur if the pain is so bad that it prevents the sufferer from using the joint regularly. If this degenerative disease affects the joints between the bones in the neck, it is called cervical osteoarthritis. This is brought about by wear and tear on the neck as we get older, so it mainly affects people from middle age onwards. The principal symptoms are pain and stiffness on the neck and, if there is pressure on the nerves in the neck, it may cause pain in the arms, shoulders, numbness and tingling in the hands and a weak grip. This sequence should be given with very light pressure.

Osteoarthritis can affect our physical and emotional well-being, leading to decreased mobility in later years.

REFLEX AREAS/POINTS TO WORK

- Entire spine
- Liver
- Thyroid
- Pituitary
- Kidneys/adrenals
- Upper lymphatics

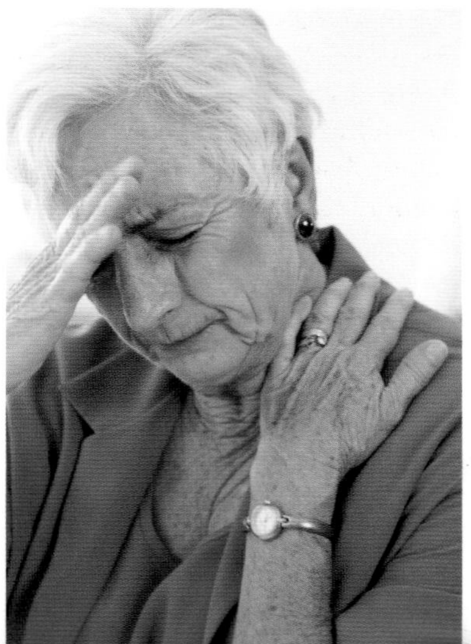

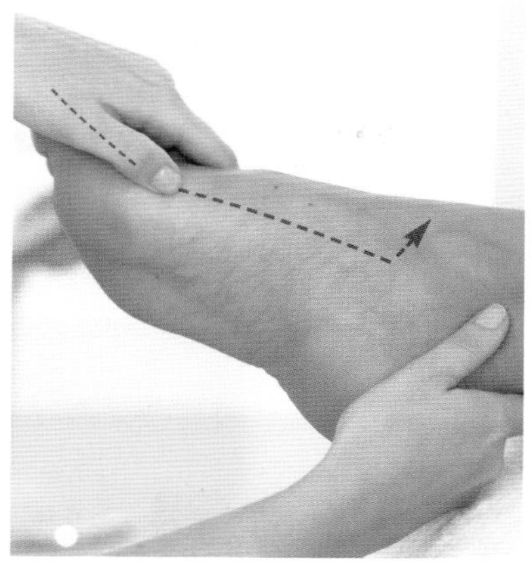

ENTIRE SPINE

Work on the medial aspect of the foot. Support the foot with one hand, and use your other thumb to make seven small steps in between the joints of the big toe, remembering that each step represents a specific vertebra. Walk towards the foot. Then take 12 gentle steps from the base of the joint of the big toe to work the thoracic vertebrae. You should end up on a bone called the navicular, which feels like a knuckle and is halfway between the bladder point and the ankle. Walk around the navicular bone, which represents lumbar one, taking five steps up to the dip in front of the ankle bone, which represents lumbar five. Repeat this movement three times.

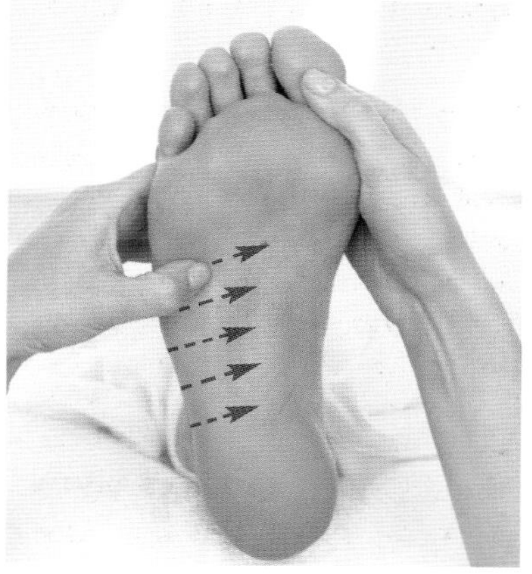

LIVER REFLEX AREA

This reflex area is only found on the right foot. Support the foot with your right hand, and place your left thumb just underneath the diaphragm line. Work slowly and precisely, horizontally across the foot, into zone five, four and just into zone three. Proceed in one direction. Continue in this manner until just above the redness of the heel and complete the movement four times.

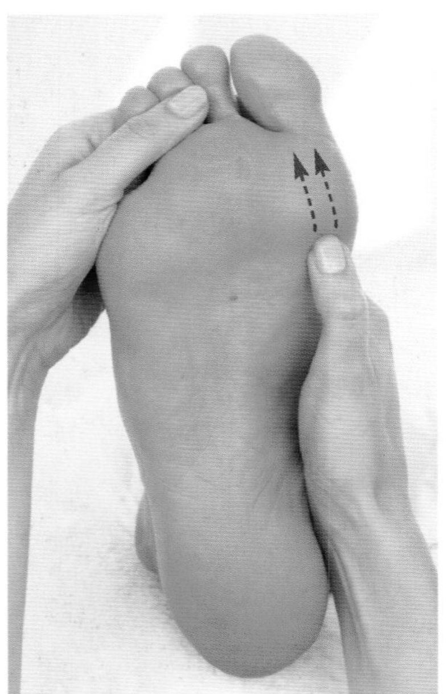

THYROID REFLEX AREA

Use your thumb to work the ball of the foot, from the diaphragm line all the way up to the neckline. Repeat this movement slowly four times over the whole area.

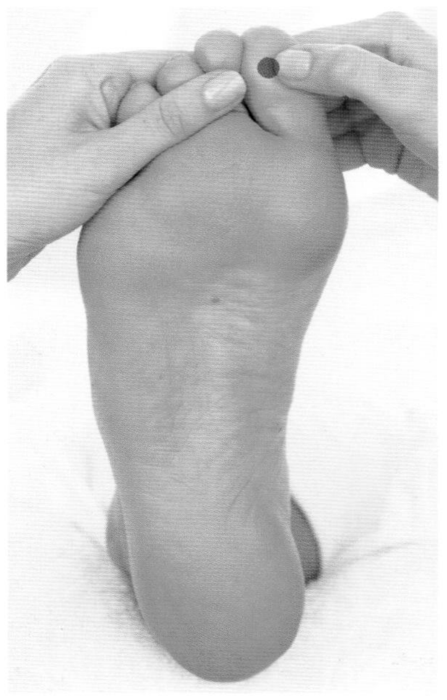

PITUITARY REFLEX POINT

Support the big toe with the fingers of one hand, and use your other thumb to make a cross to find the centre of the big toe. Place your thumb into the centre, push in and make circles for 15 seconds.

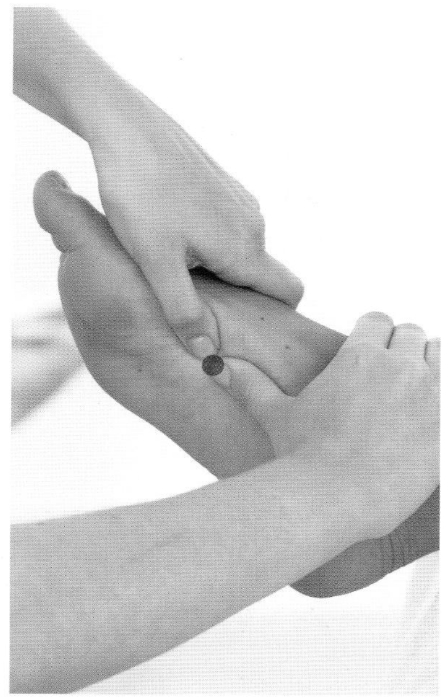

KIDNEY/ADRENAL REFLEX POINTS

You can find these reflexes in zone one, three steps down from the ball of the foot. Place your two thumbs together and gently push into the kidney/adrenal reflexes, making small circles. Work in this manner for 15 seconds.

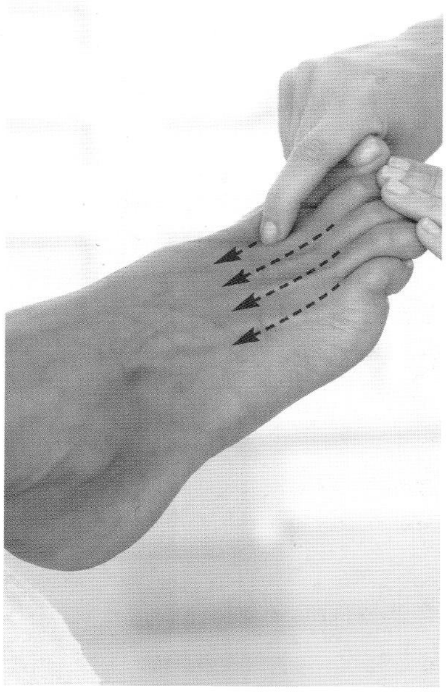

UPPER LYMPHATIC REFLEX AREA

Work on the dorsal aspect of the foot, using your index finger and thumb to walk up from the base of the toes towards the ankle in between the metatarsals. Work with a light pressure up as far as you can, then slide back to make circles lightly between the clefts of the toes. Repeat this movement five times.

Frozen shoulder

This condition is caused by inflammation and thickening of the lining of the capsule in which the joint is contained. This bursa is a small, fluid-filled sac found between muscles, between tendon and bone and between skin and bone, enabling movement to occur without friction between these surfaces. The symptoms of frozen shoulder include stiffness and pain in the shoulder, which makes normal movements of the joint difficult. In the most extreme cases the shoulder is totally immobile and the pain is severe.

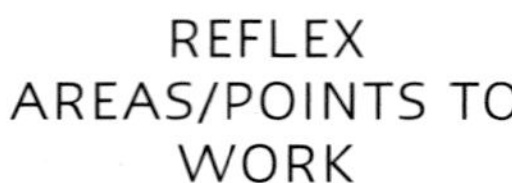

REFLEX AREAS/POINTS TO WORK

- Head
- Occipital
- Shoulder
- Elbow
- Adrenals
- Cervical vertebrae
- Thoracic vertebrae

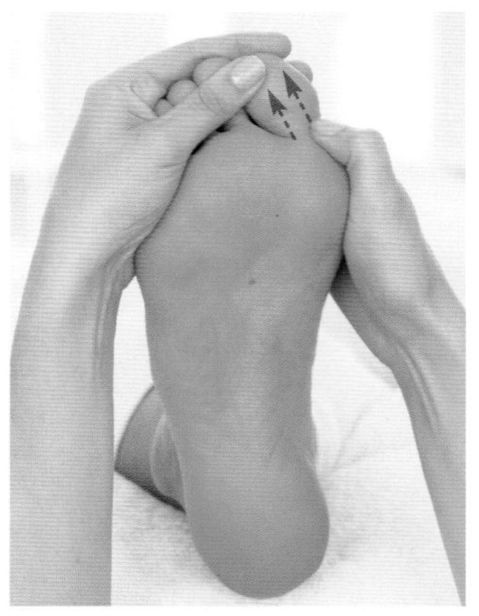

HEAD REFLEX AREA

Support the big toe with the fingers of one hand. Use your other thumb to walk up from the neckline to the top of the big toe. Repeat this movement several times in lines up the toe.

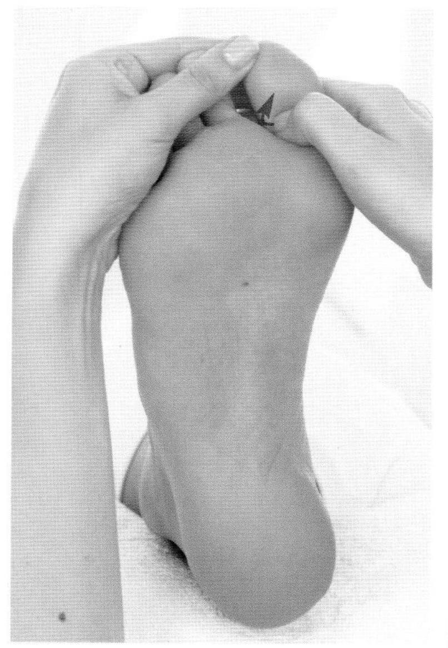

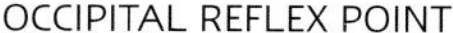

OCCIPITAL REFLEX POINT

Support the foot with one hand and gently flex back the big toe. Walk along the base of the big toe with your thumb, and hook in the crease in between the big toe and second toe. You will find a bone that juts out: place your thumb here and make gentle circles for 20 seconds to work the reflex point.

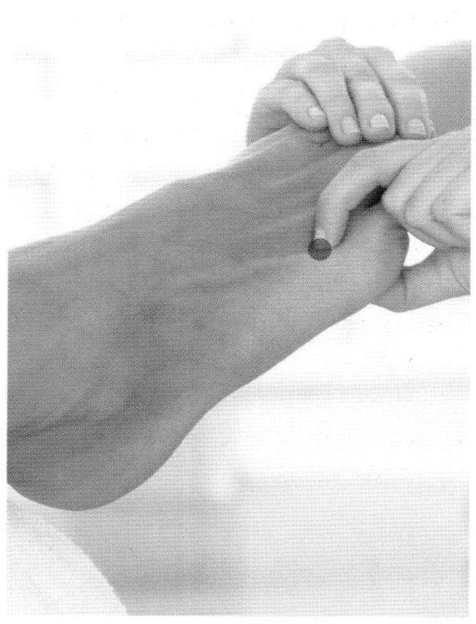

SHOULDER REFLEX POINT

You will find this reflex point on the dorsal aspect of the foot, in between the fourth and fifth metatarsals. The simplest way to find it is to place your index finger and thumb at the base of the fourth and fifth toes. Slowly walk down four steps, following the edge of the foot in a pinching movement. When you find this sensitive reflex point, stop and push in, making small circles for 15 seconds. Adjust pressure to avoid discomfort.

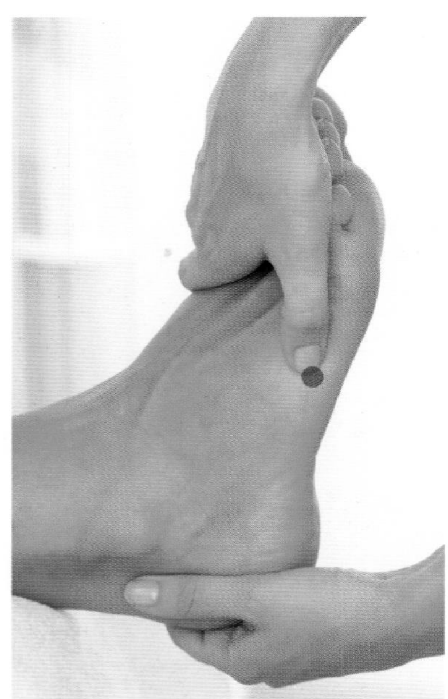

ELBOW REFLEX POINT

Use your thumb to walk three steps down the lateral aspect of the foot from the fifth toe. Push in to work the elbow reflex point, making circles for 15 seconds.

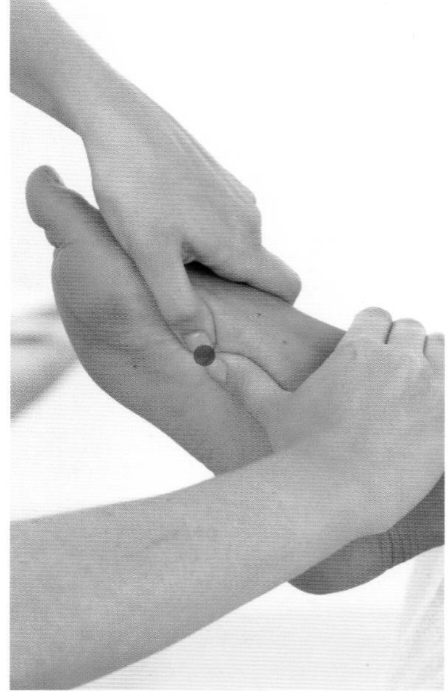

ADRENAL REFLEX POINT

You can find the adrenal reflexes in zone one, three steps down from the ball of the foot. Place your two thumbs together and gently push into the adrenal reflexes, making small circles. Work in this manner for 15 seconds.

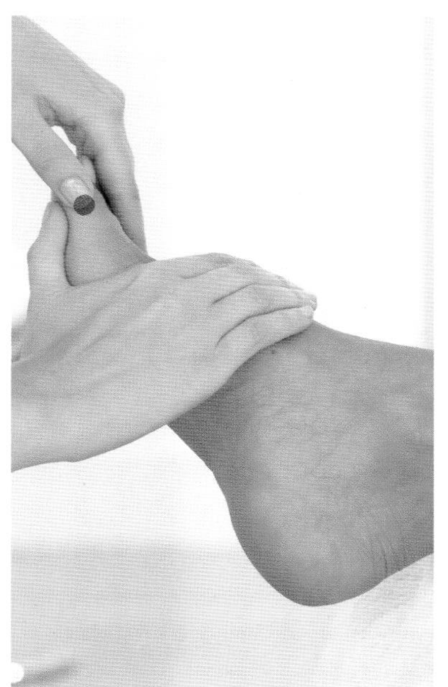
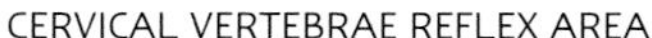

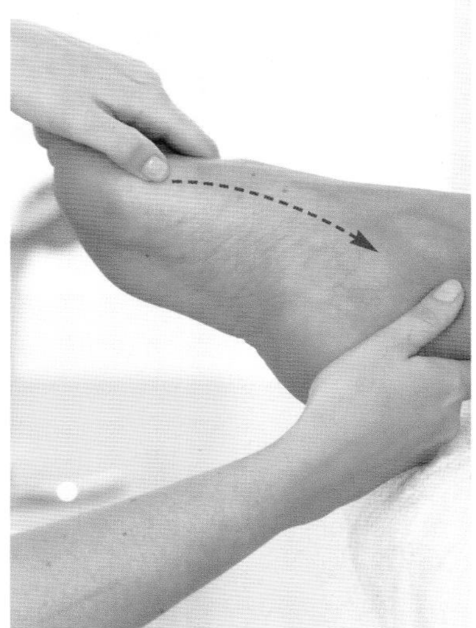

CERVICAL VERTEBRAE REFLEX AREA

This reflex area lies on the medial aspect of the big toe and in between the joints (you do not actually work on the joints, because many different factors could affect them). Support the big toe with one hand. Use the thumb of your other hand to make seven small steps, remembering that each step represents a specific vertebra. Walk towards the foot. Repeat the movement five times.

THORACIC VERTEBRAE REFLEX AREA

Support the foot and take 12 steps from the base of the joint of the big toe to work the thoracic vertebrae. You should end up on a bone called the navicular, which feels like a knuckle and is halfway between the bladder point and the ankle. Each step represents a specific vertebra and should be slow, with light to medium pressure. Repeat the movement five times.

Epilepsy

Epilepsy is the tendency to have recurrent seizures, or brief episodes of altered consciousness, caused by abnormal electrical activity in the brain. The condition usually develops in childhood, but may gradually disappear. Elderly people are at risk of developing epilepsy because they are more likely to have conditions that can cause it, such as a stroke. In most cases of epilepsy, the underlying cause is unclear, although a genetic factor may be involved. Recurrent seizures may be the result of brain damage caused by a difficult birth, a severe blow to the head, a stroke (which starves the brain of oxygen) or an infection such as meningitis. There are different types of epilepsy and different types of seizure, including the less common partial seizure, when someone may simply look blank or vacant for a few minutes or may experience odd sights or smells; and a generalized seizure, when the body stiffens and then jerks uncontrollably.`

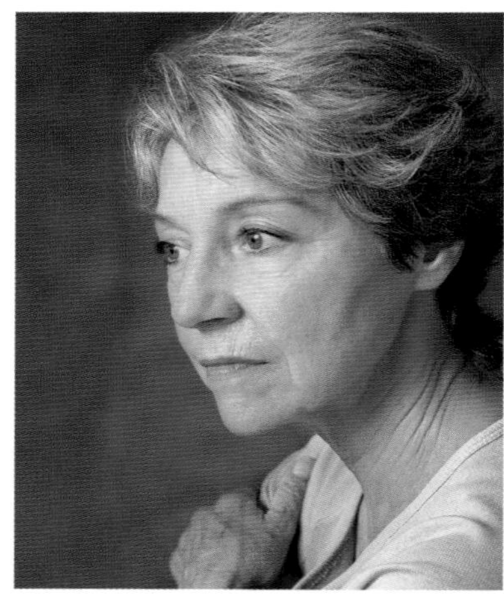

Environment and lifestyle causes include heat, lead, food allergies, alcohol and physical and emotional stress.

REFLEX AREAS/POINTS TO WORK

- Head
- Pituitary
- Thyroid
- Liver
- Adrenals
- Entire spine

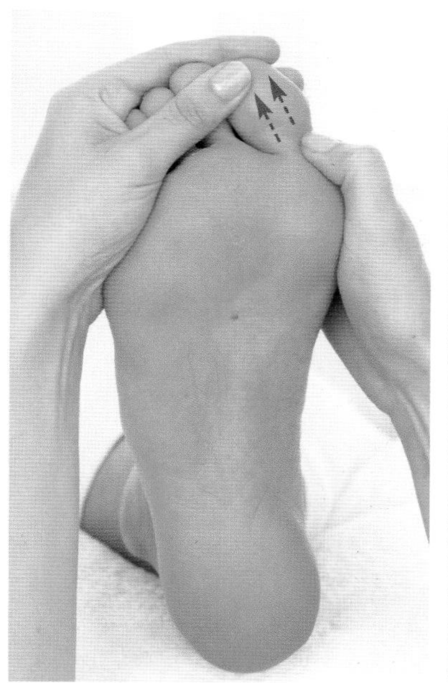

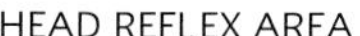

HEAD REFLEX AREA

Support the big toe with the fingers of one hand. Use your other thumb to walk up from the neckline to the top of the big toe. Repeat this several times in lines up the toe for a total of one minute.

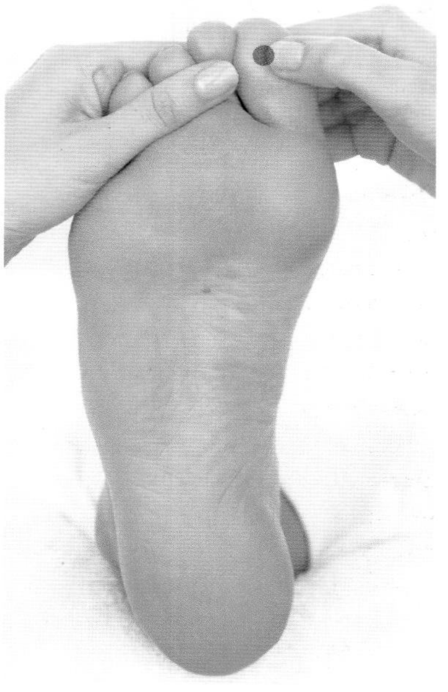

PITUITARY REFLEX POINT

Support the big toe with the fingers of one hand, and use your other thumb to make a cross to find the centre of the big toe. Place your thumb into the centre, push in and make circles for 15 seconds.

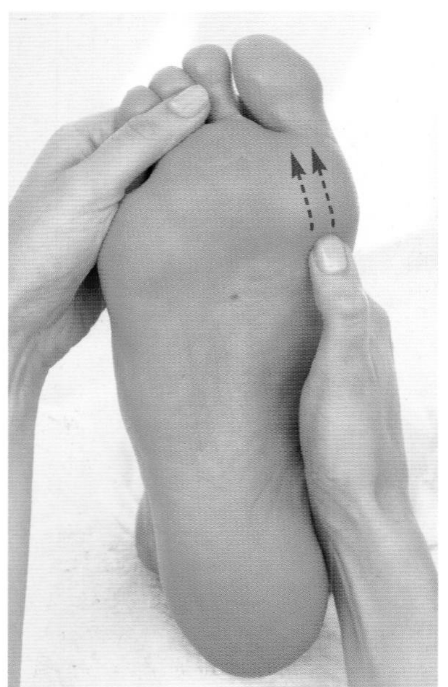

THYROID REFLEX AREA

Use your thumb to work the ball of the foot, from the diaphragm line all the way up to the neckline. Repeat this movement slowly six times over the area. Whenever you find crystals stay on the area and stimulate with circles to disperse them.

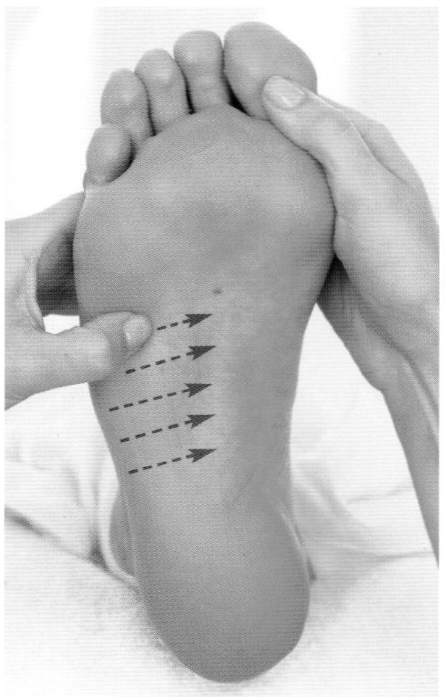

LIVER REFLEX AREA

This reflex area is only found on the right foot. Support the foot with your right hand, and place your left thumb just underneath the diaphragm line. Work slowly and precisely, horizontally across the foot, into zones five and four and just into zone three. Proceed in one direction. Continue in this manner until just above the redness of the heel. Complete the liver reflex movement five times.

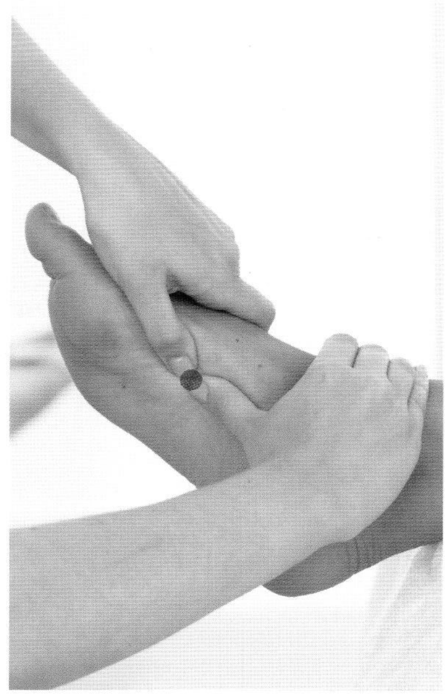

ADRENAL REFLEX POINT

You can find the adrenal reflexes in zone one, three steps down from the ball of the foot. Place your two thumbs together and gently push into the adrenal reflexes, making small circles. Work in this manner for 15 seconds.

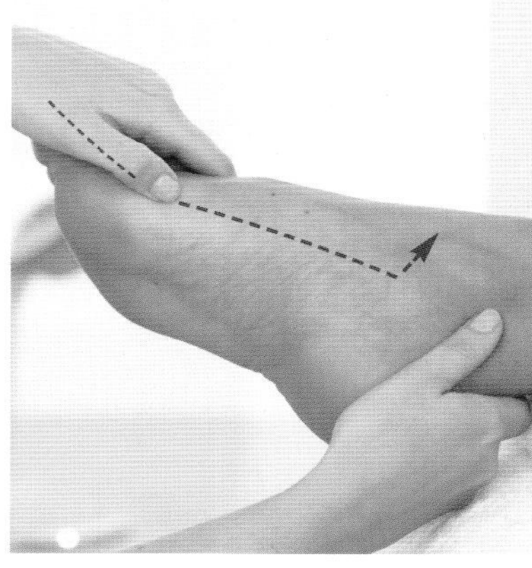

ENTIRE SPINE

Work on the medial aspect of the foot. Support the foot with one hand, and use your other thumb to make seven small steps in between the joints of the big toe, remembering that each step represents a specific vertebra. Walk towards the foot. Then take 12 gentle steps from the base of the joint of the big toe to work the thoracic vertebrae. You should end up on a bone called the navicular, which feels like a knuckle and is halfway between the bladder point and the ankle. Walk around the navicular bone, which represents lumbar one, taking five steps up to the dip in front of the ankle bone, which represents lumbar five. Repeat this movement four times.

Parkinson's disease

This degenerative disease affects the nervous system as a result of damage to nerve cells within the base of the brain. The underlying cause is unknown, but symptoms appear when there is a lack of the hormone dopamine in the brain, and this can restrict messages from one nerve cell to another. The two main theories for the onset of Parkinson's are that brain cells are destroyed by toxins in the body that the liver has been unable to remove, and that exposure to environmental toxins such as pesticides or herbicides has caused the disease. Parkinson's is more common in elderly men. The symptoms are muscle tremors, weakness and stiffness. The person may also experience trembling, shaking of the hand, arm or leg, a rigid posture, slow shuffling movements, an unbalanced walk that may break into tiny running steps and a rigid stoop. Eating, washing, dressing and other everyday activities may become very difficult for the sufferer to perform.

Parkinson's is more common in the elderly, and can make daily activities very difficult for the sufferer.

REFLEX AREAS/POINTS TO WORK

- Head
- Brain
- Liver
- Upper lymphatics
- Adrenals
- Entire spine

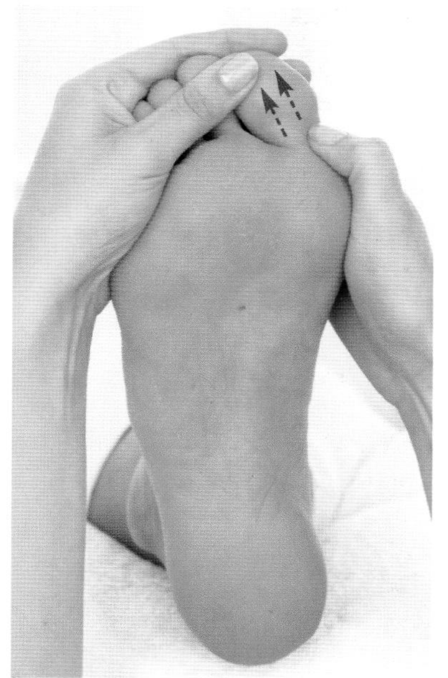

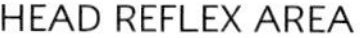

HEAD REFLEX AREA

Support the big toe with the fingers of one hand. Use your other thumb to walk up from the neckline to the top of the big toe. Repeat this several times in lines up the toe for a total of one minute.

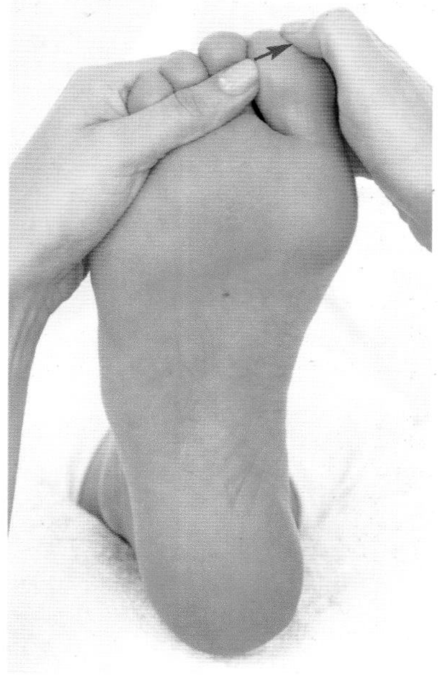

BRAIN REFLEX AREA

Support the big toe with one hand, and use your other hand to walk along the top of the big toe. Repeat this movement 12 times.

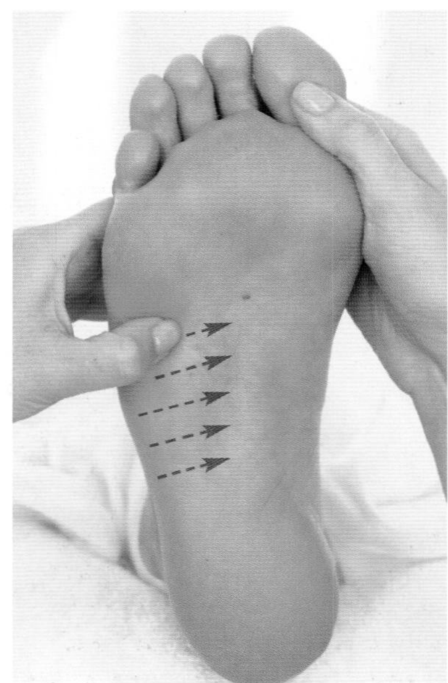

LIVER REFLEX AREA

This reflex area is only found on the right foot. Support the foot with your right hand, and place your left thumb just underneath the diaphragm line. Work slowly and precisely, horizontally across the foot, into zones five and four and just into zone three. Proceed in one direction. Continue in this manner until just above the redness of the heel. Complete the liver reflex movement five times.

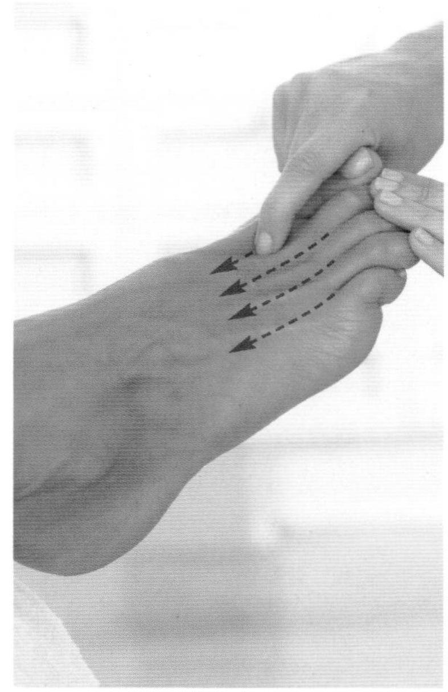

UPPER LYMPHATIC REFLEX AREA

Work on the dorsal aspect of the foot, using your index finger and thumb to walk up from the base of the toes towards the ankle in between the metatarsals. Work with a medium pressure up as far as you can, then slide back to make circles lightly between the clefts of the toes. Repeat this movement four times.

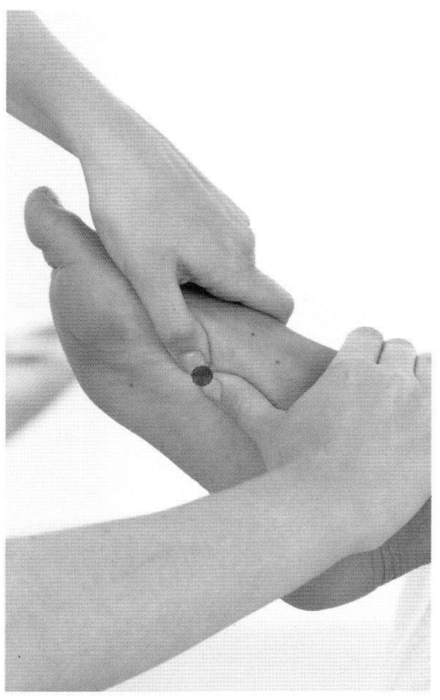

ADRENAL REFLEX POINT

You can find the adrenal reflexes in zone one, three steps down from the ball of the foot. Place your two thumbs together and gently push into the adrenal reflexes, making small circles. Work in this manner for 15 seconds.

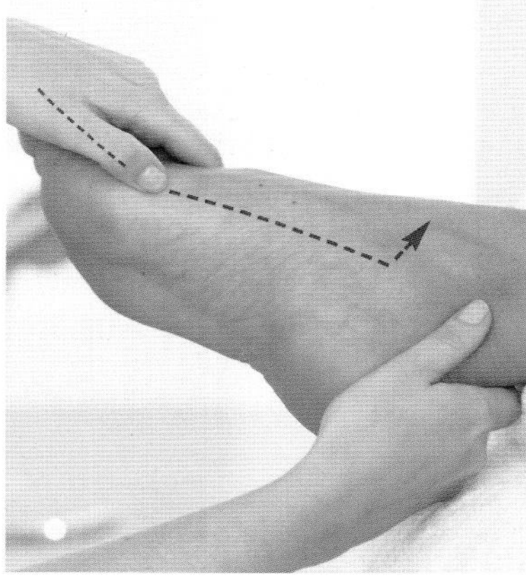

ENTIRE SPINE

Work on the medial aspect of the foot. Support the foot with one hand, and use your other thumb to make seven small steps in between the joints of the big toe, remembering that each step represents a specific vertebra. Walk towards the foot. Then take 12 gentle steps from the base of the joint of the big toe to work the thoracic vertebrae. You should end up on a bone called the navicular, which feels like a knuckle and is halfway between the bladder point and the ankle. Walk around the navicular bone, which represents lumbar one, taking five steps up to the dip in front of the ankle bone, which represents lumbar five. Repeat this movement four times.

Ménière's disease

With Ménière's disease there is an abnormal build-up of fluid in the canals of the inner ear that control balance. It can affect both ears, but in most cases just one ear is affected. Both men and women are equally at risk, and the condition often starts between the ages of 20 and 60. The main symptom is frequent severe, sudden rotational vertigo that can cause someone to fall to the ground. Other symptoms are dizziness, vertigo, aural fullness, deafness and ringing in the ear. Common triggers include salt, alcohol, caffeine and nicotine; other possible triggers include pregnancy, menstruation, allergies, visual stimuli, changes in weather pressure and stress. It is recommended that sufferers follow a diet that aims to stabilize body fluid and blood levels, so that secondary fluctuations in inner ear fluid can be avoided.

REFLEX AREAS/POINTS TO WORK

- Head
- Pituitary
- Inner ear
- Cervical vertebrae
- Liver
- Kidneys/adrenals

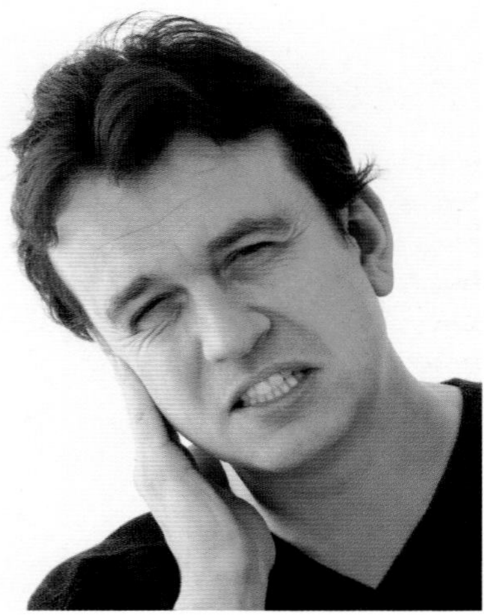

Often sufferers from Ménière's disease have low levels of manganese.

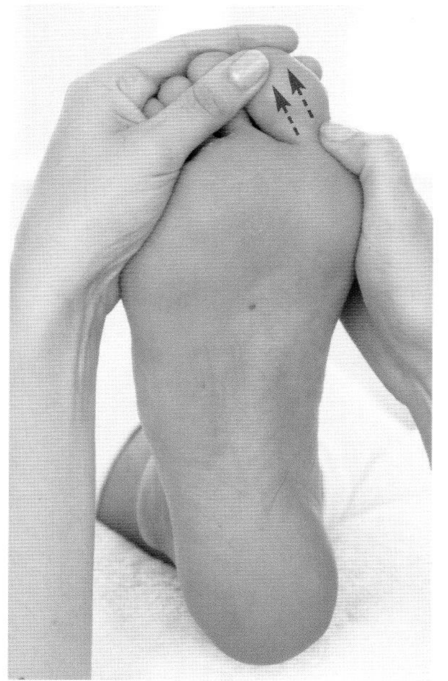

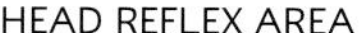

HEAD REFLEX AREA

Support the big toe with the fingers of one hand. Use your other thumb to walk up from the neckline to the top of the big toe. Repeat this several times in lines up the toe for a total of one minute.

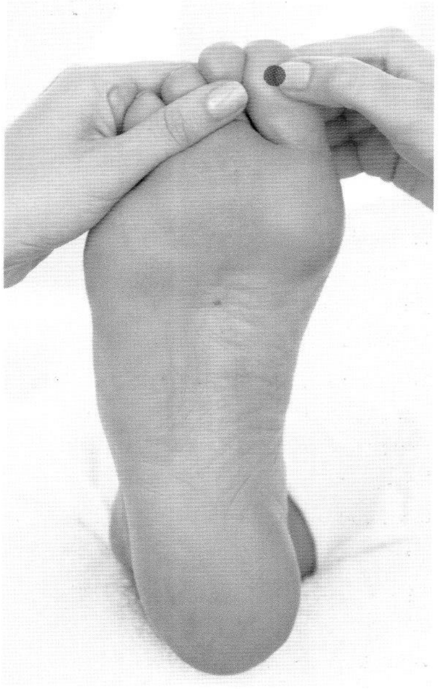

PITUITARY REFLEX POINT

Support the big toe with the fingers of one hand, and use your other thumb to make a cross to find the centre of the big toe. Place your thumb into the centre, push in and make circles for 15 seconds.

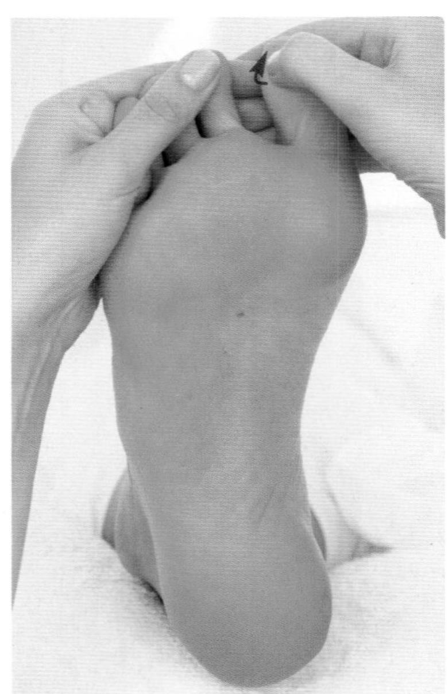

INNER EAR REFLEX POINT

Take two large steps up towards the top of the toe from the occipital reflex point. Place your thumb on the inner ear reflex and make gentle circles for ten seconds to work the point.

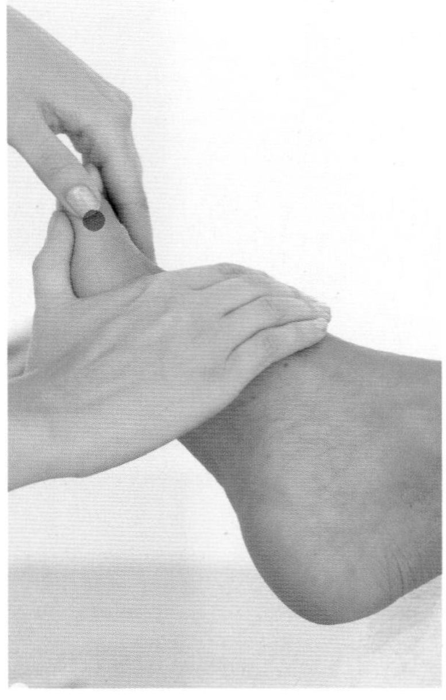

CERVICAL VERTEBRAE REFLEX AREA

This lies on the medial aspect of the big toe and in between the joints (you do not actually work on the joints because of many different factors that could affect them). Support the big toe with one hand. Use the thumb of your other hand to make seven small steps, remembering that each step represents a specific vertebra. Walk towards the foot. Repeat the movement ten times.

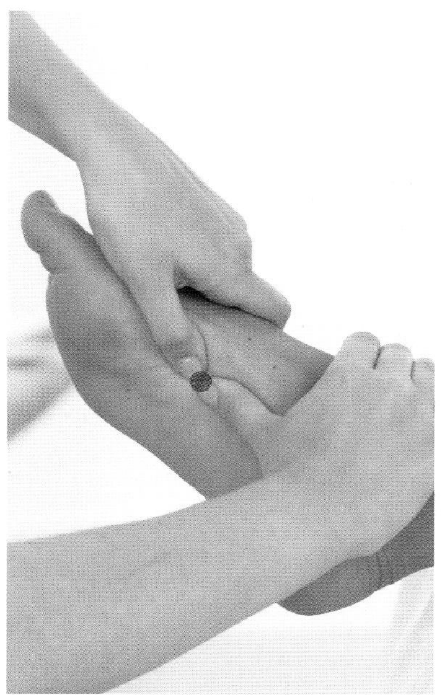

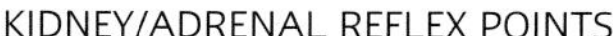

KIDNEY/ADRENAL REFLEX POINTS

You can find these reflexes in zone one, three steps down from the ball of the foot. Place your two thumbs together and gently push into the kidney/adrenal reflexes, making small circles. Work in this manner for 15 seconds.

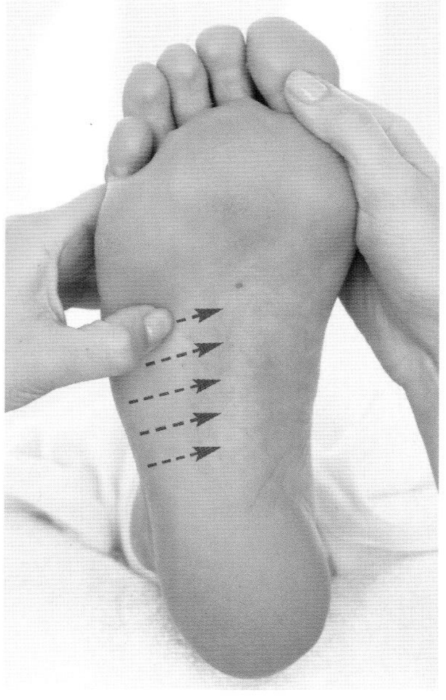

LIVER REFLEX AREA

This reflex area is only found on the right foot. Support the foot with your right hand and place your left thumb just underneath the diaphragm line. Work slowly and precisely, horizontally across the foot, into zones five and four and just into zone three. Proceed in one direction. Continue in this manner until just above the redness of the heel. Complete the liver reflex movement five times.

Multiple sclerosis

Multiple sclerosis (MS) is a debilitating disease that damages the nerve fibres in the brain, optic nerve and spinal cord. It affects various parts of the nervous system by destroying the myelin sheaths that cover the nerves and leaving scar tissue called plaques, which ultimately destroy the nerves. Multiple sclerosis is considered an auto-immune disease in which the white blood cells attack the myelin sheaths as though they were a foreign substance. The condition usually starts in early adult life and generally consists of mild relapses and long symptom-free periods throughout life, although the disease affects everyone differently. There are different stages of the condition, and symptoms vary in individuals, depending on which part of the nervous system is most affected; they may include blurred or double vision, emotional changes, slurred speech, urinary tract infections, vertigo, dizziness, clumsiness and muscle weakness.

REFLEX AREAS/POINTS TO WORK

- Entire spine
- Head
- Inner ear
- Bladder
- Adrenals
- Upper lymphatics

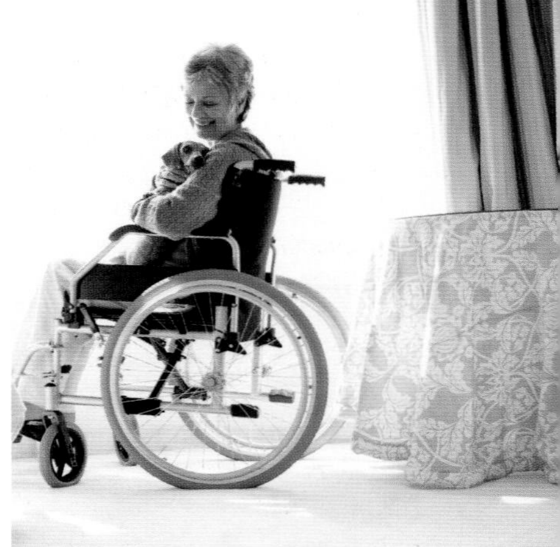

Eating essential fatty acids and receiving regular reflexology sessions have been known to help symptoms of MS.

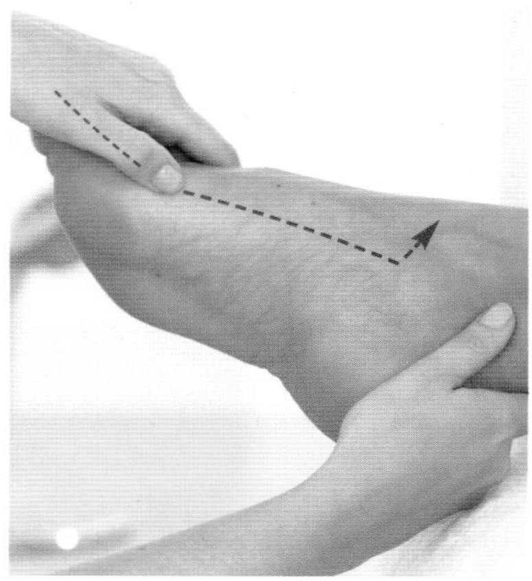

ENTIRE SPINE

Work on the medial aspect of the foot. Support the foot with one hand and use your other thumb to make seven small steps in between the joints of the big toe, remembering that each step represents a specific vertebra. Walk towards the foot. Then take 12 gentle steps from the base of the joint of the big toe to work the thoracic vertebrae. You should end up on a bone called the navicular, which feels like a knuckle and is halfway between the bladder point and the ankle. Walk around the navicular bone, which represents lumbar one, taking five steps up to the dip in front of the ankle bone, which represents lumbar five. Repeat this movement four times.

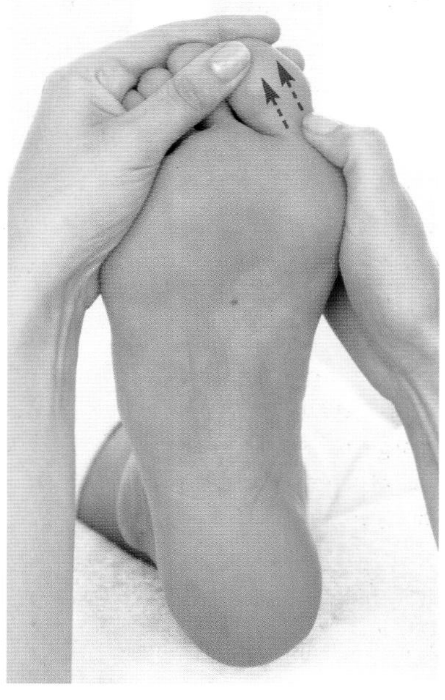

HEAD REFLEX AREA

Support the big toe with the fingers of one hand. Use your other thumb to walk up from the neckline to the top of the big toe. Repeat this several times in lines up the toe for a total of one minute.

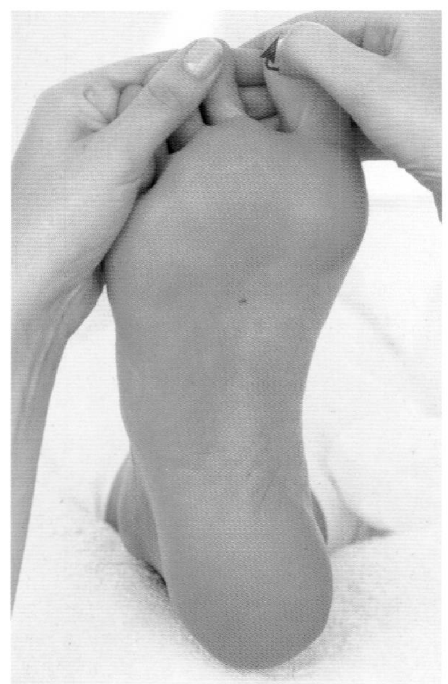

INNER EAR REFLEX POINT

Take two large steps up towards the top of the toe from the occipital reflex point. Place your thumb on the inner ear reflex and make gentle circles for 20 seconds to work the point.

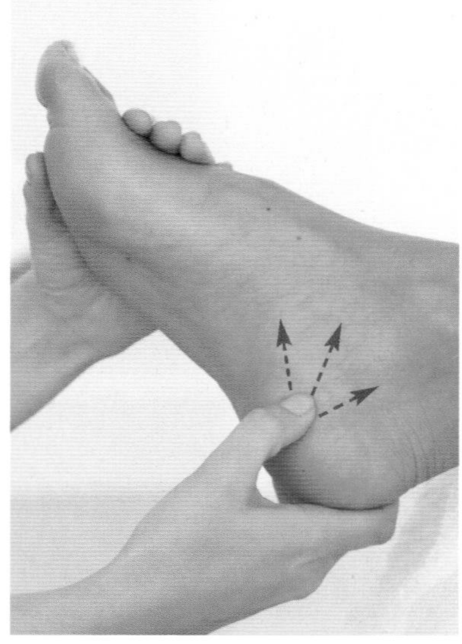

BLADDER REFLEX AREA

Work on the medial aspect of the foot. Place your thumb at the bladder point, which is at the edge of the soft area about one-third of the way from the back of the heel. Use your thumb to fan out over the area like the spokes of a bicycle wheel, always returning to the bladder point. Do this approximately 12 times.

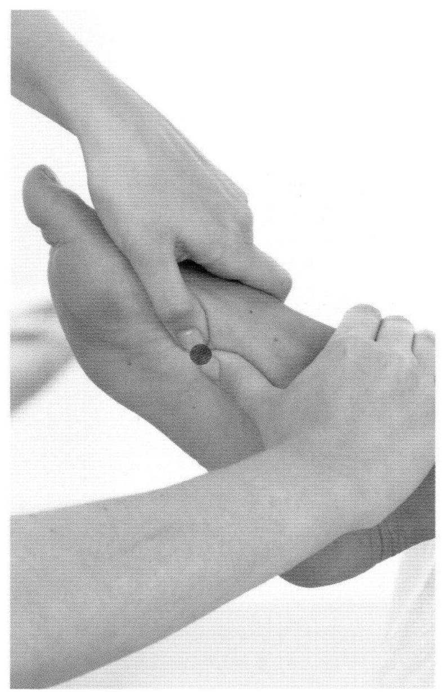

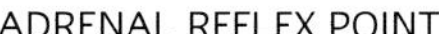

ADRENAL REFLEX POINT

You can find the adrenal reflexes in zone one, three steps down from the ball of the foot. Place your two thumbs together and gently push into the adrenal reflexes, making small circles. Work in this manner for 15 seconds.

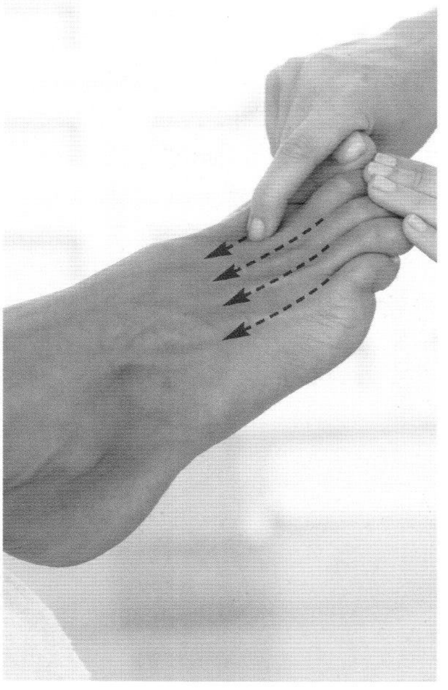

UPPER LYMPHATIC REFLEX AREA

Work on the dorsal aspect of the foot. Use your index finger and thumb to walk up from the base of the toes towards the ankle in between the metatarsals. Work with a medium pressure up as far as you can, then slide back to make circles lightly between the clefts of the toes. Repeat this movement four times.

Acne

Acne is an inflammatory skin condition that is common between the ages of 12 and 24, especially in young men, and is associated with an imbalance of hormones during puberty. Many women also suffer from premenstrual acne flare-ups that are associated with the release of the hormone progesterone after ovulation. Apart from a strong hormonal imbalance, other factors may include oily skin, a family history, stress and over-consumption of junk food and animal products. Acne can also be aggravated by certain cosmetics or by repeatedly rubbing the skin. Sugar should be eliminated to avoid outbreaks.

REFLEX AREAS/POINTS TO WORK

- Pituitary
- Ovaries/testes
- Liver
- Adrenals
- Pancreas
- Ascending colon
- Descending colon

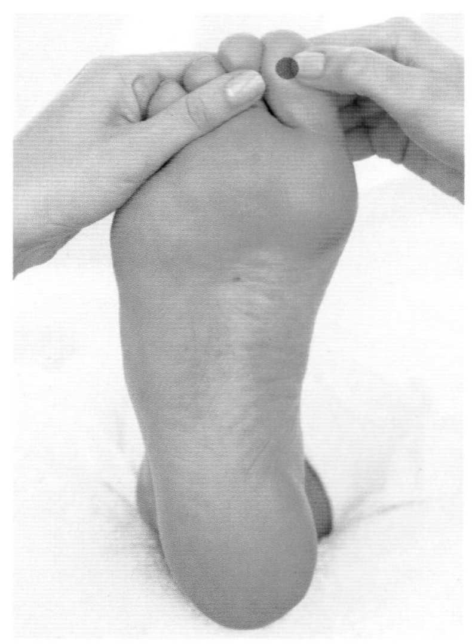

PITUITARY REFLEX POINT

Support the big toe with the fingers of one hand and use your other thumb to make a cross to find the centre of the big toe. Place your thumb into the centre, push in and make circles for 15 seconds.

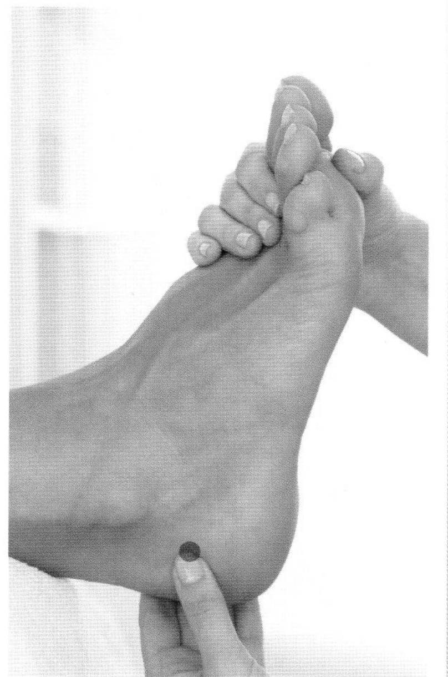

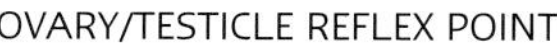

OVARY/TESTICLE REFLEX POINT

Work on the lateral side of foot. Place your index finger approximately halfway between the back of the heel and the ankle bone. Push in gently and make circles for ten seconds.

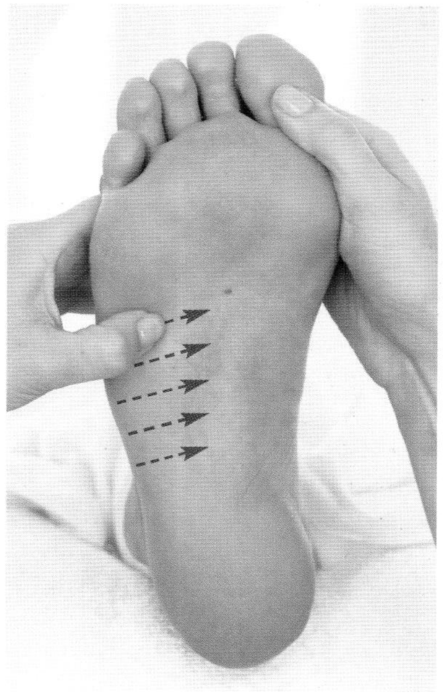

LIVER REFLEX AREA

This reflex area is only found on the right foot. Support the foot with your right hand, and place your left thumb just underneath the diaphragm line. Work slowly and precisely, horizontally across the foot, into zones five and four and just into zone three. Proceed in one direction. Continue in this manner until just above the redness of the heel. Complete the liver reflex movement six times.

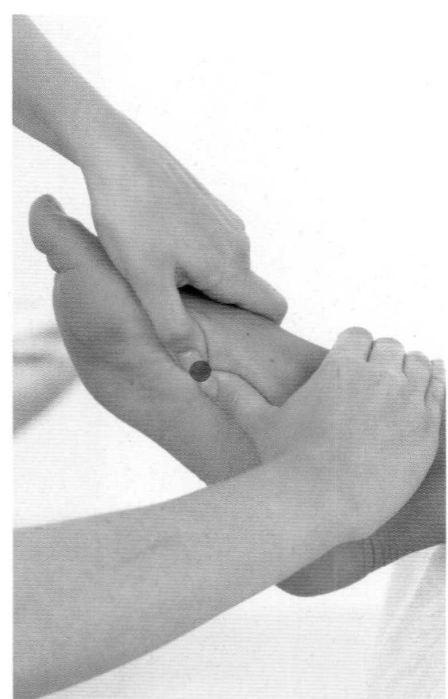

ADRENAL REFLEX POINT

You can find the adrenal reflexes in zone one, three steps down from the ball of the foot. Place your two thumbs together and gently push into the adrenal reflexes, making small circles. Work in this manner for 15 seconds.

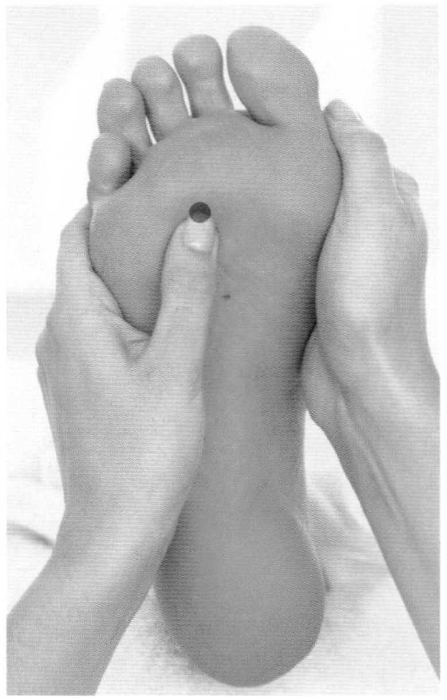

PANCREAS REFLEX POINT

This reflex point is only found on the right foot. Use your thumb and place it on the third toe, then trace a line down to below the diaphragm line. Push up into the joint and hook up for 12 seconds.

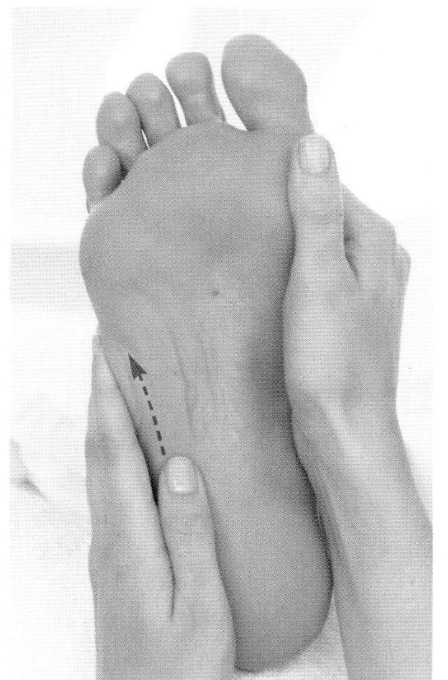

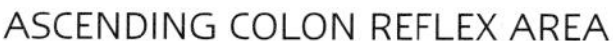

ASCENDING COLON REFLEX AREA

This reflex area is only found on the right foot. Use your left thumb to walk up zone four from the redness of the heel. Continue in this manner until you get halfway up the foot. Work the ascending colon reflex area four times in slow movements to help stimulate the peristaltic muscular action of the colon.

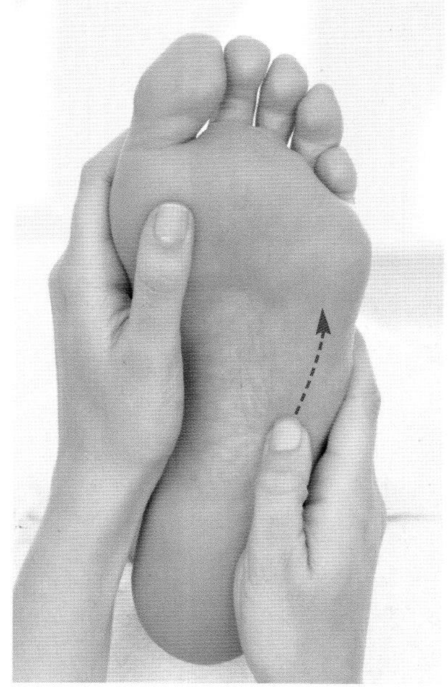

DESCENDING COLON REFLEX AREA

This reflex area is only found on the left foot. Use your right thumb to walk up zone four from the redness of the heel to work the descending colon. Continue in this manner until you arrive halfway up the foot. Work the descending colon reflex area six times and in slow movements to help stimulate the peristaltic muscular action of the colon.

Dermatitis

Inflammation of the skin that results in itching, thickening, scaling, colour changes and flaking, dermatitis often occurs as the result of allergies. Allergic or contact dermatitis may be caused by anything with which the body has had contact. The usual suspects include sensitivity to perfume, medication creams, cosmetics, glue, certain plants, and some metals found in jewellery and zippers. If the skin is in contact with the allergen, the condition will remain. Eating gluten and dairy products has been associated with making all skin conditions worse. Stress aggravates dermatitis.

REFLEX AREAS/POINTS TO WORK

- Pituitary
- Upper lymphatics
- Ascending colon
- Descending colon
- Liver
- Spleen
- Adrenals

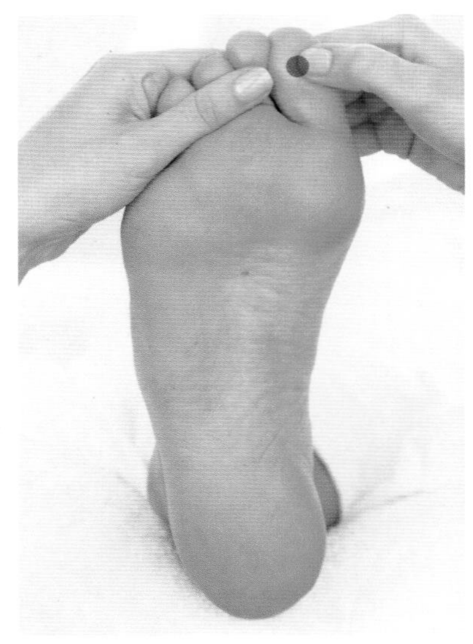

PITUITARY REFLEX POINT

Support the big toe with the fingers of one hand, and use your other thumb to make a cross to find the centre of the big toe. Place your thumb into the centre, push in and make circles for 15 seconds.

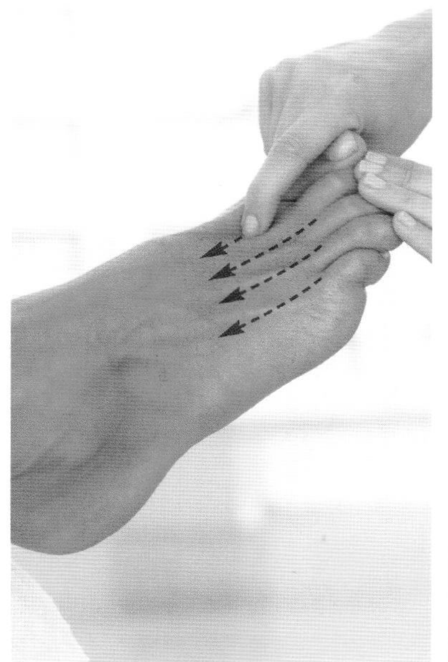

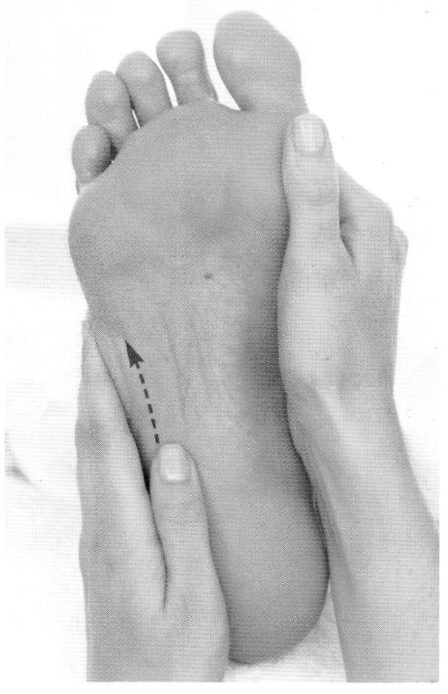

UPPER LYMPHATIC REFLEX AREA

Work on the dorsal aspect of the foot. Use your index finger and thumb to walk up from the base of the toes towards the ankle in between the metatarsals. Work with a medium pressure up as far as you can, then slide back to make circles lightly between the clefts of the toes. Repeat this movement five times.

ASCENDING COLON REFLEX AREA

This reflex area is only found on the right foot. Use your left thumb to walk up zone four from the redness of the heel. Continue in this manner until you get halfway up the foot. Work the ascending colon reflex area four times in slow movements to help to eliminate waste products effectively.

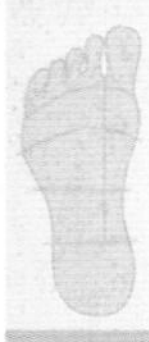

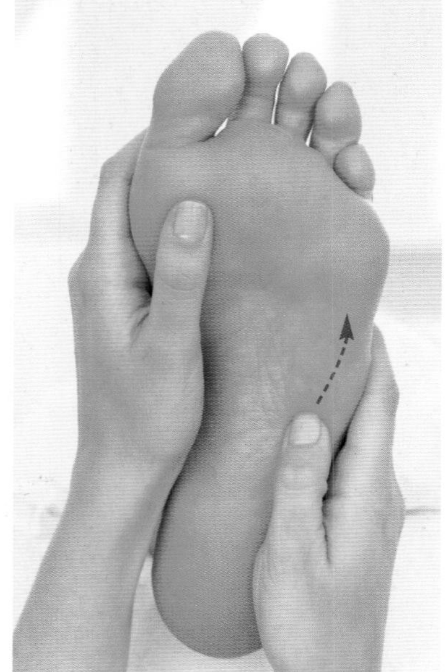

DESCENDING COLON REFLEX AREA

This reflex area is only found on the left foot. Use your right thumb to walk up zone four from the redness of the heel to work the descending colon. Continue in this manner until you arrive halfway up the foot. Work the descending colon reflex area six times and in slow movements to help stimulate the peristaltic muscular action of the colon.

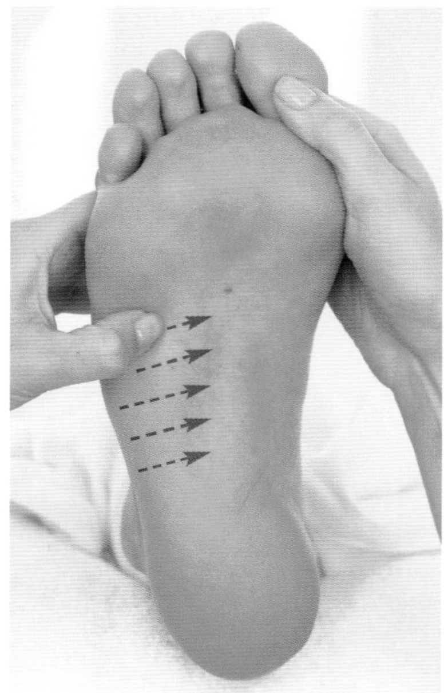

LIVER REFLEX AREA

This reflex area is only found on the right foot. Support the foot with your right hand and place your left thumb just underneath the diaphragm line. Work slowly and precisely, horizontally across the foot, into zones five and four and just into zone three. Proceed in one direction. Continue in this manner until just above the redness of the heel. Complete the liver reflex movement six times.

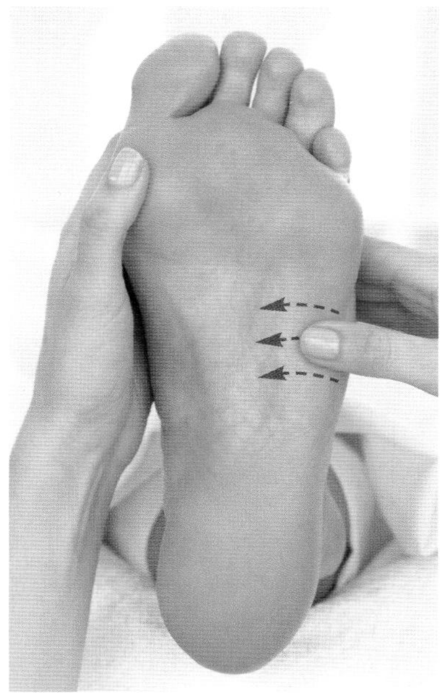
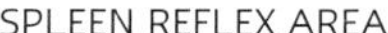

SPLEEN REFLEX AREA

This reflex area is only found on the left foot. Support the foot with your left hand, and place your right thumb just underneath the diaphragm line. Work slowly and precisely, horizontally across the foot, into zones five and four and just into zone three. Proceed in one direction. Continue in this manner for four horizontal lines, completing the spleen reflex six times.

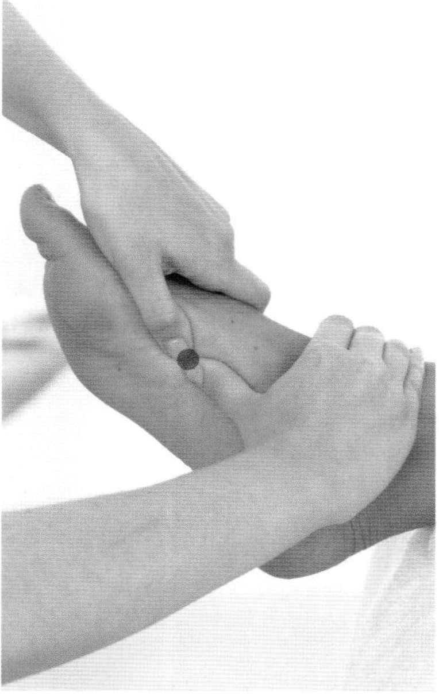

ADRENAL REFLEX POINT

You can find the adrenal reflexes in zone one, three steps down from the ball of the foot. Place your two thumbs together and gently push into the adrenal reflexes, making small circles. Work in this manner for 20 seconds.

Boils

Boils are round, pus-filled lumps on the skin, which result from inflammation and infection caused by bacteria. This disorder is common among children and young adults. Boils affect the deepest portion of the hair follicle and can appear on the scalp, under the arms, on the buttocks and the face. They are often red, tender and painful and symptoms may include itching, localized swelling and pain. Boils can heal within a month, but are contagious because the pus can contaminate nearby skin, causing new boils. They are often an indication that the sufferer has a lowered immune system as a result of poor nutrition, diabetes mellitus, the use of immunosuppressive drugs or suffering from an illness. An onion poultice is good for boils because it reduces pain and draws toxins from the infected area: place a finely chopped onion between two pieces of cloth and put it on the affected area of the body to draw out impurities.

REFLEX AREAS/POINTS TO WORK

- Adrenals
- Pituitary
- Upper lymphatics
- Pancreas
- Spleen
- Entire spine

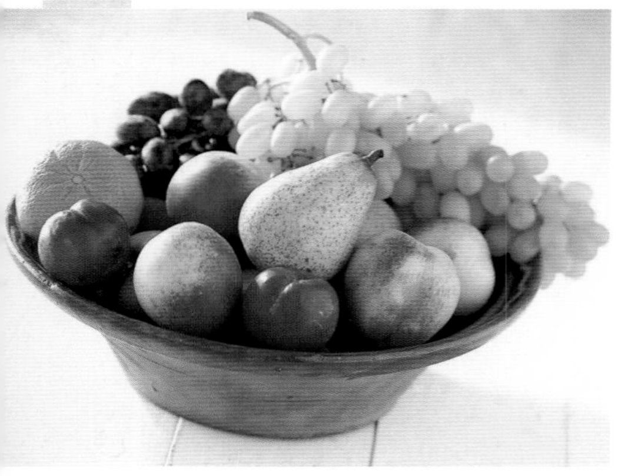

A nutritious diet is one aspect of a healthy immune system. Replace sugar with fresh fruit to help eliminate boils.

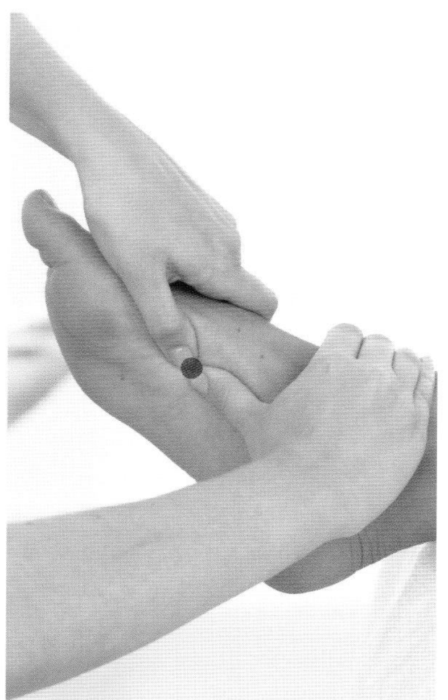

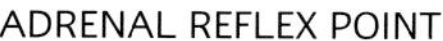

ADRENAL REFLEX POINT

You can find the adrenal reflexes in zone one, three steps down from the ball of the foot. Place your two thumbs together and gently push into the adrenal reflexes, making small circles. Work in this manner for 20 seconds.

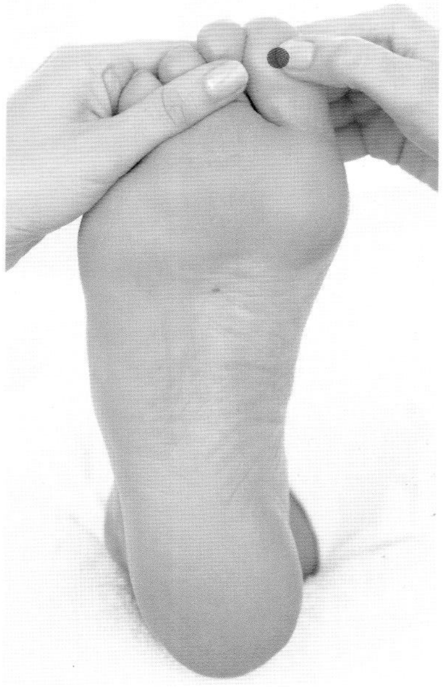

PITUITARY REFLEX POINT

Support the big toe with the fingers of one hand, and use your other thumb to make a cross to find the centre of the big toe. Place your thumb into the centre, push in and make circles for 20 seconds.

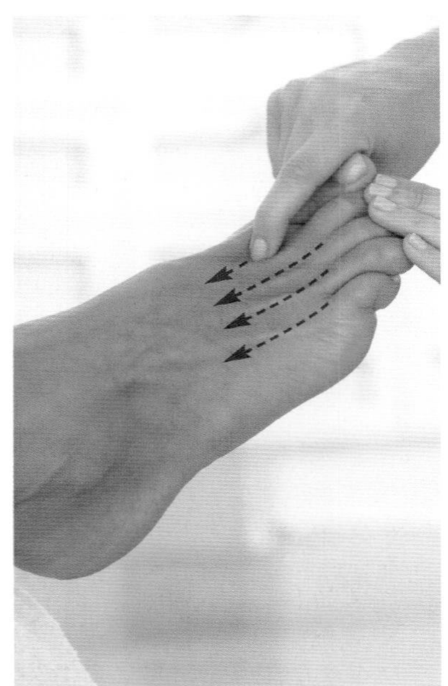

UPPER LYMPHATIC REFLEX AREA

Work on the dorsal aspect of the foot. Use your index finger and thumb to walk up from the base of the toes towards the ankle in between the metatarsals. Work with medium pressure up as far as you can, then slide back to make circles lightly between the clefts of the toes. Repeat this movement six times.

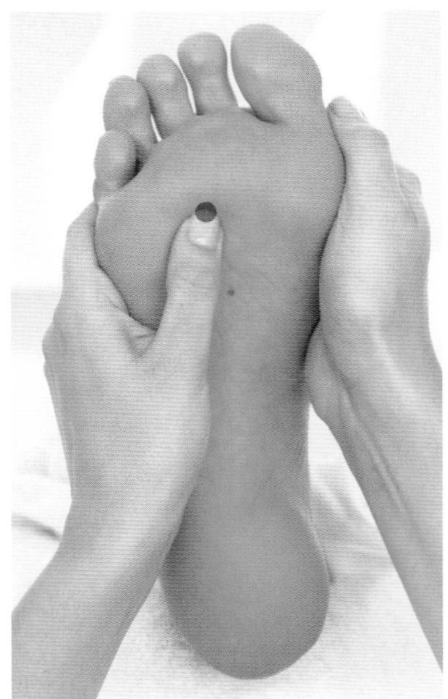

PANCREAS REFLEX POINT

This reflex point is only found on the right foot. Place your thumb on the third toe and trace a line down to below the diaphragm line. Push up into the joint and hook up for ten seconds.

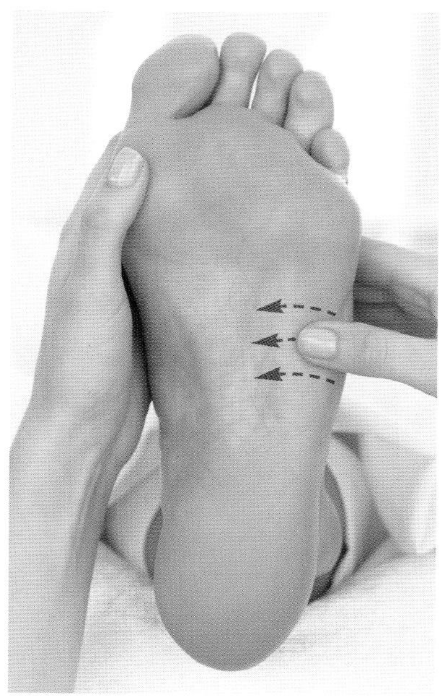

SPLEEN REFLEX AREA

This reflex area is only found on the left foot. Support the foot with your left hand and place your right thumb just underneath the diaphragm line. Work slowly and precisely, horizontally across the foot, into zones five and four and just into zone three. Proceed in one direction. Continue in this manner for four horizontal lines. Complete the spleen reflex six times.

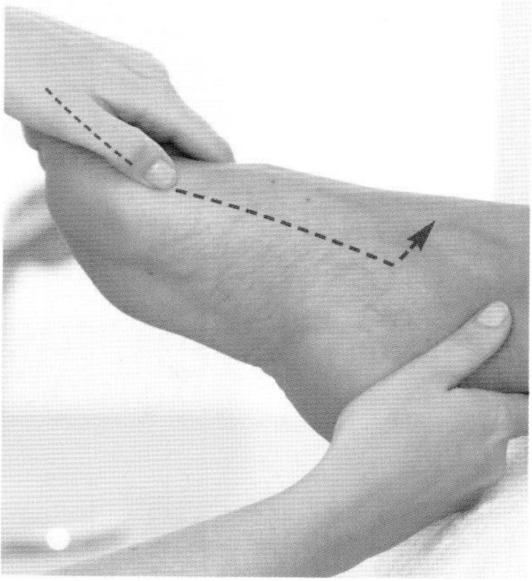

ENTIRE SPINE

Work on the medial aspect of the foot. Support the foot with one hand, and use your other thumb to make seven small steps in between the joints of the big toe, remembering that each step represents a specific vertebra. Walk towards the foot. Then take 12 gentle steps from the base of the joint of the big toe to work the thoracic vertebrae. You should end up on a bone called the navicular, which feels like a knuckle and is halfway between the bladder point and the ankle. Walk around the navicular bone, which represents lumbar one, taking five steps up to the dip in front of the ankle bone, which represents lumbar five. Repeat this movement five times.

Psoriasis

This skin condition appears as patches of silvery scales or red areas on the arms, elbows, knees, legs, ears, scalp and back. It generally affects young adults between the ages of 15 and 25 and can be triggered by stress. The colon should be kept clean with a diet of 50 per cent of raw foods, because an unhealthy colon has been linked to psoriasis. The condition normally follows a pattern of occasional flare-ups followed by periods of remission. Psoriasis is often hereditary and is linked to a rapid growth of cells in the skin's outer layer, causing patches that spread over a large area.

REFLEX AREAS/POINT TO WORK

- Pituitary
- Stomach
- Liver
- Ascending colon
- Descending colon
- Entire spine
- Kidneys/adrenals

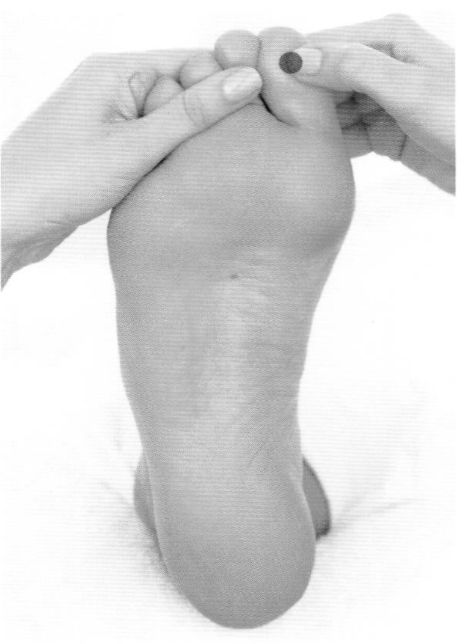

PITUITARY REFLEX POINT

Support the big toe with the fingers of one hand, and use your other thumb to make a cross to find the centre of the big toe. Place your thumb into the centre, push in and make circles for 15 seconds.

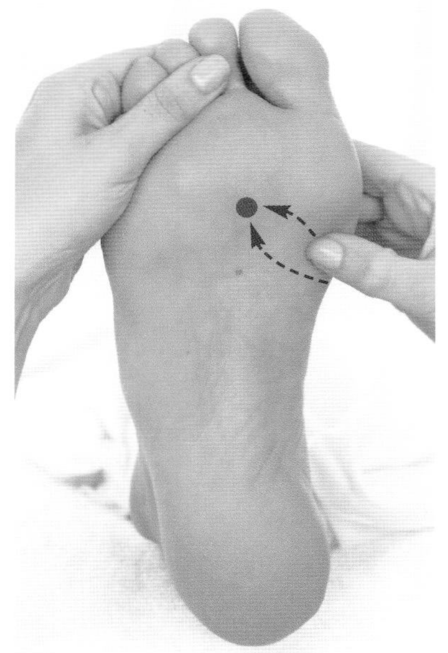

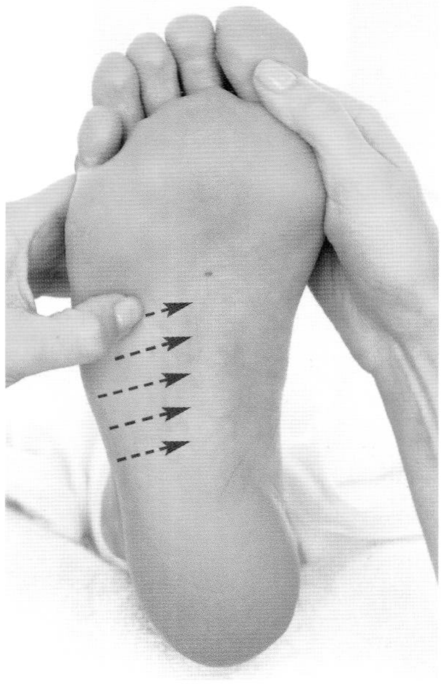

STOMACH REFLEX AREA

You will find this reflex area just under the ball of the foot. Support the foot with one hand, and place your other thumb below the thyroid reflex area. Gently work up laterally to the solar plexus reflex, making small circles. Repeat this movement six times.

LIVER REFLEX AREA

This reflex area is only found on the right foot. Support the foot with your right hand, and place your left thumb just underneath the diaphragm line. Work slowly and precisely, horizontally across the foot, into zones five and four and just into zone three. Proceed in one direction. Continue in this manner until just above the redness of the heel. Complete the liver reflex movement six times.

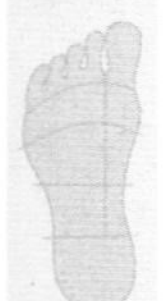

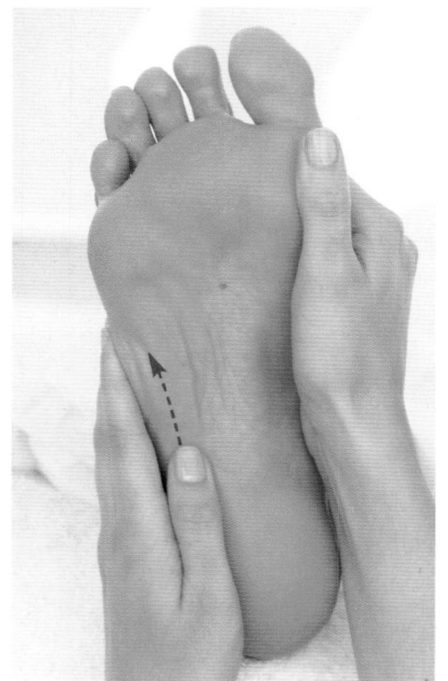

ASCENDING COLON REFLEX AREA

This reflex area is only found on the right foot. Use your right thumb to walk up zone four from the redness of the heel. Continue in this manner until you get to halfway up the foot. Work the ascending colon reflex area six times and in slow movements to help keep the colon clean.

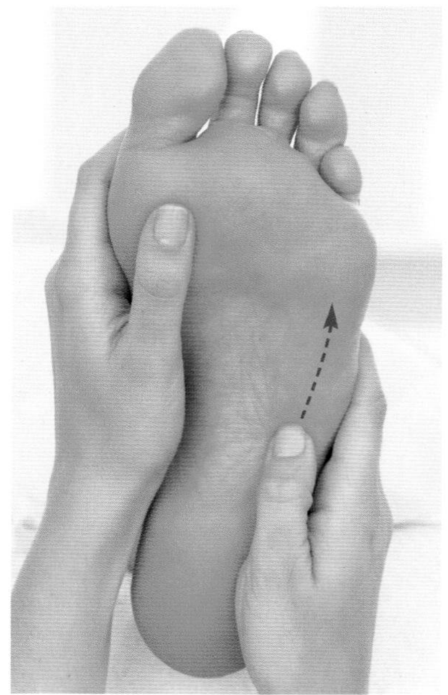

DESCENDING COLON REFLEX AREA

This reflex area is only found on the left foot. Use your right thumb to walk up zone four from the redness of the heel to work the descending colon. Continue in this manner until you arrive halfway up the foot. Work the descending colon reflex area six times and in slow movements to help stimulate the peristaltic muscular action of the colon.

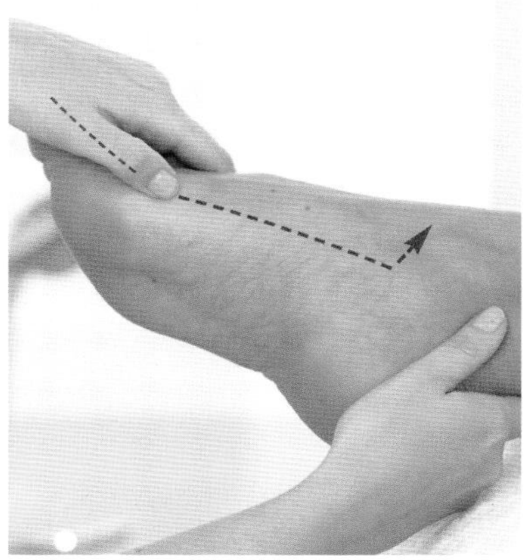

ENTIRE SPINE

Work on the medial aspect of the foot. Support the foot with one hand, and use your other thumb to make seven small steps in between the joints of the big toe, remembering that each step represents a specific vertebra. Walk towards the foot. Then take 12 gentle steps from the base of the joint of the big toe to work the thoracic vertebrae. You should end up on a bone called the navicular, which feels like a knuckle and is halfway between the bladder point and the ankle. Walk around the navicular bone, which represents lumbar one, taking five steps up to the dip in front of the ankle bone, which represents lumbar five. Repeat this movement five times.

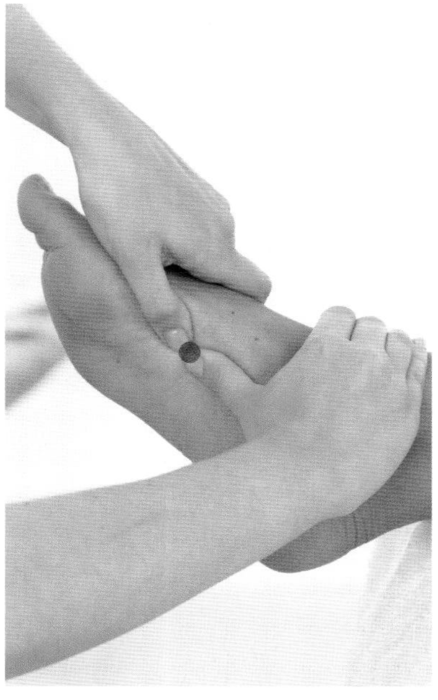

KIDNEY/ADRENAL REFLEX POINTS

You can find these reflexes in zone one, three steps down from the ball of the foot. Place your two thumbs together and gently push into the kidney/adrenal reflexes, making small circles. Work in this manner for 20 seconds.

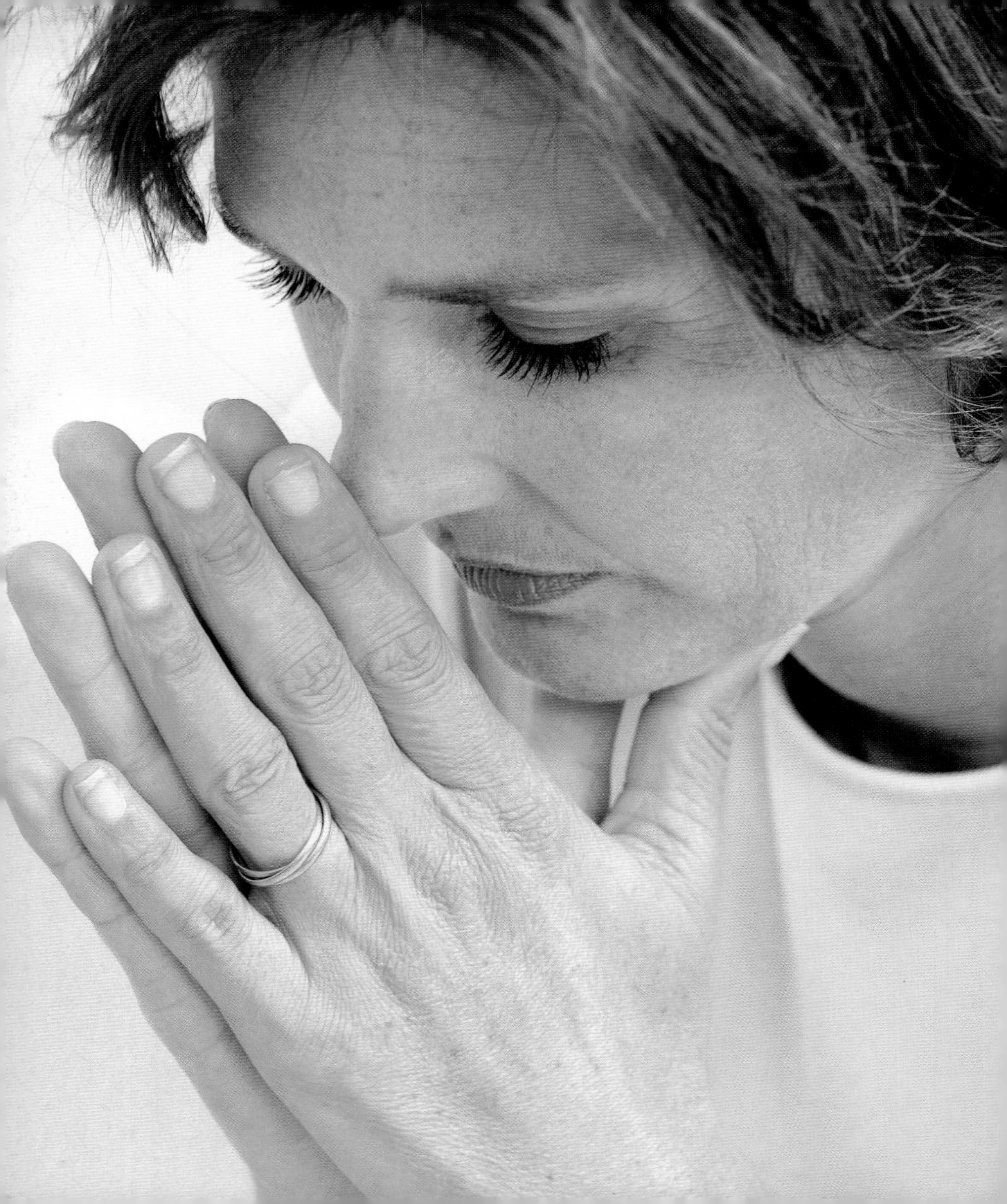

PART 6

Specialized reflexology

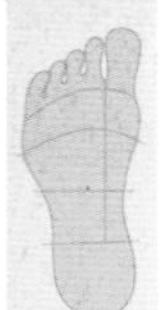

How to use this part

This part of the book shows you how specialized foot reflexology treatments can help with particular stages in life, from pregnancy and childhood to the golden years; it also looks specifically at reflexology for women, for men and for couples, as well as at how to combat stress. Choose a sequence that will meet your client's needs. Each sequence should take 15 minutes to help to maximize the potential benefits. Always start and finish treatments witih relaxation techniques.

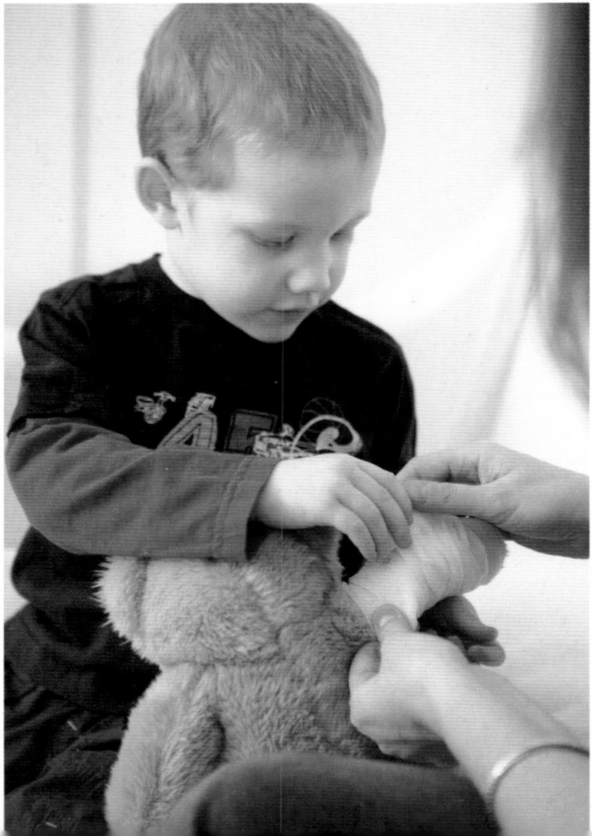

Small children often like to hold their favourite toy during a treatment.

Moods and emotions

First, we will look at the way reflexology can help us cope with situations that we feel we can't control. Sometimes we have to be our own best friend, checking that we are looking after ourselves properly. Are we eating sufficient healthy foods? Allowing ourselves relaxation time without feeling guilty? Taking time out to treat ourselves? Putting our own needs first occasionally is not a selfish act.

Illness is a natural expression of what is happening inside the body. Many factors can bring about disease, and the most important of all is state of mind. Emotions can harm the hormonal system, damage the digestion, tamper with body temperature and exacerbate anxiety. Drugs may mask the symptoms, but if your moods and emotions are responsible for your condition, then you need to take control. If someone has a negative mindset, a busy mind or is suffering from anxiety, grief, insomnia, fear, nightmares, post-traumatic stress disorder or hypertension, gentle reflexology is a safe, effective way to calm the mind, and has no unpleasant side-effects.

LIFESTYLE TIPS

Many disorders can be directly related to stress, which is a breeding ground for disease, and may be exacerbated by its effects. During a stressful period the body can become depleted of essential vitamins and minerals, so you need to focus on healthy eating and exercise to rid the body of the stress hormones and unused glucose. Avoid processed foods and chocolate, junk and snack foods, fried foods, sugars, artificial sweeteners, carbonated soft drinks and excessive quantities of red meat. A diet rich in raw fresh fruit and vegetables with plenty of herbal teas and mineral water is best. Reflexology encourages the body to relax, enabling all the functions and systems in the body to work more efficiently.

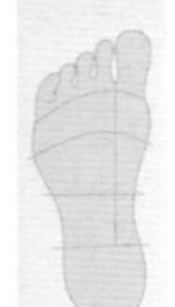

Stress

Stress relates to any reaction to a physical, emotional or mental stimulus that affects the body's natural balance. Stress is often seen as a psychological or mental problem, but it has a number of very damaging physical effects. The symptoms of stress include high blood pressure, high cholesterol levels, diabetes, headaches, chronic fatigue syndrome, memory loss and depression. Stress often affects the appetite, causing indigestion or bad food reactions in the body, leading to constipation or diarrhoea because the digestive system either slows or shuts down. Caffeine can contribute to nervousness and insomnia. Identify the source of stress, because this can be the first step in managing it. Get onto a programme of physical exercise to clear the mind, regulate deep breathing and keep stress under control.

REFLEX AREAS/POINTS TO WORK

- Diaphragm
- Thyroid
- Pituitary
- Entire spine
- Kidneys/adrenals
- Pancreas

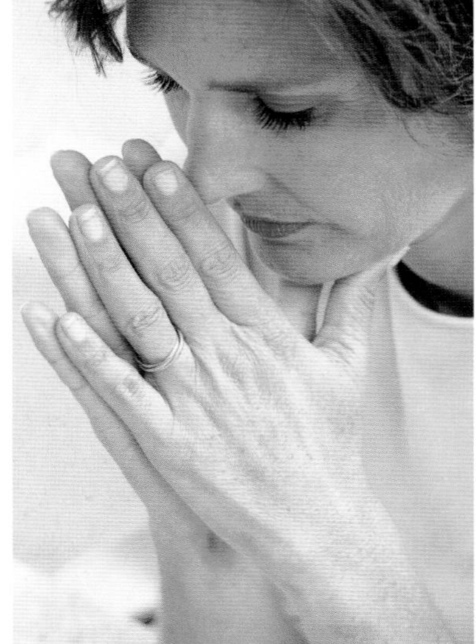

Severe stress can have a profound negative affect on menstrual cycles and menopausal symptoms.

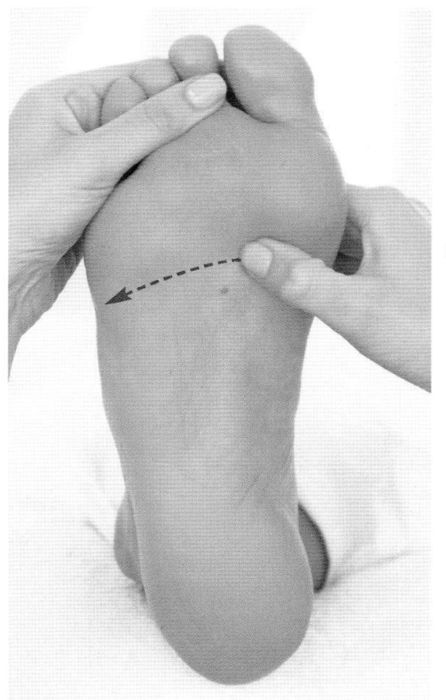

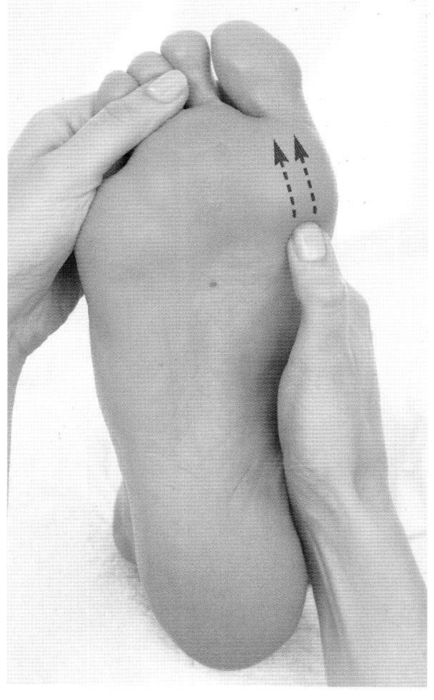

DIAPHRAGM REFLEX AREA

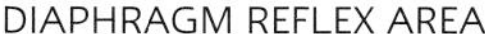

Flex the foot back with one hand to create skin tension. Use the thumb of your other hand to work under the metatarsal heads, across from the lateral to the medial aspect of the foot. Use slow steps and repeat this movement eight times.

THYROID REFLEX AREA

Use one thumb to work the ball of the foot from the diaphragm line all the way up to the neckline. Repeat this movement slowly six times over the area. Optimum functioning of the thyroid can help with energy levels.

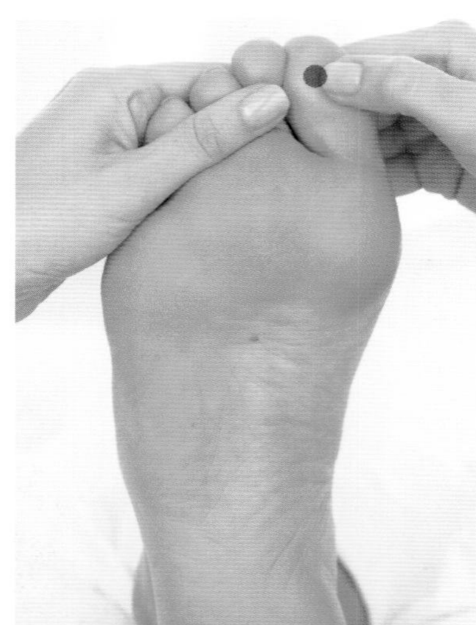

PITUITARY REFLEX POINT

Support the big toe with the fingers of one hand, and use your other thumb to make a cross to find the centre of the big toe. Place your thumb into the centre, push in and make circles for 15 seconds.

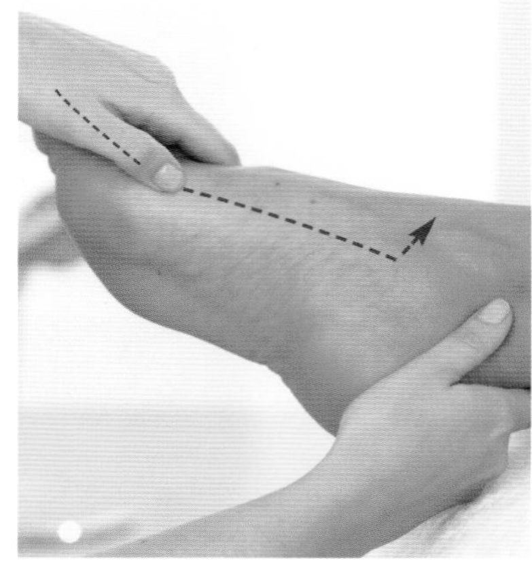

ENTIRE SPINE

Work on the medial aspect of the foot. Support the foot with one hand, and use your other thumb to walk gently seven steps in between the joints of the big toe, remembering that each step represents a specific vertebra. Walk towards the foot. Then take 12 gentle steps underneath the bone from the base of the joint of the big toe to work the thoracic vertebrae. You should end up on a bone called the navicular, which feels like a knuckle and is halfway between the bladder point and the ankle. Walk around the navicular bone, which represents lumbar one, taking five steps up to the dip in front of the ankle bone, which represents lumbar five. Repeat this movement gently five times.

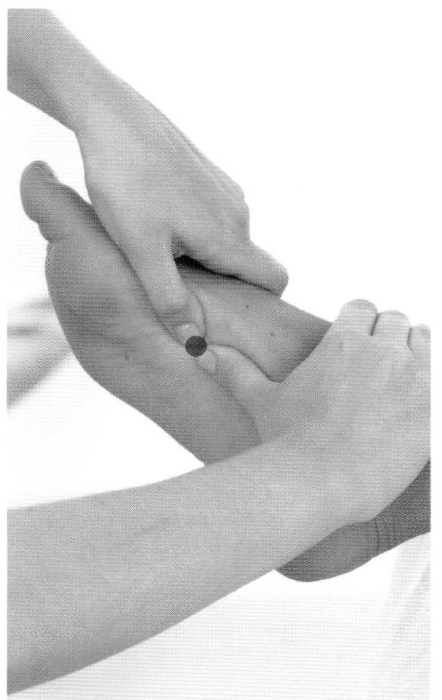

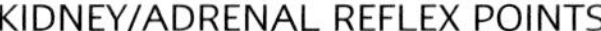

KIDNEY/ADRENAL REFLEX POINTS

You can find these reflexes in zone one, three steps down from the ball of the foot. Place your two thumbs together and gently push into the kidney/adrenal reflexes, making small circles. Work in this manner for 20 seconds.

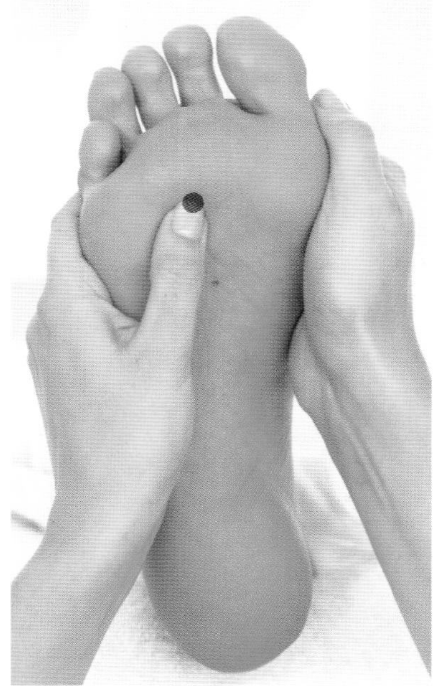

PANCREAS REFLEX POINT

This reflex point is only found on the right foot. Place your thumb on the third toe and trace a line down to below the diaphragm line. Push up into the joint and make small circles for 15 seconds.

Depression

People with depression tend to find that the disease affects their whole body, including their sleep patterns, the way they feel about themselves, what they eat and how they react to life itself. They lose interest in the people and things around them and find it hard to experience pleasure. The common symptoms are backache, chronic fatigue, changes in appetite and sleep patterns, digestive disorders, restlessness, quickness to anger and a feeling of worthlessness. Exercise helps because it releases endorphins, the body's feel-good hormones, which produce a natural high.

REFLEX AREAS/POINTS TO WORK

- Head
- Hypothalamus
- Entire spine
- Thyroid
- Liver
- Ascending colon
- Descending colon

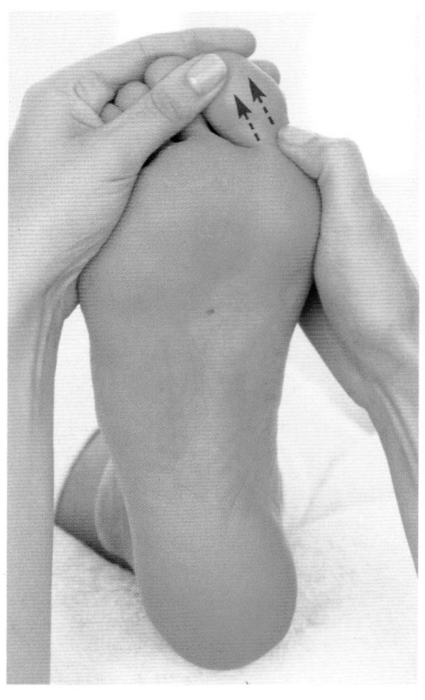

HEAD REFLEX AREA

Support the big toe with the fingers of one hand. Use your other thumb to walk up from the neckline to the top of the big toe. Repeat this several times in lines up the toe, for a total of one minute.

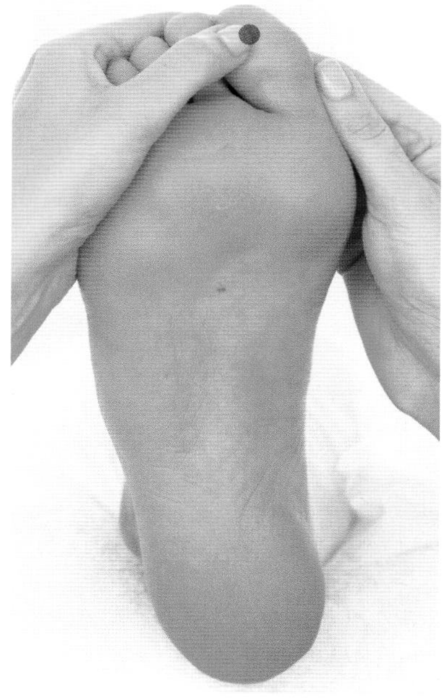

HYPOTHALAMUS REFLEX POINT

Support the big toe with the fingers of one hand, and use your other thumb to make a cross to find the centre of the big toe. Now move your thumb one step up towards the tip of the big toe and take a small step laterally. Hook in for ten seconds.

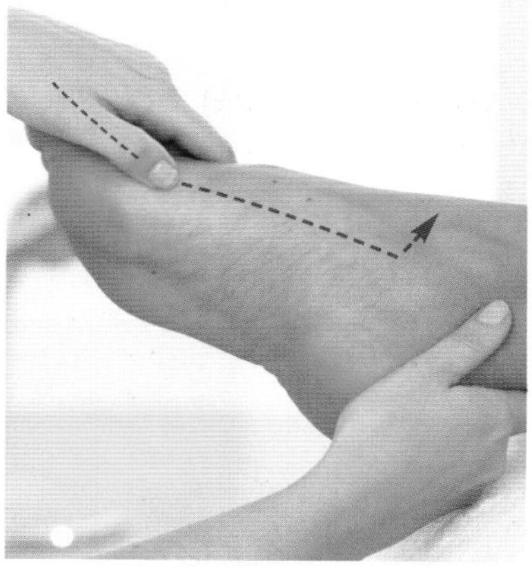

ENTIRE SPINE

Work on the medial aspect of the foot. Support the foot with one hand, and use your other thumb to walk gently seven steps in between the joints of the big toe, remembering that each step represents a specific vertebra. Walk towards the foot. Then take 12 gentle steps underneath the bone from the base of the joint of the big toe to work the thoracic vertebrae. You should end up on a bone called the navicular, which feels like a knuckle and is halfway between the bladder point and the ankle. Walk around the navicular bone, which represents lumbar one, taking five steps up to the dip in front of the ankle bone, which represents lumbar five. Repeat this movement gently five times.

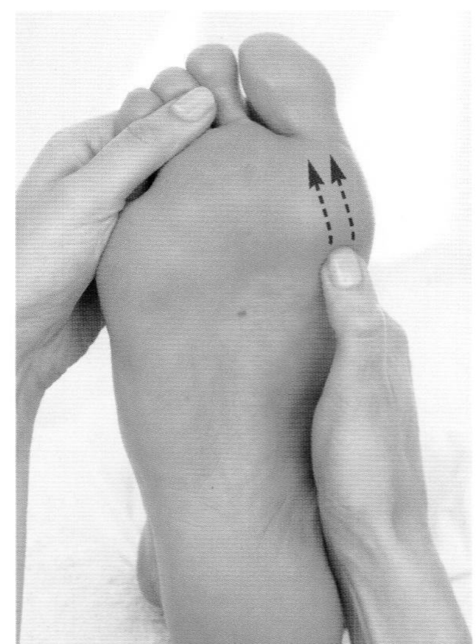

THYROID REFLEX AREA

Use the thumb of one hand to work the ball of the foot from the diaphragm line all the way up to the neckline. Repeat this movement slowly six times over the area. The energy needed to get on with the day can be restored in the thyroid.

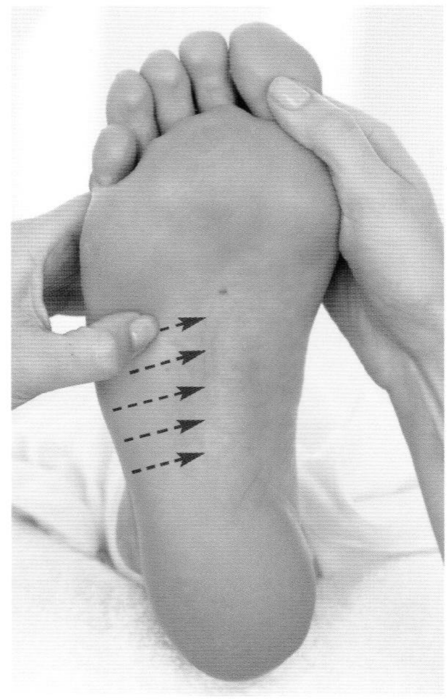

LIVER REFLEX AREA

This reflex area is only found on the right foot. Support the foot with your right hand, and place your left thumb just underneath the diaphragm line. Work slowly and precisely, horizontally across the foot, into zones five and four and just into zone three. Proceed in one direction. Continue in this manner until just above the redness of the heel. Complete the liver reflex movement six times.

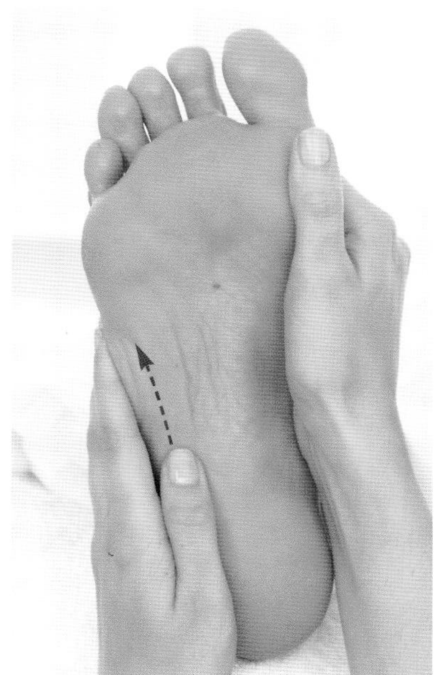

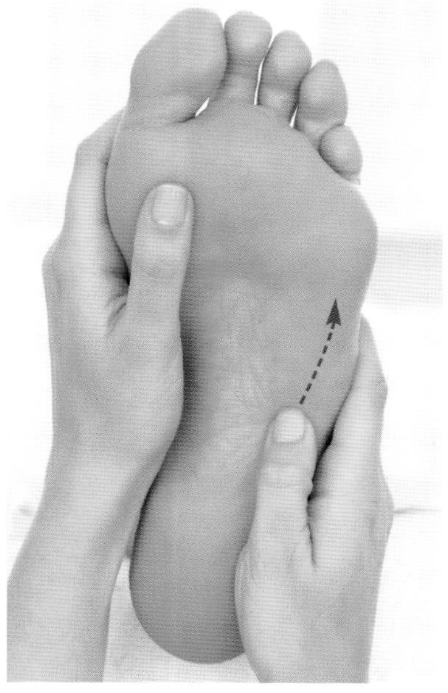

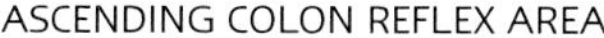

ASCENDING COLON REFLEX AREA

This reflex area is only found on the right foot. Use your left thumb to walk up zone four from the redness of the heel. Continue in this manner until you get halfway up the foot. Work the ascending colon reflex area four times in slow movements to help rid the colon of waste products.

DESCENDING COLON REFLEX AREA

This reflex area is only found on the left foot. Use your right thumb to walk up zone four from the redness of the heel to work this part of the colon. Continue in this manner until you arrive halfway up the foot. Work this reflex area six times and in slow movements to help stimulate the peristaltic muscular action of the colon.

Anxiety disorder

Anxiety can manifest itself as a panic attack and can affect all ages. It is usually abrupt, short and intense, and happens when the body's natural fight-or-flight responses activate at the wrong time. All the stress responses go into overdrive, which can be distressing and disturbing for the person having the attack. The sufferer is often overwhelmed by a sense of impending disaster, or may feel they are having a heart attack or stroke. Other symptoms include dizziness, heart palpitations, sweating, nausea, difficulty in breathing or thinking clearly, and a feeling of unreality. Avoid stress, sugar, processed foods, caffeinated products, excess alcohol and recreational drugs. Keep a nutritional diary, because an allergy to some foods can set off a panic attack. Use hand reflexology relaxation techniques during an attack.

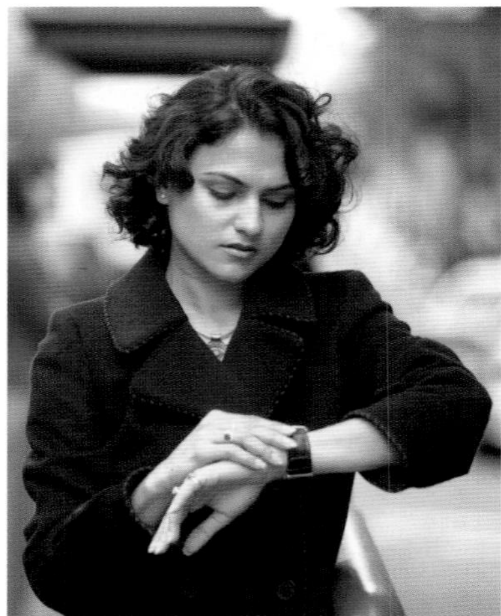

Panic attacks can affect the sufferer anywhere, at any time.

REFLEX AREAS/POINTS TO WORK

- Head
- Pituitary
- Diaphragm
- Lungs
- Kidneys/adrenals
- Thoracic vertebrae

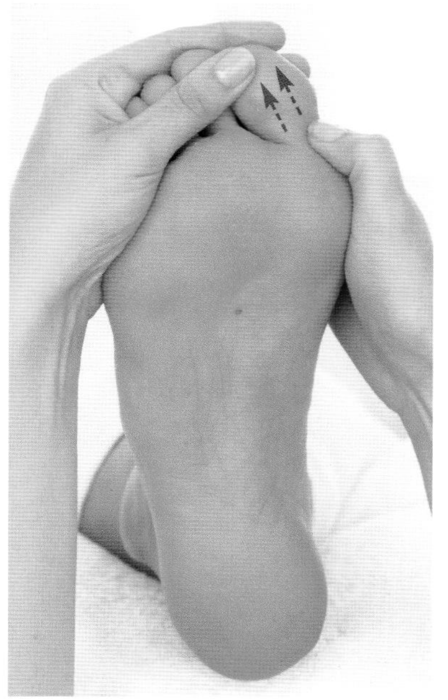

HEAD REFLEX AREA

Support the big toe with the fingers of one hand. Use your other thumb to walk up from the neckline to the top of the big toe. Repeat this several times in lines up the toe for a total of one minute.

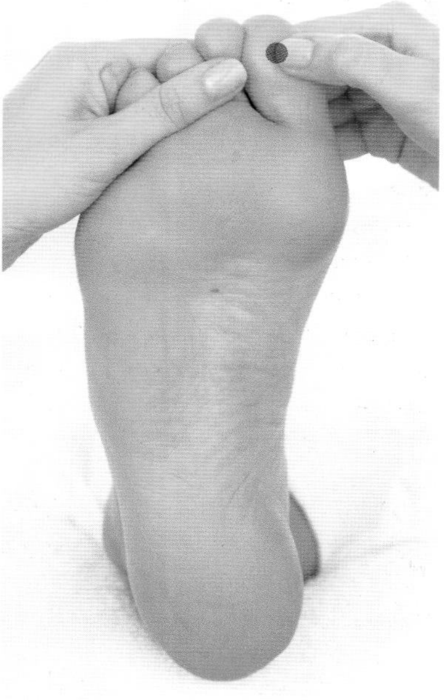

PITUITARY REFLEX POINT

Support the big toe with the fingers of one hand, and use your other thumb to make a cross to find the centre of the big toe. Place your thumb into the centre, push in and make circles for 15 seconds.

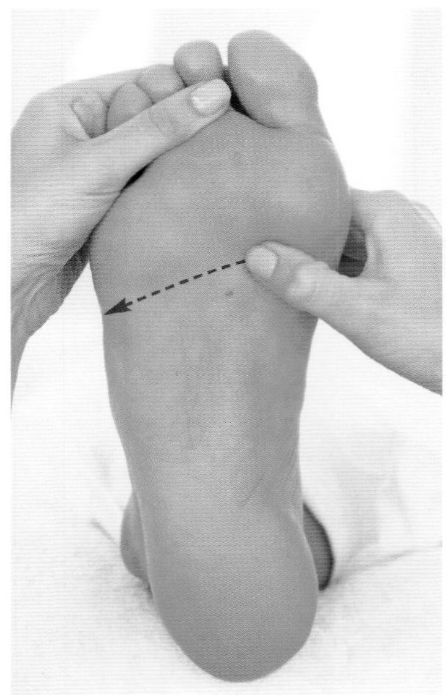

DIAPHRAGM REFLEX AREA

Flex the foot back with one hand to create skin tension. Use the thumb of your other hand to work under the metatarsal heads, across from the lateral to the medial aspect of the foot. Use slow steps and repeat this movement eight times.

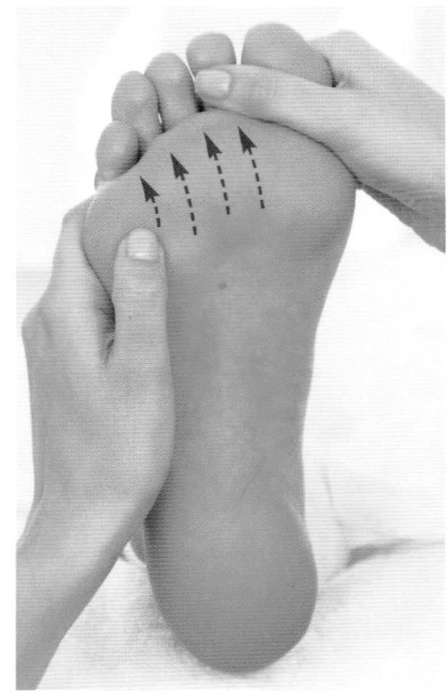

LUNG REFLEX AREA

Flex the foot back with your hand to create skin tension. Use the thumb of your other hand to work up from the diaphragm line to the eye/ear general area. You should be working in between the metatarsals. Repeat this process five times, making sure that you have worked in between all the metatarsals.

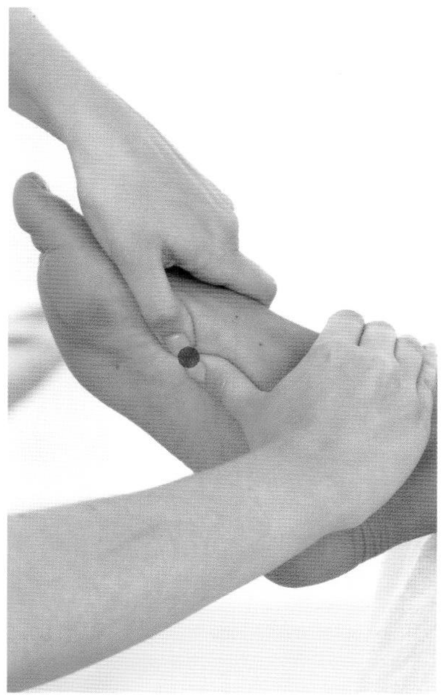

KIDNEY/ADRENAL REFLEX POINTS

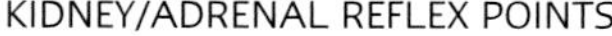

You can find these reflexes in zone one, three steps down from the ball of the foot. Place your two thumbs together and gently push into the kidney/adrenal reflexes, making small circles. Work in this manner for 20 seconds.

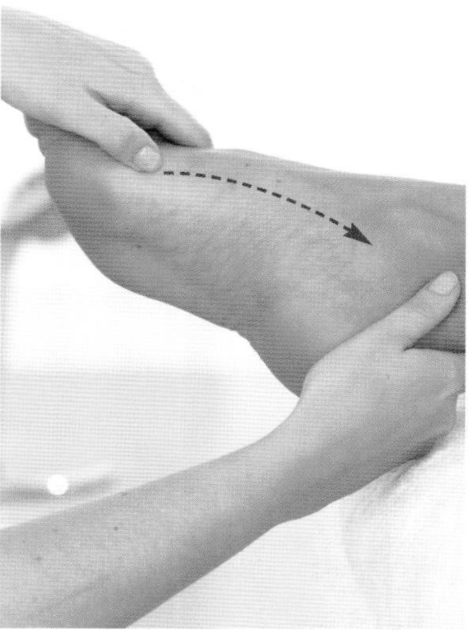

THORACIC VERTEBRAE REFLEX AREA

Support the foot and take 12 steps from the base of the joint of the big toe to work the thoracic vertebrae. You should end up on a bone called the navicular, which feels like a knuckle and is halfway between the bladder point and the ankle. Each step represents a specific vertebra and should be slow, with light to medium pressure. Repeat this movement three times to access spinal nerves.

REFLEXOLOGY FOR WOMEN

Women suffer from many conditions that are related to their hormones, and if this system is not functioning well, it can create a domino effect throughout the body. More women than men have digestive problems, because the digestive system

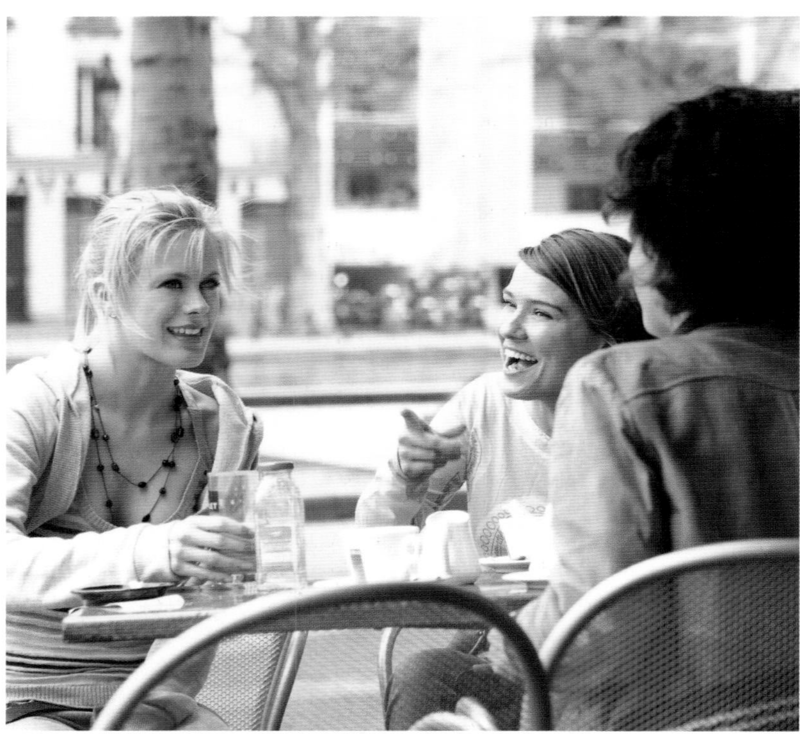

Reflexology can provide help for a number of ailments and symptoms that many women may suffer.

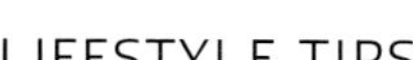

LIFESTYLE TIPS

Being overweight can alter menstrual cycles by causing excessive production of oestrogen, which interferes with the normal feedback system of the hormonal cycle. Fat manufactures and stores oestrogen, so if you suffer from a disorder that is affected by excess oestrogen (such as endometriosis or fibroids), it is best to lose weight to reduce oestrogen levels.

Regular eating is important for stabilizing blood-sugar levels, as low blood sugar affect levels of progesterone. Eating more wholewheat bread, oats, rye and brown rice every two hours can help stabilize blood-sugar levels, putting less strain on the hormones. When blood sugar crashes it can raise adrenaline levels, affecting mood and your response to stress.

slows down during menstruation as the level of the hormone progesterone relaxes the muscle tissues in the body. Premenstrual syndrome-related headaches (see page 270) are another common reason to visit the doctor.

Too much oestrogen in the body is associated with polycystic ovarian syndrome, fibroids (see page 278) and endometriosis (see page 274), so it is wise to avoid the steroids found in milk and meat and the synthetic oestrogen found in soft plastics. Hormones affect our moods and emotions and the way we react to other people. The key in reflexology for women is to focus on the body's hormonal and nervous systems.

Premenstrual syndrome (PMS)

Up to 70 per cent of all women suffer from some form of PMS. One reason for this is an imbalance of hormones: too much oestrogen and inadequate levels of progesterone. Premenstrual syndrome affects women between one and two weeks before menstruation, when hormone levels are changing. There are many symptoms, including muscle cramps, anxiety, mood swings, headaches, clumsiness, backache, acne, breast tenderness, depression, insomnia, constipation and water retention. Eat plenty of fresh fruit and vegetables, organic grains, nuts, fish, organic chicken and turkey, to help keep your liver free of excess toxins. Eliminate salt from the diet to reduce water retention. Avoid caffeine, because it depletes nutrients from the body, is associated with increased levels of anxiety and is linked to breast tenderness. Drinking chamomile tea will help to increase levels of glycine in the body; this amino acid is known to relieve muscle spasms (including menstrual cramps) by relaxing the uterus.

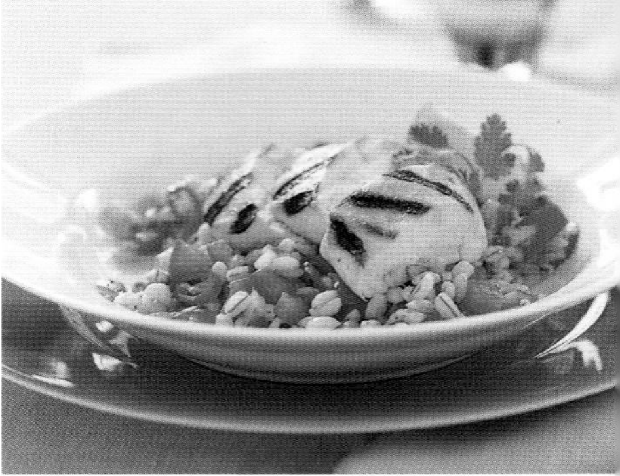

Plenty of fresh organic vegetables and fish can help to balance hormone levels and prevent PMS.

REFLEX AREAS/POINTS TO WORK

- Pituitary
- Thyroid
- Pancreas
- Adrenals
- Ovaries
- Entire spine

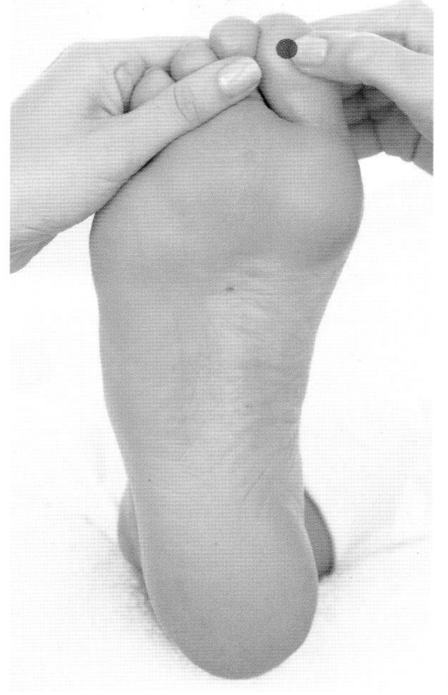

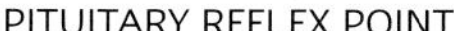

PITUITARY REFLEX POINT

Support the big toe with the fingers of one hand, and use your other thumb to make a cross to find the centre of the big toe. Place your thumb into the centre, push in and make circles for 15 seconds.

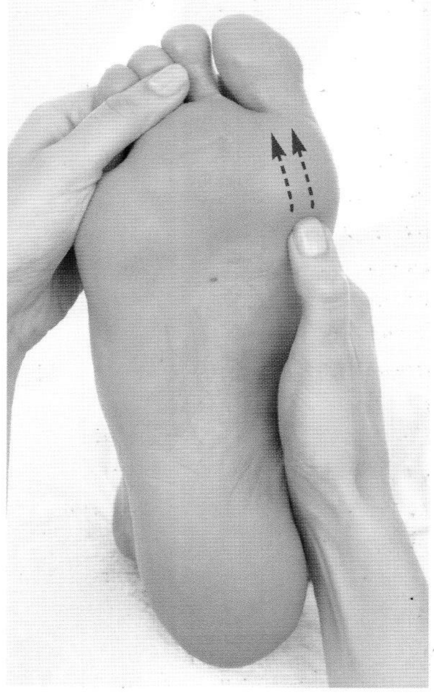

THYROID REFLEX AREA

Use the thumb of one hand to work the ball of the foot, from the diaphragm line all the way up to the neckline. Repeat this movement slowly six times over the area.

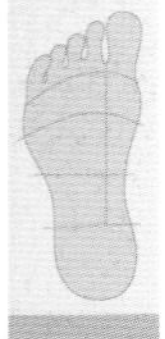

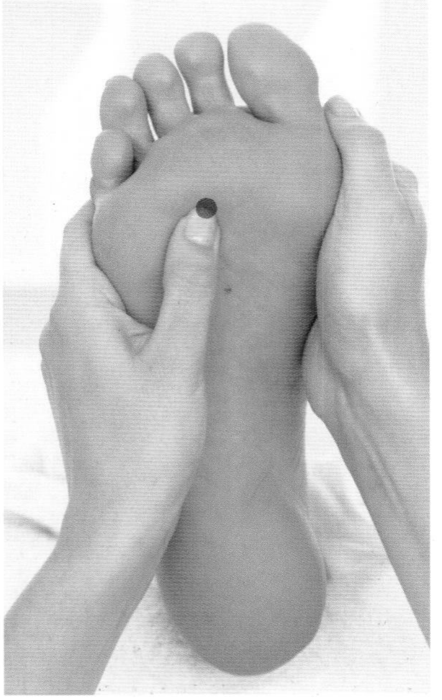

PANCREAS REFLEX POINT

This reflex point is only found on the right foot. Use your thumb and place it on the third toe, tracing a line down to below the diaphragm line. Push up into the joint, making small circles for 12 seconds.

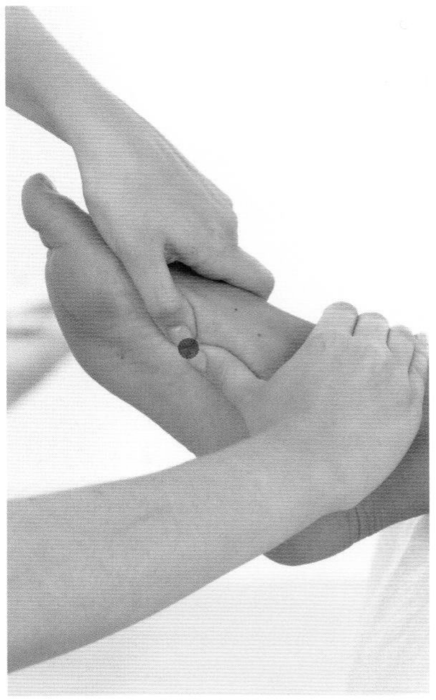

ADRENAL REFLEX POINT

You can find the adrenal reflexes in zone one, three steps down from the ball of the foot. Place your two thumbs together and gently push into the adrenal reflexes, making small circles. Work in this manner for 15 seconds.

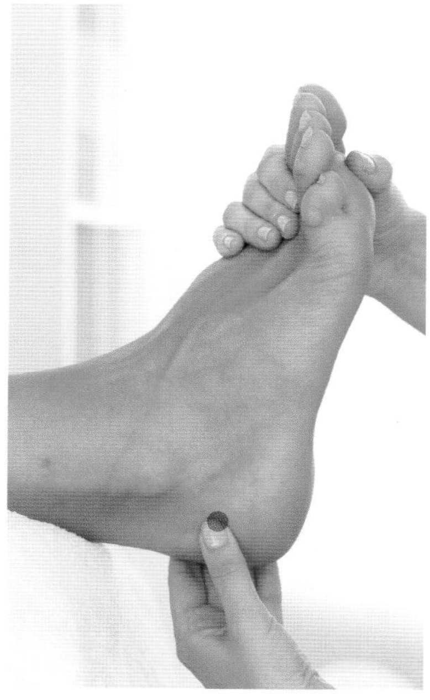

OVARY REFLEX POINT

Work on the lateral aspect of foot. Place your index finger approximately halfway between the back of the heel and the ankle bone. Push in gently, making circles for 20 seconds.

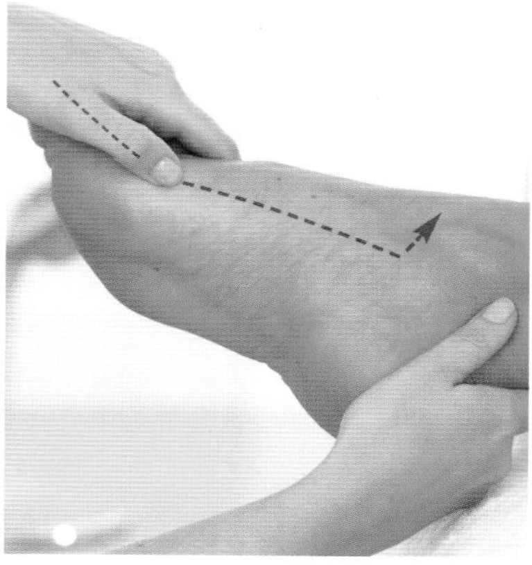

ENTIRE SPINE

Work on the medial aspect of the foot. Support the foot with one hand, and use your other thumb to walk gently seven steps in between the joints of the big toe, remembering that each step represents a specific vertebra. Walk towards the foot. Then take 12 gentle steps underneath the bone from the base of the joint of the big toe to work the thoracic vertebrae. You should end up on a bone called the navicular, which feels like a knuckle and is halfway between the bladder point and the ankle. Walk around the navicular bone, which represents lumbar one, taking five steps up to the dip in front of the ankle bone, which represents lumbar five. Repeat this movement gently five times.

Endometriosis

This is a disorder that affects women aged 20–40; no one knows what causes it. Cells from the lining of the uterus grow elsewhere in the body – most commonly in the abdominal cavity. These implants still respond to hormonal changes controlling menstruation, which means that they bleed each month, causing adhesions. Common symptoms include excessive pain, abnormal/heavy menstrual bleeding, lower back pain, nausea, diarrhoea and constipation and, in some cases, rectal bleeding. Using tampons can encourage 'reflux menstruation', which may make endometriosis worse.

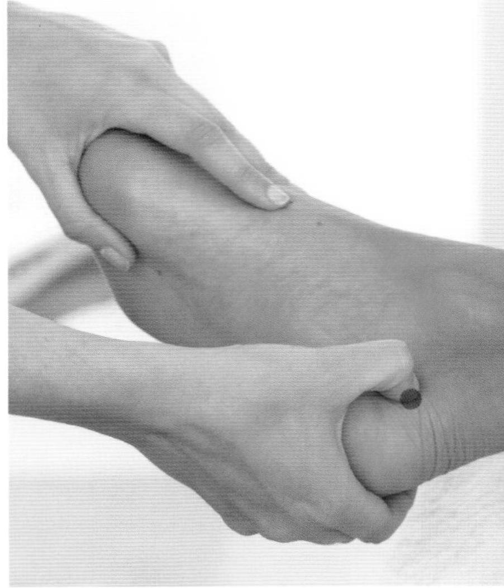

UTERUS REFLEX POINT

Work on the medial aspect of foot. Place your index finger approximately halfway between the back of the heel and the ankle bone. Push in gently, making circles for 20 seconds.

REFLEX AREAS/POINTS TO WORK

- Uterus
- Ovaries
- Ascending colon
- Descending colon
- Pituitary
- Adrenals
- Thoracic and lumbar vertebrae

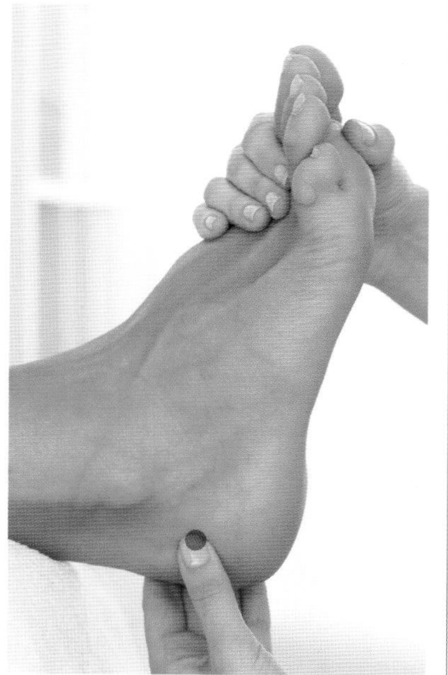

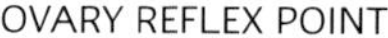

OVARY REFLEX POINT

Work on the lateral aspect of foot. Place your index finger approximately halfway between the back of the heel and the ankle bone.. Push in gently, making circles for 20 seconds.

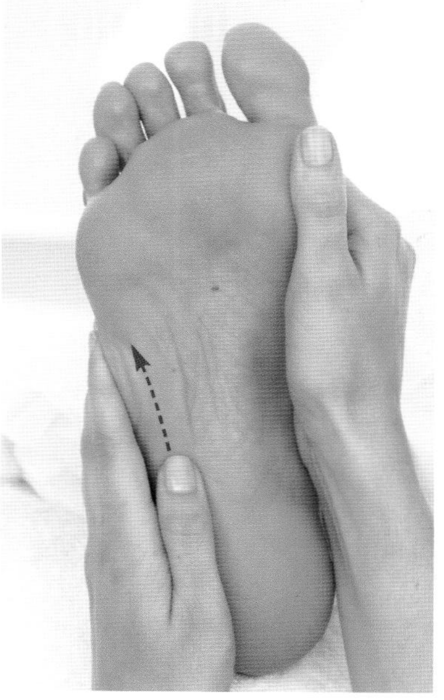

ASCENDING COLON REFLEX AREA

This reflex area is only found on the right foot. Use your left thumb to walk up zone four from the redness of the heel. Continue in this manner until you get halfway up the foot. Work the ascending colon reflex area four times in slow movements to help the colon eliminate excess hormones that could play havoc withn the body.

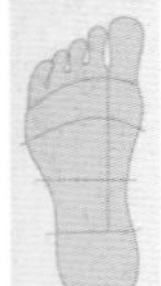

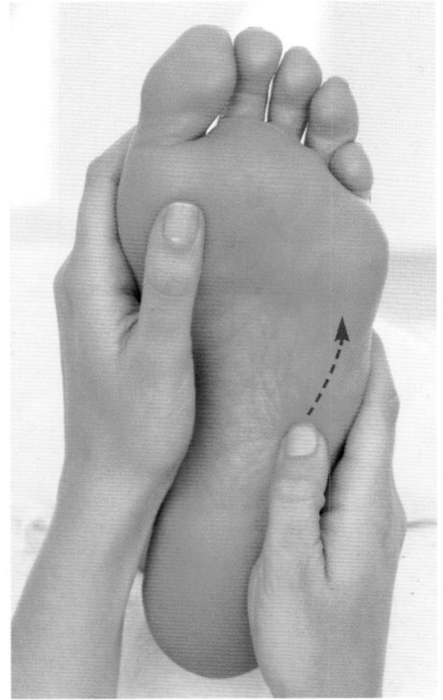

DESCENDING COLON REFLEX AREA

This reflex area is only found on the left foot. Use your right thumb to walk up zone four from the redness of the heel, to work this part of the colon. Continue in this manner until you arrive halfway up the foot. Work this reflex area six times and in slow movements to help stimulate the peristaltic muscular action of the colon.

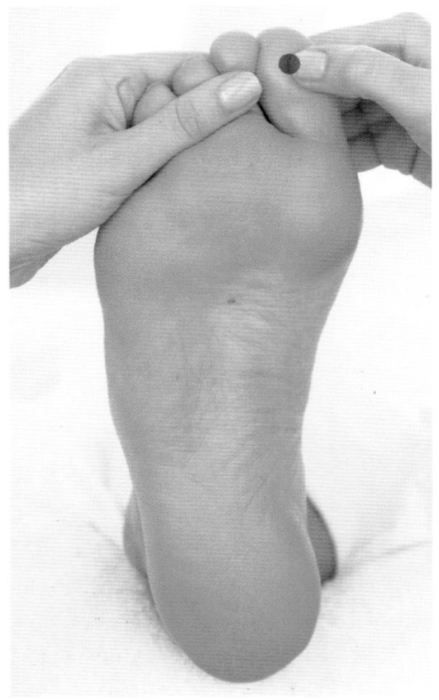

PITUITARY REFLEX POINT

Support the big toe with the fingers of one hand, and use your other thumb to make a cross to find the centre of the big toe. Place your thumb into the centre, push in and make circles for 15 seconds to help balance hormone levels.

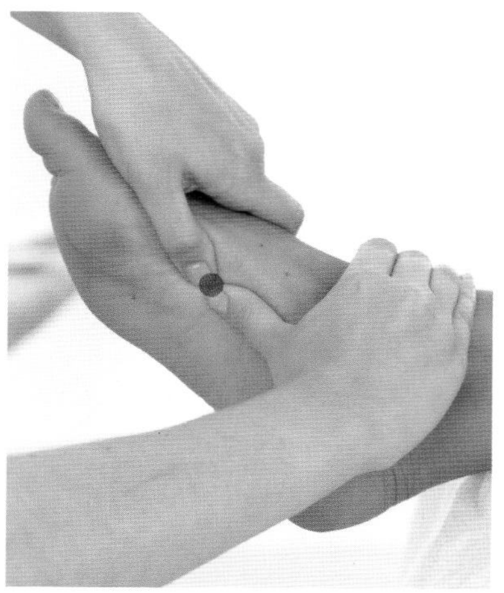

ADRENAL REFLEX POINT

You can find the adrenal reflexes in zone one, three steps down from the ball of the foot. Place your two thumbs together and gently push into the adrenal reflexes, making small circles. Work in this manner for 15 seconds to help ease pain.

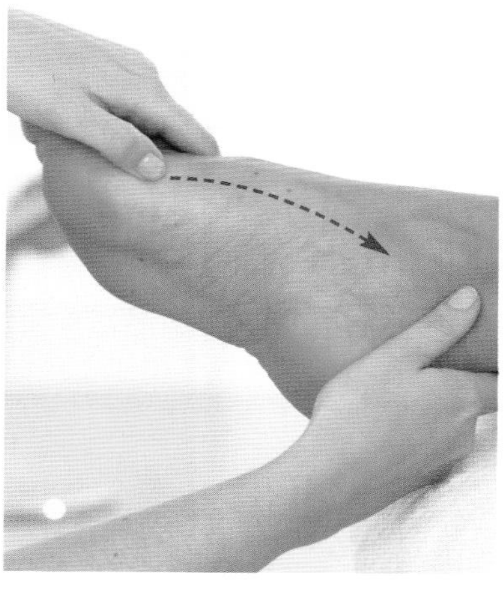

THORACIC AND LUMBAR VERTEBRAE REFLEX AREA

This lies on the medial aspect of the foot. Support the foot with one hand. Use your other thumb to take 12 gentle steps underneath the bone from the base of the joint of the big toe to work the thoracic vertebrae. You should end up on a bone called the navicular, which feels like a knuckle and is halfway between the the bladder point and the ankle. Walk around the navicular bone, which represents lumbar one, taking five steps up to the dip in front of the ankle bone, which represents lumbar five. Repeat this movement four times.

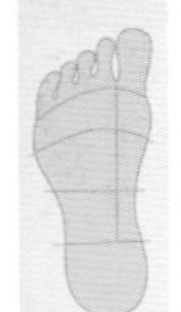

Fibroids

Uterine fibroids are non-cancerous tumours of the uterus. They are made up of bundles of abnormal muscle cells that can form on both the interior wall and the exterior wall of the uterus. They tend to affect women in their late thirties and usually shrink after the menopause. A lot of women who develop fibroids are not aware of them until a pelvic examination occurs. If fibroids grow to a large size, they can affect the periods, making them heavy, frequent or painful. Other symptoms include anaemia (because of a significant loss of blood), bleeding between periods, increased vaginal discharge and painful sexual intercourse. The use of the oral contraceptive pill has been associated with the development of fibroids.

REFLEX AREAS/POINTS TO WORK

- Sacrum
- Bladder
- Lumbar vertebrae
- Uterus
- Pituitary
- Adrenals

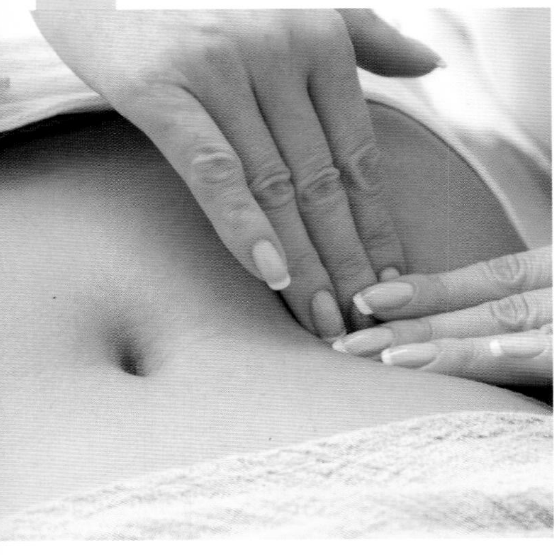

Always have digestive problems diagnosed because they could mask gynaecological disorders such as fibroids.

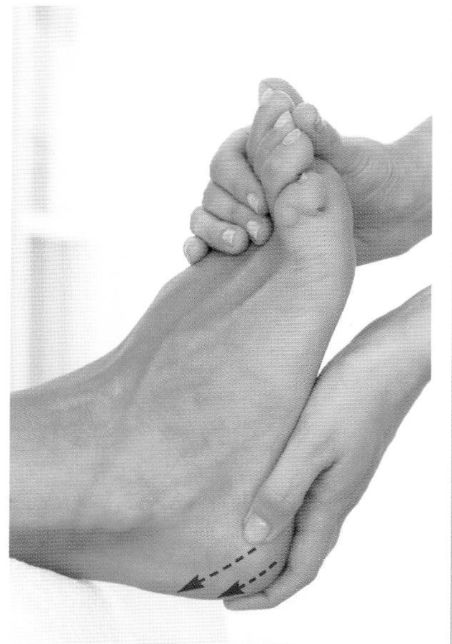

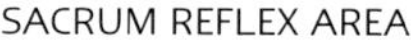

SACRUM REFLEX AREA

Work on the lateral aspect of the foot. Place your thumb at the back quadrant of the heel and walk with slow, precise movements for 25 seconds. Repeat this until you have covered this section of the heel, always keeping low to avoid going over the ovary or testicle reflex point.

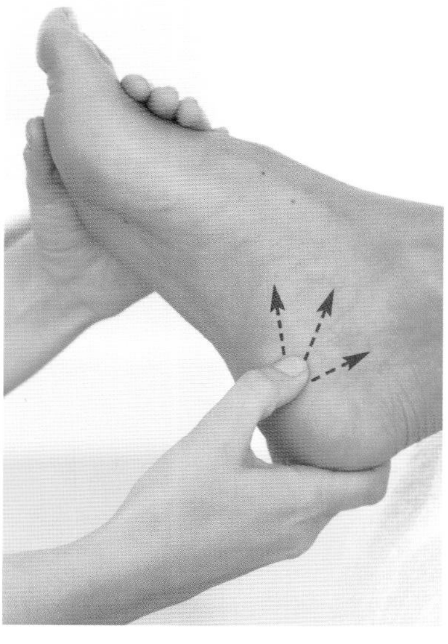

BLADDER REFLEX AREA

Work on the medial aspect of the foot. Place your thumb at the bladder point, which is at the edge of the soft area about one-third of the way from the back of the heel. Use your thumb to fan out over the area, like the spokes of a bicycle wheel, always returning to the bladder point. Work on this area ten times.

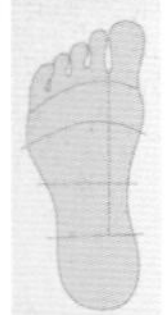

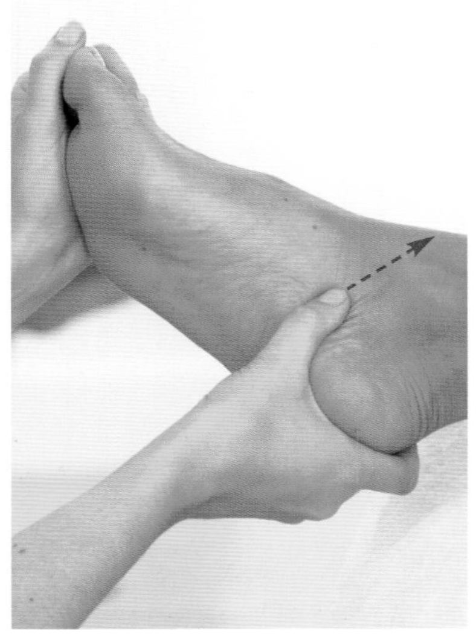

LUMBAR VERTEBRAE REFLEX AREA

This area lies on the medial aspect of the foot. Support the foot with one hand. Place your thumb on a bone called the navicular, which feels like a knuckle and is halfway between the bladder point and the ankle. Walk around the navicular bone, which represents lumbar one, taking five steps up to the dip in front of the ankle bone, which represents lumbar five. Repeat this movement four times.

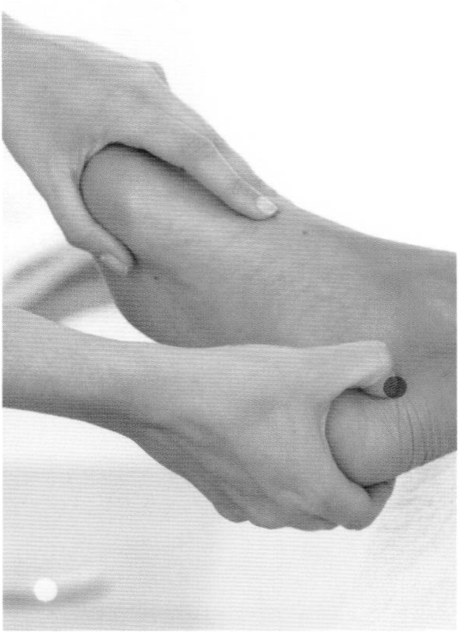

UTERUS REFLEX POINT

Working on the medial aspect of foot, place your index finger approximately halfway between the back of the heel and the ankle bone. Push in gently, making circles for 15 seconds.

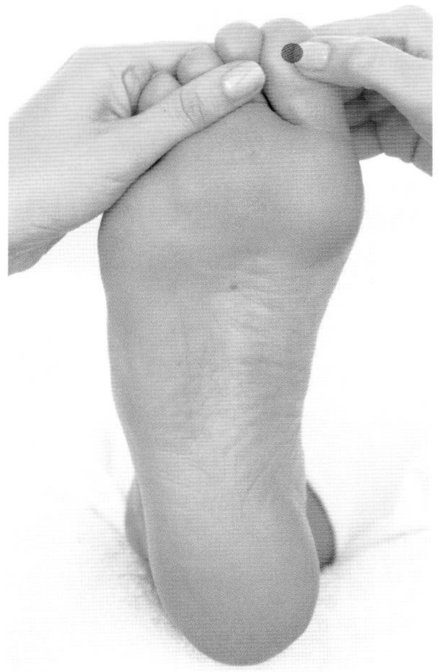

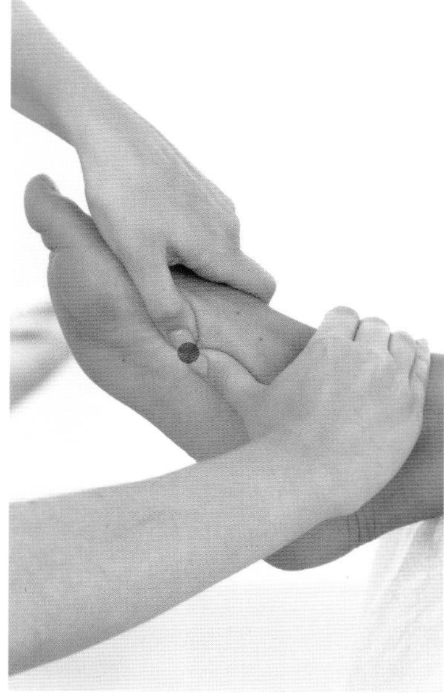

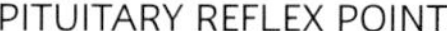

PITUITARY REFLEX POINT

Support the big toe with the fingers of one hand, and use your other thumb to make a cross to find the centre of the big toe. Place your thumb into the centre, push in and make circles for 15 seconds.

ADRENAL REFLEX POINT

You can find the adrenal reflexes in zone one, three steps down from the ball of the foot. Place your two thumbs together and gently push into the adrenal reflexes, making small circles. Work in this manner for 15 seconds.

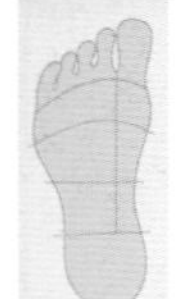

Menopause

This indicates the end of a woman's fertility and occurs when a woman stops ovulating and menstruating each month. It normally happens around the age of 50, but some women have been diagnosed with an early menopause in their twenties. Oestrogen production falls dramatically after the menopause, and oestrogen is needed for normal cell functioning in the skin, arteries, heart, bladder and liver, and for proper bone formation. Women become more at risk of suffering osteoporosis and cardiovascular disease at this time. To help optimize your health, get regular exercise and reduce your intake of dairy products and red meat, as these encourage hot flushes and calcium loss from the bones.

REFLEX AREAS/POINTS TO WORK

- Hypothalamus/pituitary
- Thyroid
- Parathyroids
- Liver
- Kidneys/adrenals
- Entire spine

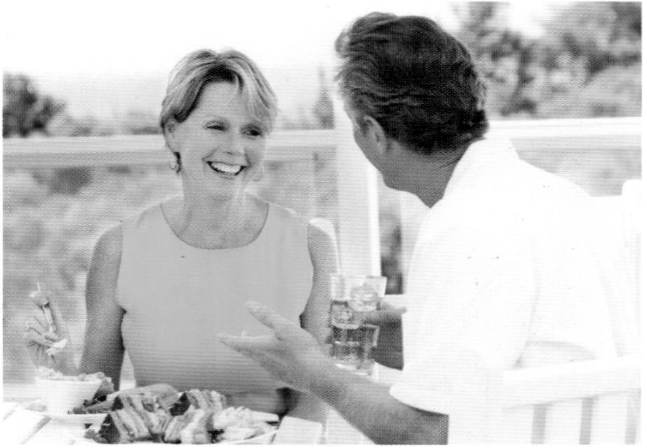

A healthy diet and exercise helps to ease menopausal symptoms.

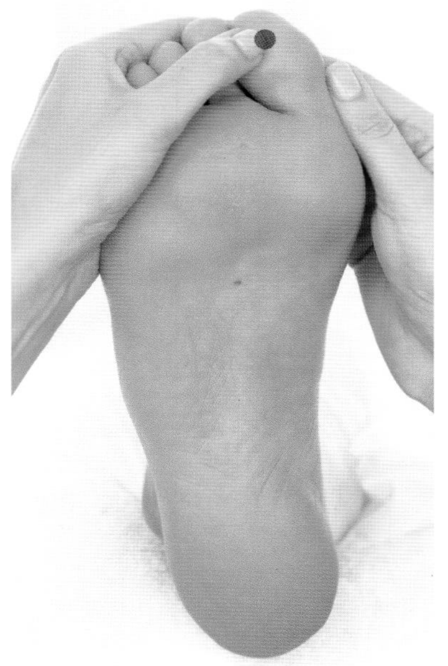

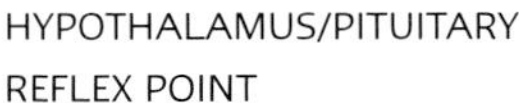

HYPOTHALAMUS/PITUITARY REFLEX POINT

Support the big toe with the fingers of one hand and find the centre of the big toe. Place one thumb on the centre of the big toe for the pituitary gland. Place your other thumb one step up from the pituitary and one small step laterally. Place both thumbs together and make circles for 30 seconds.

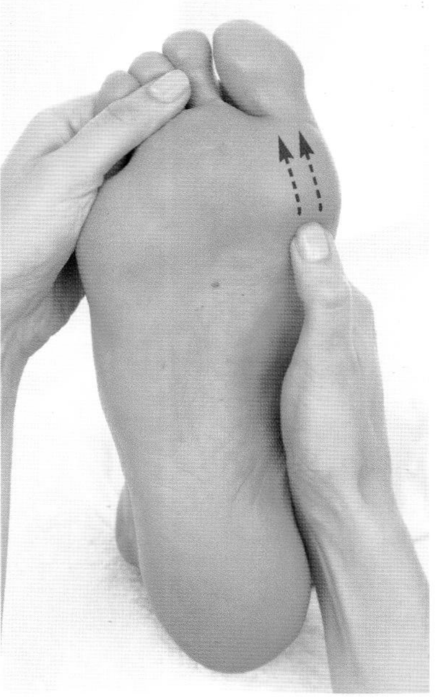

THYROID REFLEX AREA

Use the thumb of one hand to work the ball of the foot, from the diaphragm line all the way up to the neckline. Repeat this movement slowly six times over the area. The thyroid produces calcitonin, a hormone that helps support healthy bones.

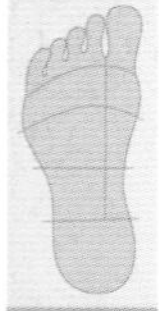

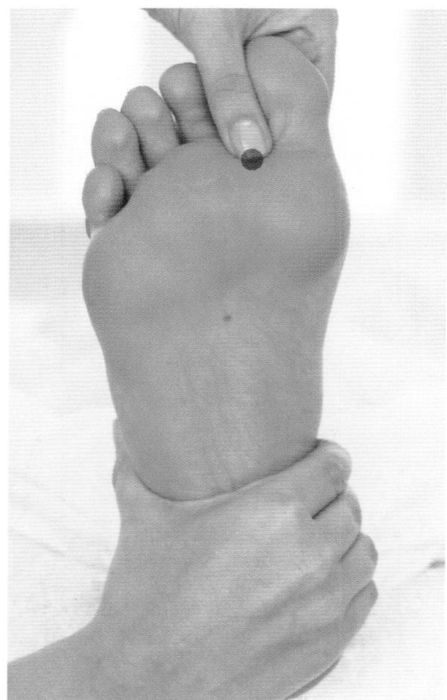

PARATHYROID REFLEX POINT

You can find this point in between the big toe and the second toe. Use your index finger and thumb to pinch a section of skin between the first and second toes. Hold the pressure and gently make circles for 15 seconds.

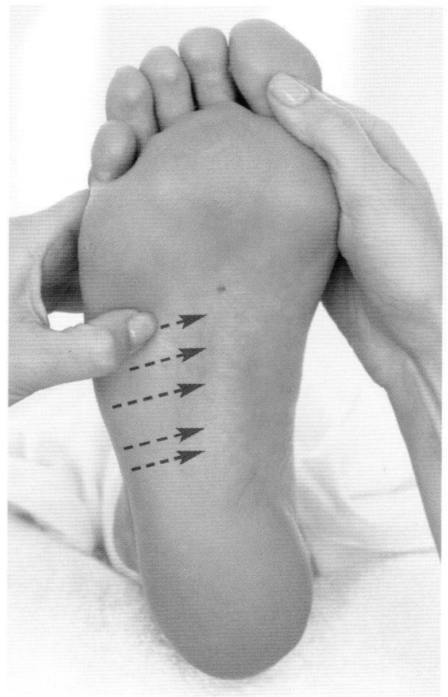

LIVER REFLEX AREA

The liver reflex area is only found on the right foot. Support the foot with your right hand, and place your left thumb just underneath the diaphragm line. Work slowly and precisely, horizontally across the foot, into zones five and four and just into zone three. Proceed in one direction. Continue in this manner until just above the redness of the heel, completing the liver reflex six times.

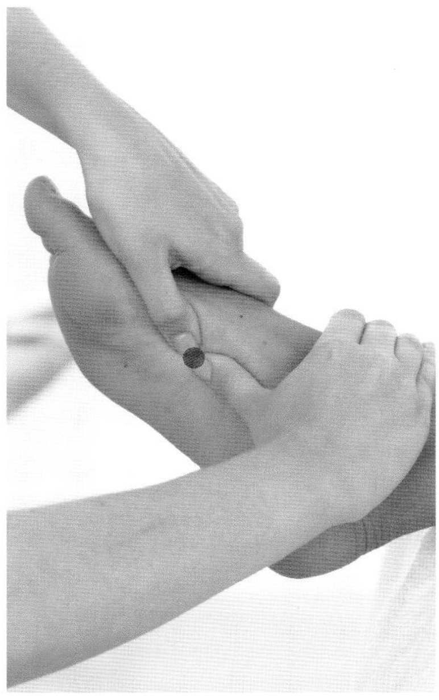

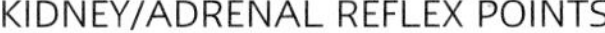

KIDNEY/ADRENAL REFLEX POINTS

You can find these reflexes in zone one, three steps down from the ball of the foot. Place your two thumbs together and gently push into the kidney/adrenal reflexes, making small circles. Work in this manner for 15 seconds.

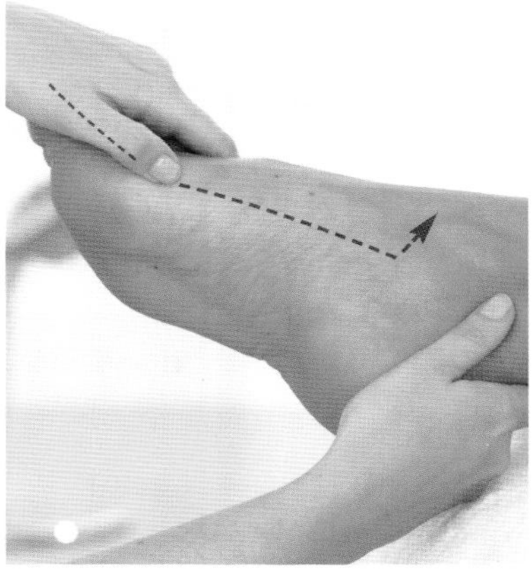

ENTIRE SPINE

Work on the medial aspect of the foot. Support the foot with one hand, and use your other thumb to walk gently seven steps in between the joints of the big toe, remembering that each step represents a specific vertebra. Walk towards the foot. Then take 12 gentle steps underneath the bone from the base of the joint of the big toe to work the thoracic vertebrae. You should end up on a bone called the navicular, which feels like a knuckle and is halfway between the bladder point and the ankle. Walk around the navicular bone, which represents lumbar one, taking five steps up to the dip in front of the ankle bone, which represents lumbar five. Repeat this movement gently three times.

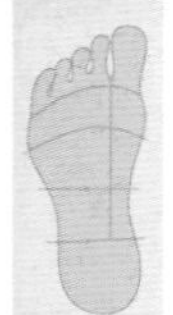

REFLEXOLOGY FOR MEN

Some scientists have observed that cells from male and female organisms differ in ways that result not from hormones, but from foundation stones such as chromosomes. This means that all the organs and parts of the body have the potential to respond differently between the sexes. Reflexology for men should not focus solely on male diseases such as those affecting the reproductive organs – impotence (see page 288), enlarged prostate (see page 292), prostatitis (see page 296) and infertility (see page 300) – but also on the way that many diseases express themselves differently in men.

The China Reflexology Association found that reflexology is an excellent therapy for treating men with sexual dysfunction, including impotence, premature ejaculation and ejaculation deficiencies. Its 1996 *China Reflexology Symposium Report* described a study on 37 men who were treated with reflexology; it was 87.5 per cent effective for impotence and 100 per cent effective for other conditions.

LIFESTYLE TIPS

Impotence is a common disorder that can be made worse by the stress surrounding the condition, as well as by the effects of lifestyle choices. As our bodies age, the sex organs can take longer to respond, so consider changing the way you make love. As sexual functions alter, you may need a longer period of stimulation to achieve an erection. Arteriosclerosis is a disease that affects the nerves that govern sexual arousal and the blood supply to the penis; eating a diet low in fats can help to reverse this clogging of the blood vessels. If you are concerned, there are many therapy options that can be discussed with your doctor.

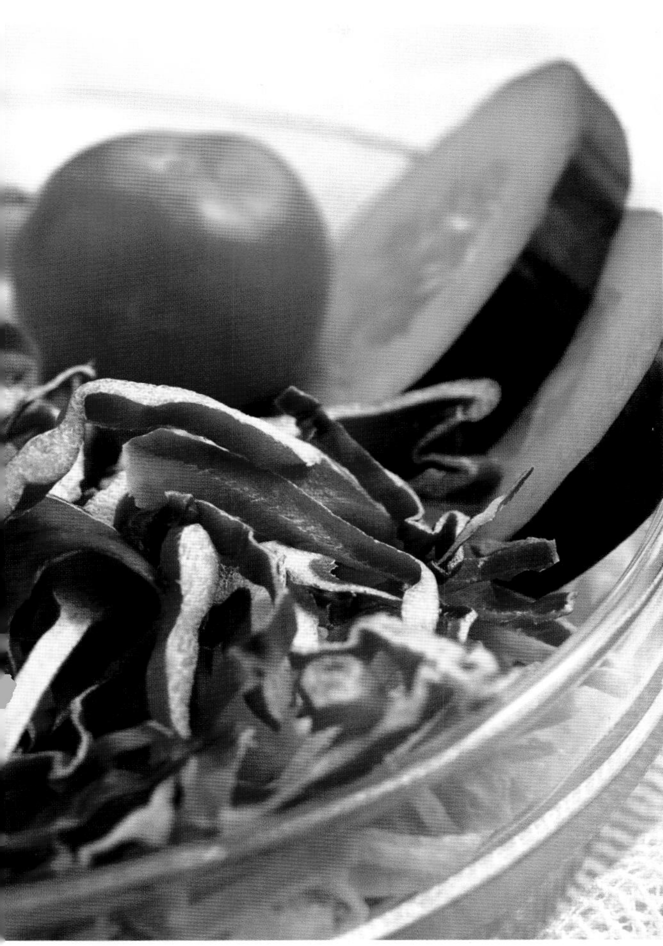

A low-fat diet rich in raw fruit and vegetables can benefit male sexual performance and fertility.

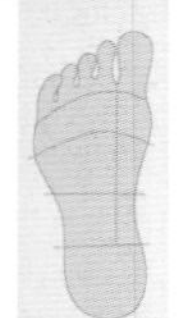

Impotence

Impotence is characterized by an inability to achieve or maintain an erection adequate for sexual intercourse. Around 2.3 million men in the UK and 30 million men in the US suffer from erection problems, and around one in three men over 60 is affected by a degree of impotence. Erections result from a combination of brain stimuli, blood vessel and hormonal actions and nerve function. Some diseases and factors that can contribute to impotence include atherosclerosis (hardening of the arteries), high blood pressure, diabetes, alcohol, cigarettes and a history of sexually transmitted disease. Impotence may also be a side-effect of certain medications, such as antidepressants, antihistamines and ulcer medication. It can also sometimes have psychological roots. Avoid stress, cigarette smoke, animal fats, sugar, fried and junk food; stay away from alcohol, because it not only affects sexual function, but may cause the male equivalent of the menopause. Reflexology can help improve impotence.

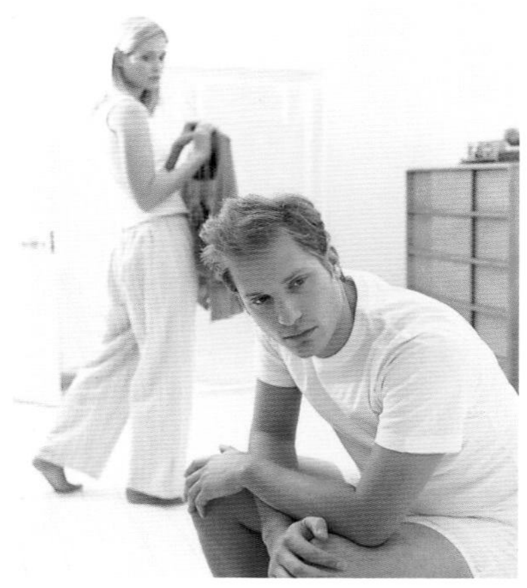

Always look into the side-effects of any medication you are taking as some can cause impotence.

REFLEX AREAS/POINTS TO WORK

- Prostate
- Testes
- Thoracic and lumbar vertebrae
- Adrenals
- Diaphragm
- Lungs

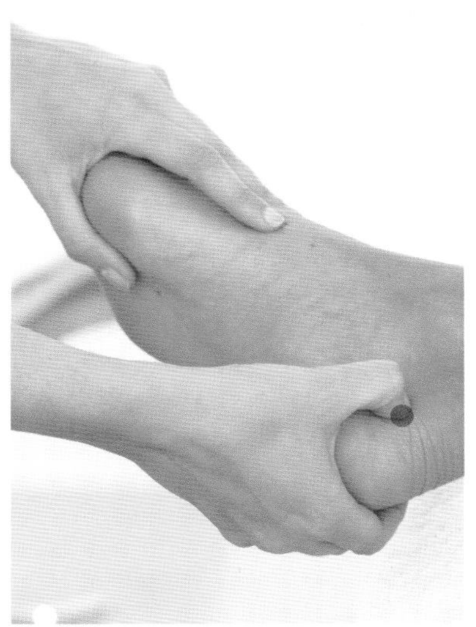

PROSTATE REFLEX POINT

Work on the medial aspect of foot. Place your index finger approximately halfway between the back of the heel and the ankle bone. Push in gently, making circles for 20 seconds.

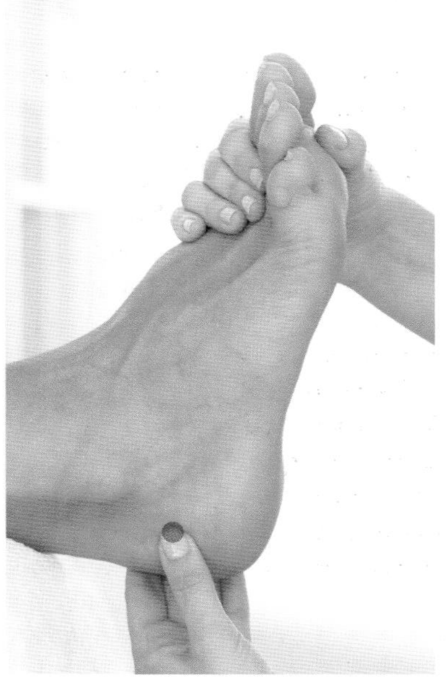

TESTES REFLEX POINT

Work on the lateral aspect of foot. Place your index finger approximately halfway between the back of the heel and the ankle bone. Push in gently, making circles for ten seconds.

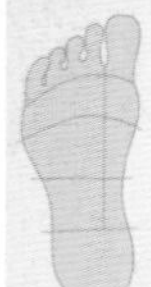

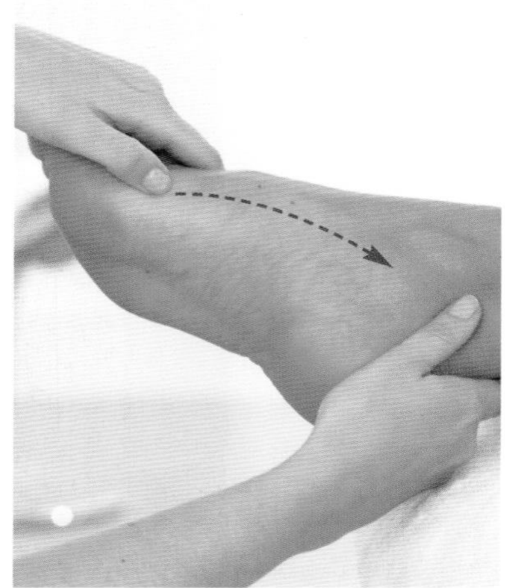

THORACIC AND LUMBAR VERTEBRAE REFLEX AREA

Work on the medial aspect of the foot. Support the foot with one hand. Use your other thumb to take 12 gentle steps underneath the bone from the base of the joint of the big toe to work the thoracic vertebrae. You should end up on a bone called the navicular, which feels like a knuckle and is halfway between the bladder point and the ankle. Walk around the navicular bone, which represents lumbar one, taking five steps up to the dip in front of the ankle bone, which represents lumbar five. Repeat this movement four times.

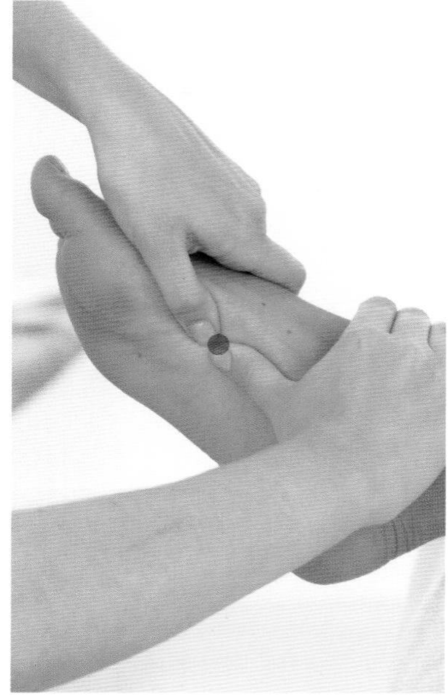

ADRENAL REFLEX POINT

You can find the adrenal reflexes in zone one, three steps down from the ball of the foot. Place your two thumbs together and gently push into the adrenal reflexes, making small circles. Work in this manner for 15 seconds.

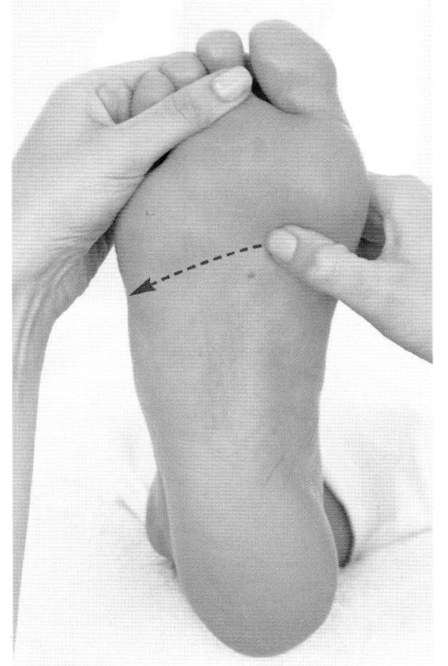

DIAPHRAGM REFLEX AREA

Support the foot with one hand, and use the thumb of your other hand to work under the metatarsal heads, across from the medial to the lateral aspect of the foot. Use slow steps and repeat this movement eight times.

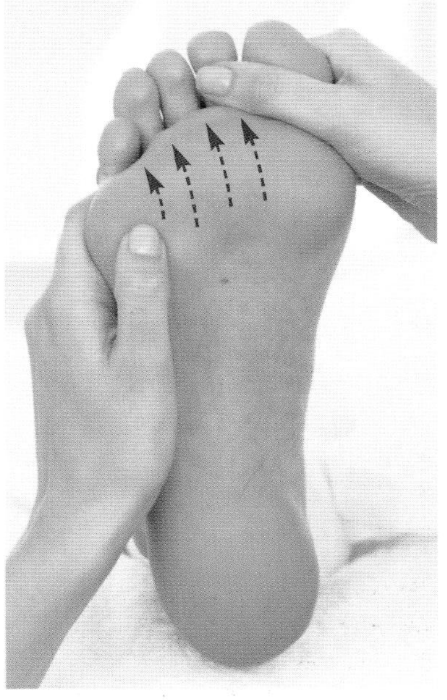

LUNG REFLEX AREA

Flex the foot back with your hand to create skin tension. Use the thumb of your other hand to work up from the diaphragm line to the eye/ear general area. You should be working in between the metatarsals. Repeat this process five times, making sure you have worked in between all the metatarsals, dispersing any crystals.

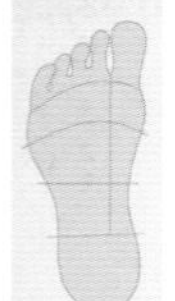

Enlarged prostate

This condition, which is also called benign prostatic hypertrophy, is the gradual enlargement of the prostate gland. It may be due to hormonal changes as the result of ageing, as a man's testosterone levels gradually decline. It affects more than half of all men over 50, and 75 per cent of men over the age of 70. The condition is non-cancerous, but can cause unpleasant symptoms, including difficulty in urinating, getting up frequently at night to urinate, blood in the urine, pain and burning, difficulty in starting and stopping urination, bladder infections and damage to the kidneys. Lifestyle choices to reduce blood cholesterol levels are recommended, because research has shown a connection between prostate disorders and high cholesterol, so plenty of the following foods should be included in the diet: carrots, bananas, apples, cold-water fish, garlic, tomatoes and olive oil. Regular reflexology treatments will also help to reduce stress and sustained tension, which contribute to high blood cholesterol levels.

REFLEX AREAS/POINTS TO WORK

- Pituitary
- Prostate
- Bladder
- Liver
- Kidneys/adrenals
- Thoracic and lumbar vertebrae

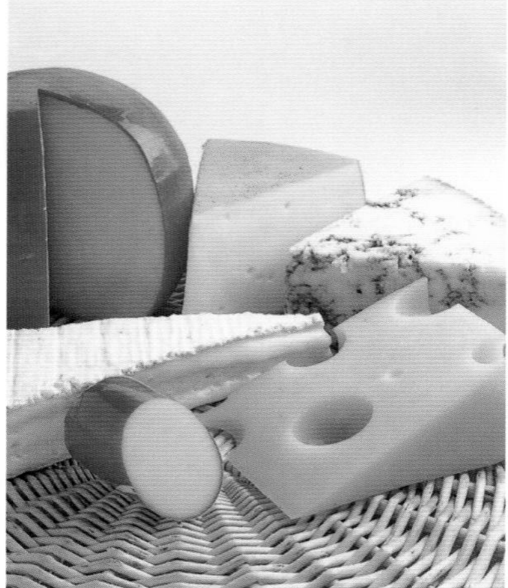

High-cholesterol foods such as cheese should be avoided since high cholesterol may be linked to prostate disorders.

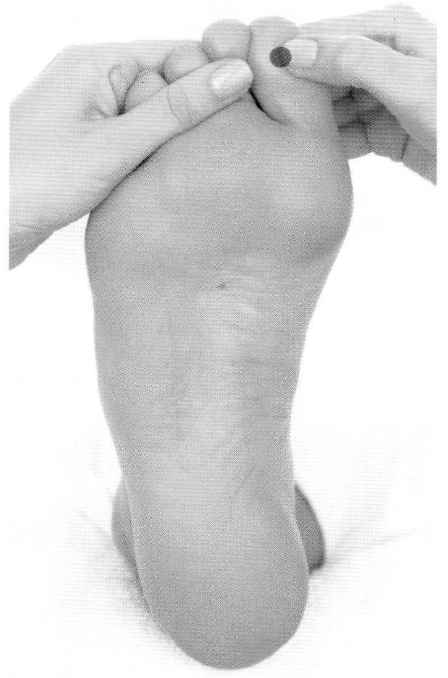

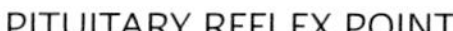

PITUITARY REFLEX POINT

Support the big toe with the fingers of one hand, and use your other thumb to make a cross to find the centre of the big toe. Place your thumb into the centre, push in and make circles for 15 seconds.

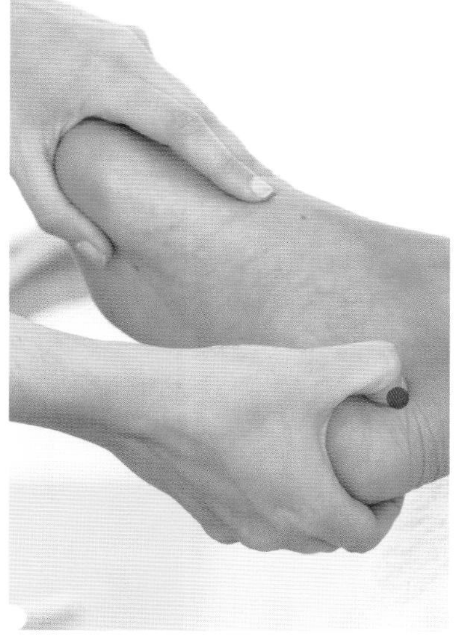

PROSTATE REFLEX POINT

Work on the medial aspect of foot. Place your index finger approximately halfway between the back of the heel and the ankle bone. Push in gently, making circles for 20 seconds.

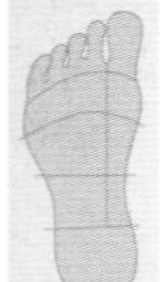

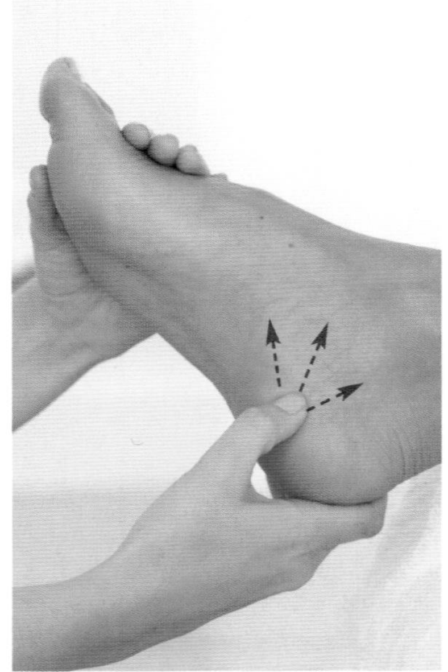

BLADDER REFLEX AREA

Work on the medial aspect of the foot, placing your thumb at the bladder point, which is at the edge of the soft area about one-third of the way from the back of the heel. Use your thumb to fan out over the area, like the spokes of a bicycle wheel, always returning to the bladder point. Work on this area ten times.

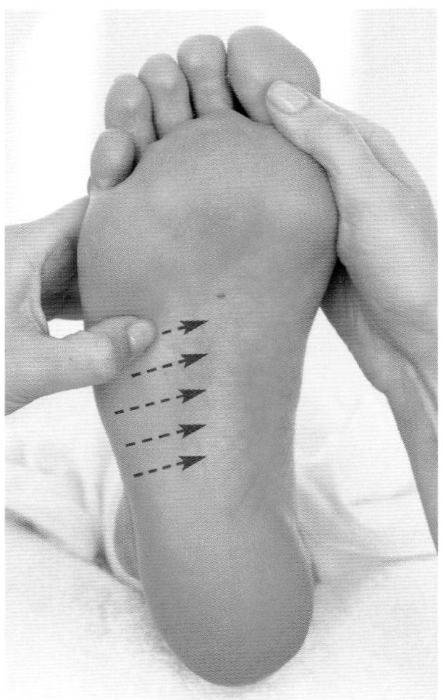

LIVER REFLEX AREA

This reflex area is only found on the right foot. Support the foot with your right hand, and place your left thumb just underneath the diaphragm line. Work slowly and precisely, horizontally across the foot, into zones five and four and just into zone three. Proceed in one direction. Continue in this manner until just above the redness of the heel. Complete the liver reflex movement six times.

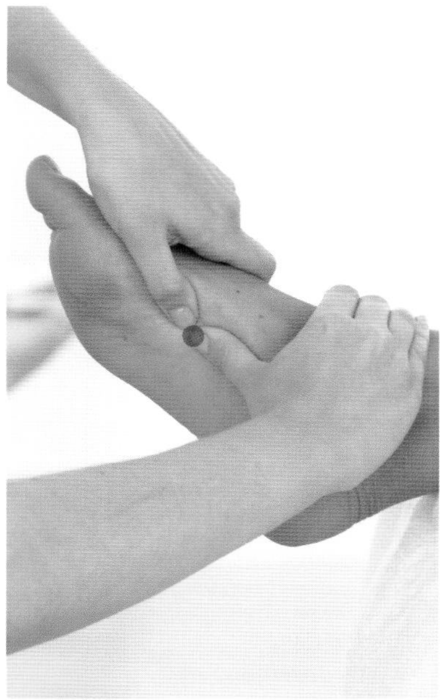

KIDNEY/ADRENAL REFLEX POINTS

You can find these reflexes in zone one, three steps down from the ball of the foot. Place your two thumbs together and gently push into the kidney/adrenal reflexes, making small circles. Work in this manner for 15 seconds.

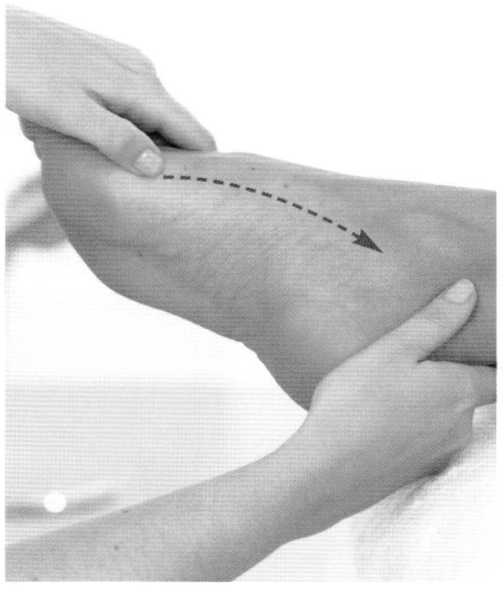

THORACIC AND LUMBAR VERTEBRAE REFLEX AREA

This lies on the medial aspect of the foot. Support the foot with one hand. Use your other thumb to take 12 gentle steps underneath the bone from the base of the joint of the big toe to work the thoracic vertebrae. You should end up on a bone called the navicular, which feels like a knuckle and is halfway between the bladder point and the ankle. Walk around the navicular bone, which represents lumbar one, taking five steps up to the dip in front of the ankle bone, which represents lumbar five. Repeat this movement four times.

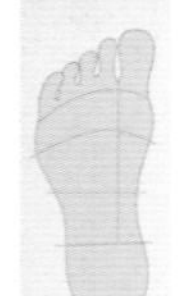

Prostatitis

Prostatitis is inflammation of the prostate gland and is common in men of all ages. The usual causes are bacteria that invade the prostate, or hormonal changes that occur with age. The prostate is a male sex gland and its function is to squeeze fluid during ejaculation (prostate fluid makes up the bulk of semen). The main symptoms of prostatitis include urine retention (which can affect the bladder and kidneys), pain between the scrotum and rectum, fever, a burning sensation when urinating and a feeling of fullness in the bladder. Increase your intake of zinc, because zinc helps with all prostate problems.

REFLEX AREAS/POINTS TO WORK

- Lymphatics
- Pituitary
- Prostate
- Thoracic and lumbar vertebrae
- Bladder
- Ureter tube
- Kidneys/adrenals

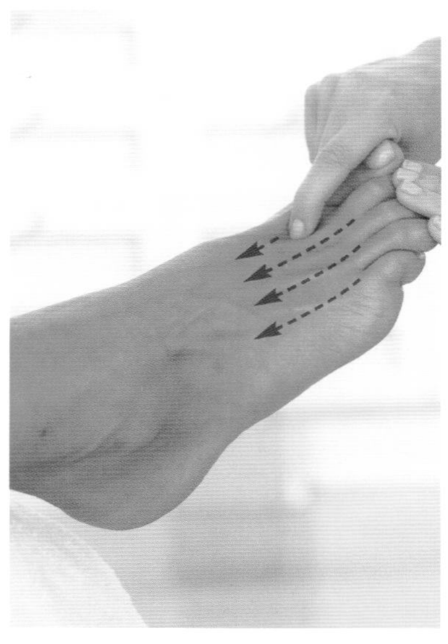

UPPER LYMPHATIC REFLEX AREA

Work on the dorsal aspect of the foot. Use your index finger and thumb to walk up from the base of the toes towards the ankle, in between the metatarsals. Work with a medium pressure up as far as you can, then slide back to make circles lightly between the clefts of the toes. Repeat this movement six times to strengthen the body's immune system.

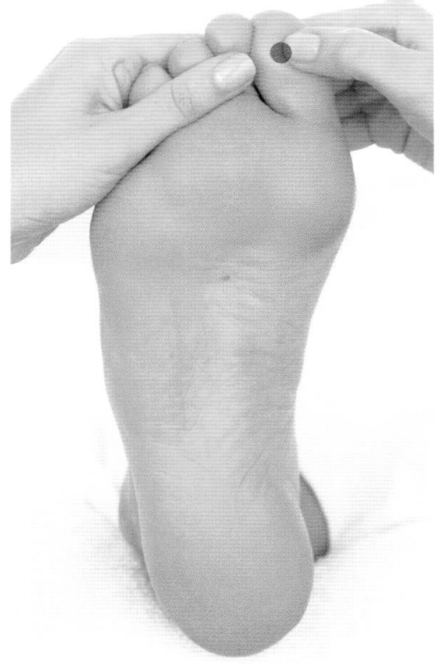

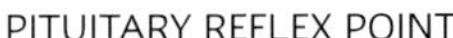

PITUITARY REFLEX POINT

Support the big toe with the fingers of one hand, and use your other thumb to make a cross to find the centre of the big toe. Place your thumb into the centre, push in and make circles for 15 seconds.

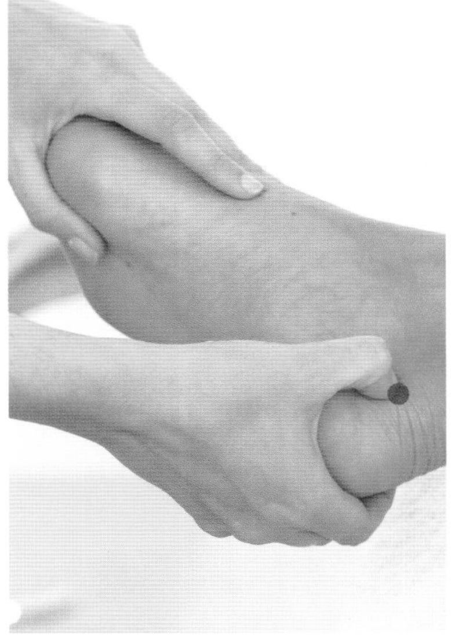

PROSTATE REFLEX POINT

Work on the medial aspect of foot. Place your index finger approximately halfway between the back of the heel and the ankle bone. Push in gently and make circles for 20 seconds.

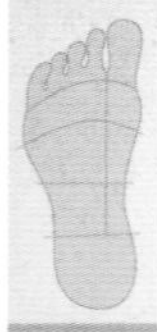

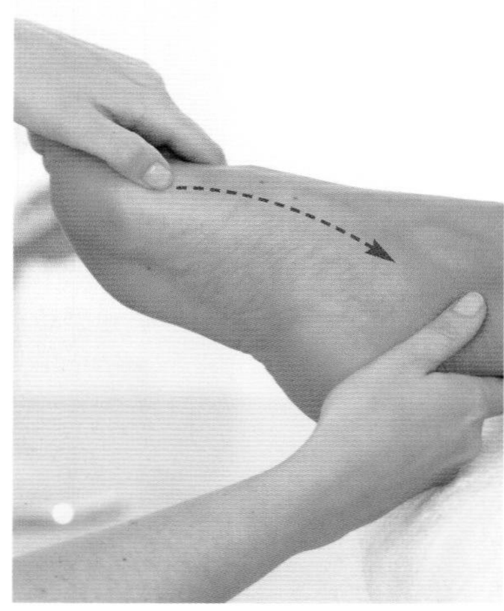

THORACIC AND LUMBAR VERTEBRAE REFLEX AREA

This lies on the medial aspect of the foot. Support the foot with one hand. Use your other thumb to take 12 gentle steps underneath the bone from the base of the joint of the big toe to work the thoracic vertebrae. You should end up on a bone called the navicular, which feels like a knuckle and is halfway between the bladder point and the ankle. Walk around the navicular bone, which represents lumbar one, taking five steps up to the dip in front of the ankle bone, which represents lumbar five. Repeat this movement four times.

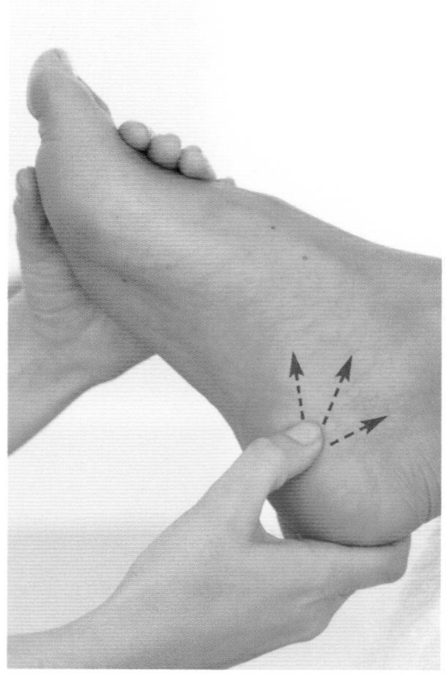

BLADDER REFLEX AREA

Work on the medial aspect of the foot, placing your thumb at the bladder point, which is at the edge of the soft area about one-third of the way from the back of the heel. Use your thumb to fan out over the area, like the spokes of a bicycle wheel, always returning to the bladder point. Work on this area ten times.

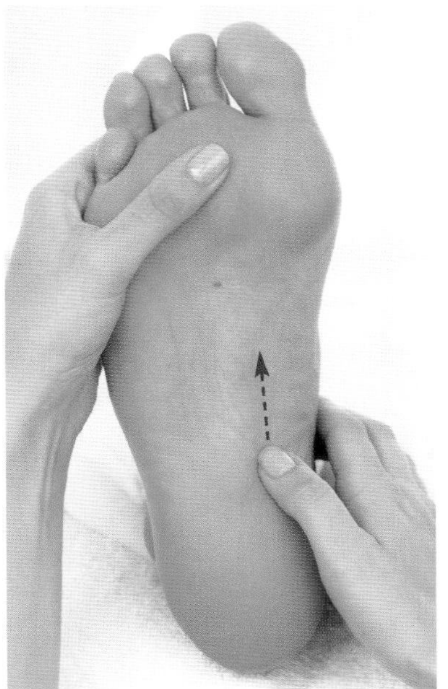

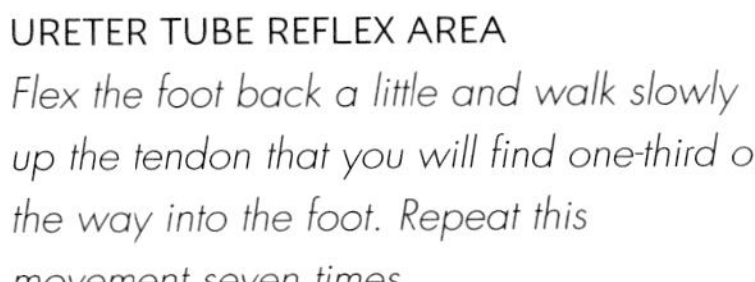

URETER TUBE REFLEX AREA

Flex the foot back a little and walk slowly up the tendon that you will find one-third of the way into the foot. Repeat this movement seven times.

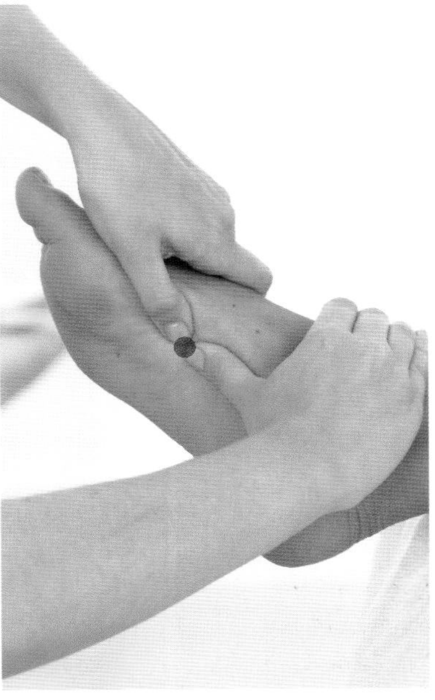

KIDNEY/ADRENAL REFLEX POINTS

The adrenals lie on the kidney and you will find these reflexes at the top of the ureter tube reflex area. When you have reached the top of the ureter tube reflex, place your two thumbs together and gently push into the kidney/adrenal reflexes, making small circles. Work in this manner for ten seconds. These are naturally sensitive reflexes, so your pressure should be soft to help reduce blood pressure.

Infertility in men

This is usually the result of a low number of sperm or abnormal sperm. Around one in five couples experiences infertility, and sperm factors account for about 40 per cent of all cases. A variety of factors can influence this, including exposure to excessive heat, toxins or radiation, testicular injury, disorder of the hormones, recent illness or a long bout of fever, testicular mumps and alcohol consumption. Some causes of sperm inadequacy (exposure to heat, endocrine disorders and recent illness) may be reversible. Men should have a general endocrine examination to see if there are any abnormalities; the examination may reveal hypothyroidism (an underactive thyroid), hyperthyroidism (an overactive thyroid) or a problem with the pituitary gland. Overwork and stress can also affect fertility. Testosterone is made in the body from cholesterol, and very low cholesterol diets can lower testosterone levels. However, antioxidant nutrients such as vitamin E may help to protect so-called 'good' cholesterol from being damaged.

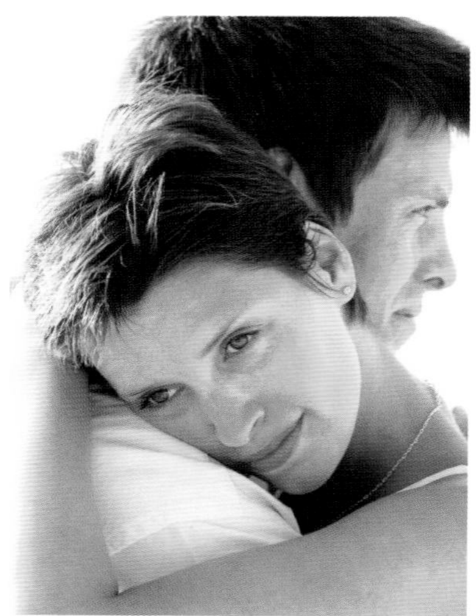

It can take some couples up to three years to conceive naturally. Eating a healthy diet is important if you are trying for a baby.

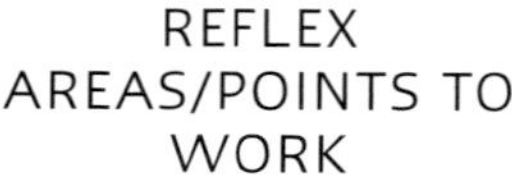

REFLEX AREAS/POINTS TO WORK

- Pituitary
- Testes
- Vas deferens
- Thyroid
- Liver
- Adrenals

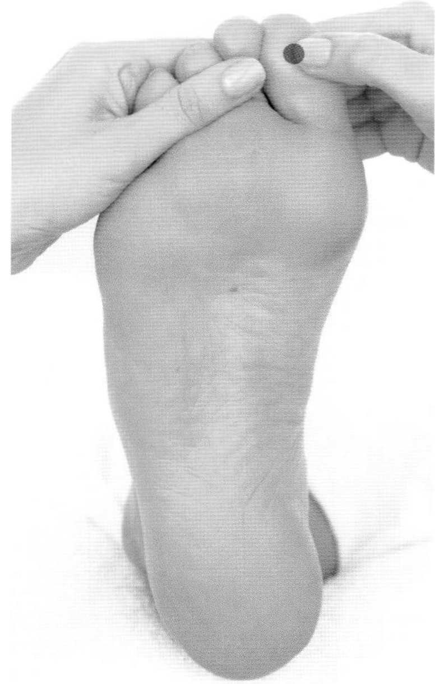

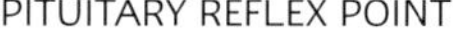

PITUITARY REFLEX POINT

Support the big toe with the fingers of one hand, and use your other thumb to make a cross to find the centre of the big toe. Place your thumb into the centre, push in and make circles for 15 seconds.

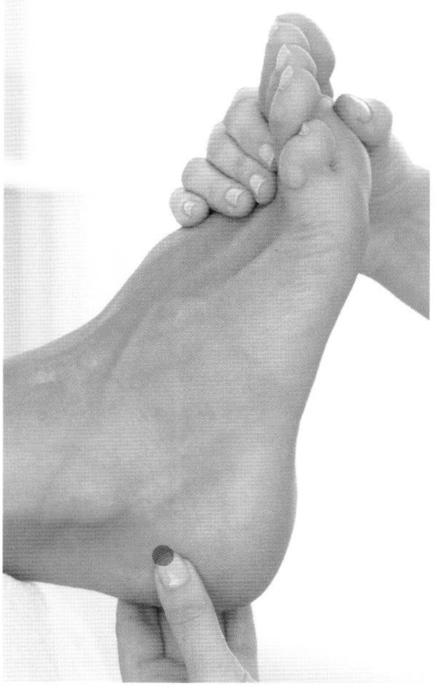

TESTES REFLEX POINT

Work on the lateral aspect of foot. Place your index finger approximately halfway between the back of the heel and the ankle bone. Push in gently and make circles for 15 seconds.

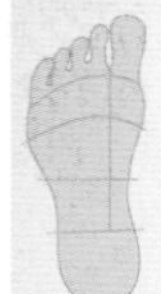

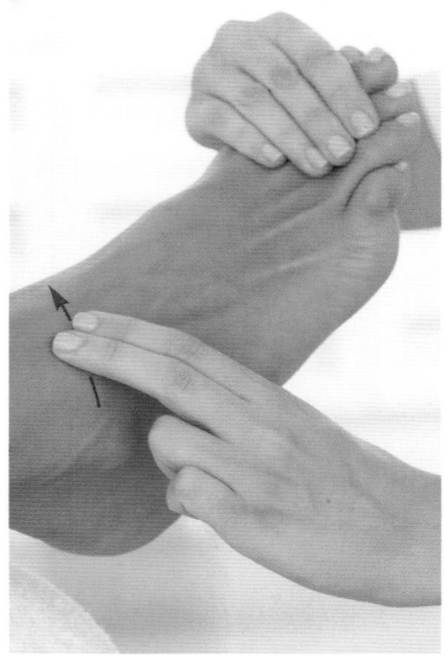

VAS DEFERENS REFLEX AREA

You will find this reflex area across the top of the foot. Use your index and middle fingers to walk from the lateral to the medial aspect of the foot, connecting anklebone to anklebone, and back again. Continue in this manner 12 times.

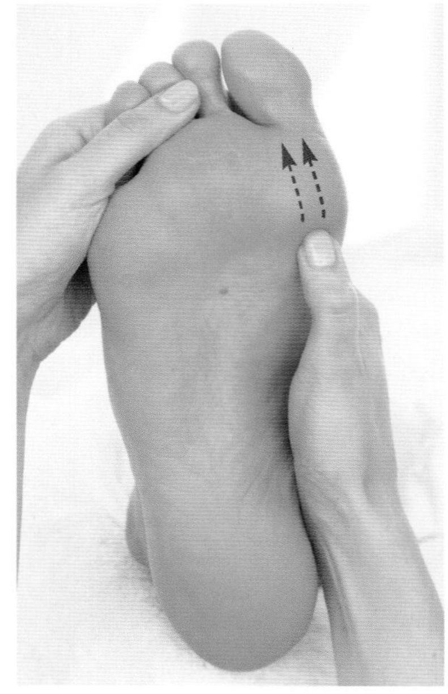

THYROID REFLEX AREA

Use the thumb to work the ball of the foot from the diaphragm line all the way up to the neckline. Repeat this movement slowly six times over the area, dispersing crystals where you find them.

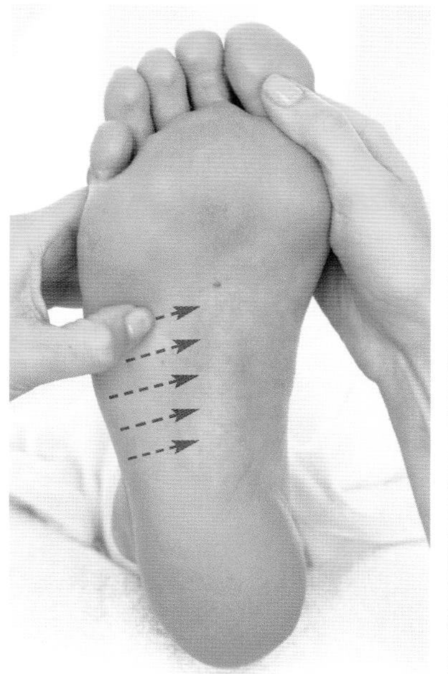

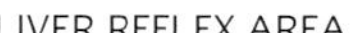

LIVER REFLEX AREA

This reflex area is only found on the right foot. Support the foot with your right hand, and place your left thumb just underneath the diaphragm line. Work slowly and precisely, horizontally across the foot, into zones five and four and just into zone three. Proceed in one direction. Continue in this manner until just above the redness of the heel. Complete the liver reflex movement six times.

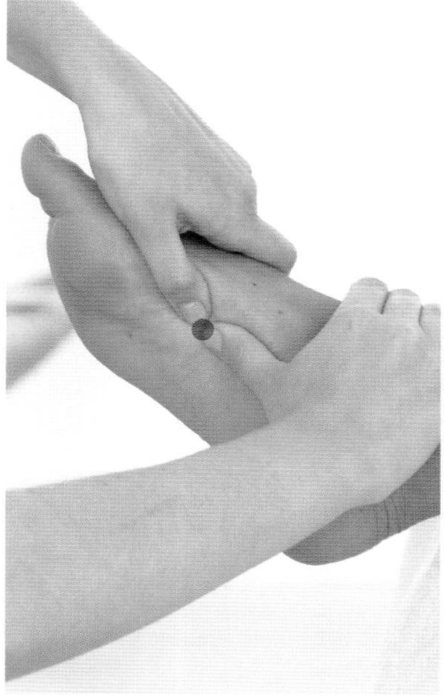

ADRENAL REFLEX POINT

You can find the adrenal reflexes in zone one, three steps down from the ball of the foot. Place your two thumbs together and gently push into the adrenal reflexes, making small circles. Work in this manner for 15 seconds.

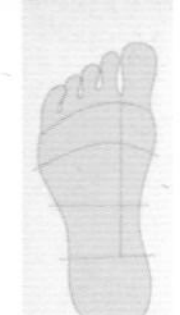

PREGNANCY

Reflexology and pregnancy go very well together, and there is much research to support this. Reflexology can help to balance the hormones, regulate periods and ovulation, ease pregnancy-related problems, achieve a natural labour and reduce labour time. Most of the problems that occur during pregnancy are the result of hormonal changes within the body, vitamin and mineral deficiencies and a

Reflexology can help with pregnancy related problems such as tiredness, lower back pain and sleep patterns.

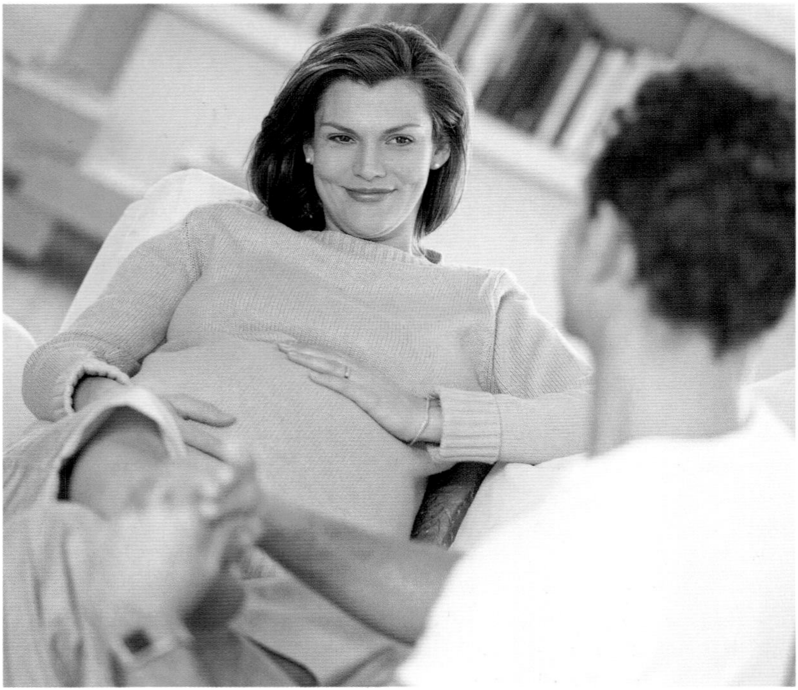

LIFESTYLE TIPS

Fertility declines in both sexes after the ages of 25–30 and, because people are delaying starting a family until their thirties, infertility is becoming increasingly common. Here are some suggestions to help with conception. Cut out tobacco and caffeine, because these make it difficult for the body to nurture an embryo. Get hair analysis to identify any mineral deficiencies (such as zinc) and any toxins in the body. Be aware that digestive diseases like coeliac disease and inflammatory bowel disease could be the basis of malabsorption, causing a deficiency in vitamins and minerals. Cut out alcohol consumption, as one drink per day reduces the chances of conceiving by 50 per cent. Alcohol can delay ovulation; it also prevents the liver from working properly, which could affect blood-sugar balance and the elimination of toxins and old hormones from the body. Alcohol is also a supertoxin, which can block the body's absorption of essential fatty acids, vitamins and essential nutrients.

redistribution of weight because of the inevitable weight gain. Weight is an important factor in ovulation: a woman needs 18 per cent body fat to ovulate, which is why women with eating disorders may find it difficult to conceive.

Reflexology has been used successfully by women who wish to get pregnant and give birth to a healthy baby. I suggest you treat them with a holistic approach in their pre-conception care programme: healthy snacking stabilizes blood sugar (low blood sugar affects progesterone levels). High levels of protein are needed to conceive, while zinc is important for both sexes. Avoid high doses of vitamin C as it dries cervical fluid, thus preventing the sperm from reaching the egg.

Infertility in women

Infertility is the failure to conceive after a year or more of regular sexual activity during the time of ovulation. It can also refer to a woman not being able to carry a pregnancy to term. The most common causes of female infertility include ovulation failure or defect, blocked Fallopian tubes, endometriosis (see page 274) and uterine fibroids (see page 278). Some women develop antibodies to their partner's sperm, and sexually transmitted diseases cause some cases of infertility. Synthetic oestrogens, which are stored in the fat cells, can also disrupt the hormonal balance and have been associated with infertility, breast cancer, low sperm counts in men and the early onset of puberty; they are found in tap water containing residues of the oral-contraceptive pill and HRT, steroids in non-organic meat, milk and dairy produce, some toiletries, detergents and soft plastics.

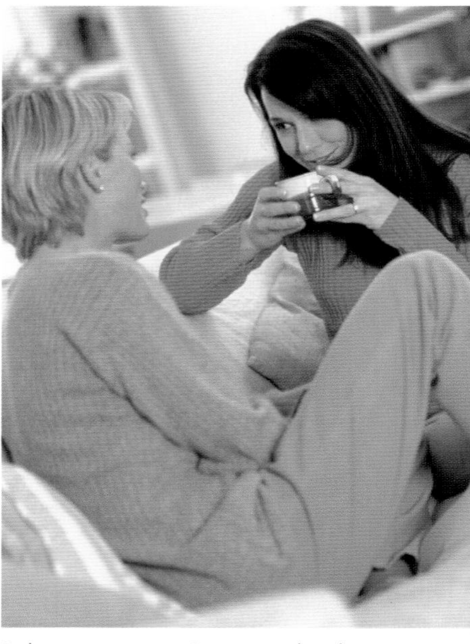

Balance in a woman's emotional and physical well-being is extremely important in the attempt to conceive.

REFLEX AREAS/POINTS TO WORK

- Pituitary
- Thyroid
- Ovaries
- Fallopian tubes
- Thoracic and lumbar vertebrae
- Lymphatics

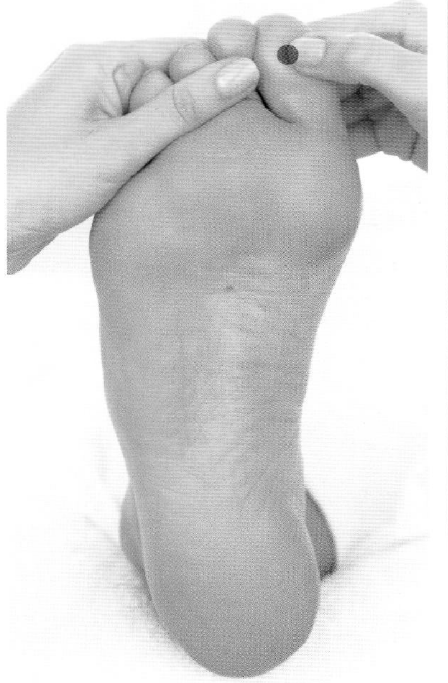

PITUITARY REFLEX POINT

Support the big toe with the fingers of one hand, and use your other thumb to make a cross to find the centre of the big toe. Place your thumb into the centre, push in and make circles for 15 seconds.

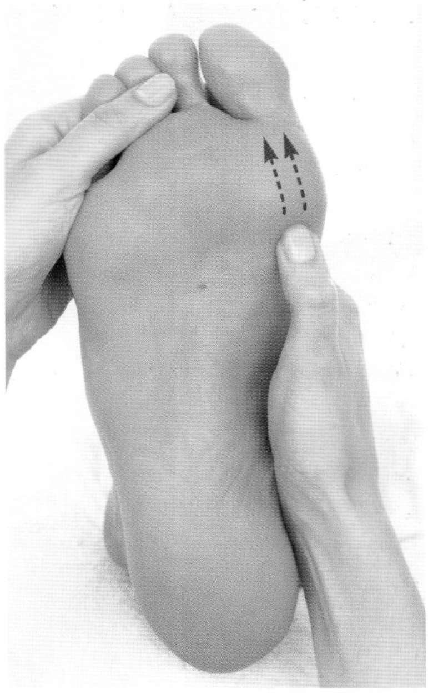

THYROID REFLEX AREA

Use your thumb to work the ball of the foot from the diaphragm line all the way up to the neckline. Repeat this movement slowly six times over the area to assist in balancing the hormones.

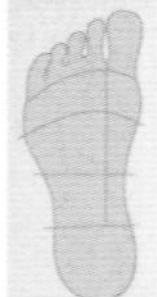

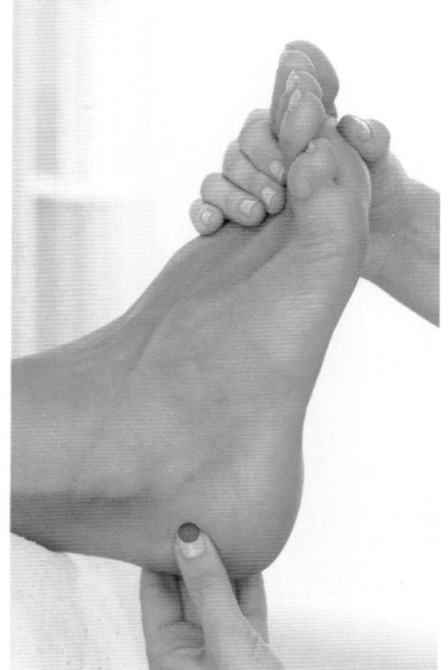

OVARY REFLEX POINT

Work on the lateral aspect of foot. Place your index finger approximately halfway between the back of the heel and the ankle bone. Push in gently and make circles for 15 seconds.

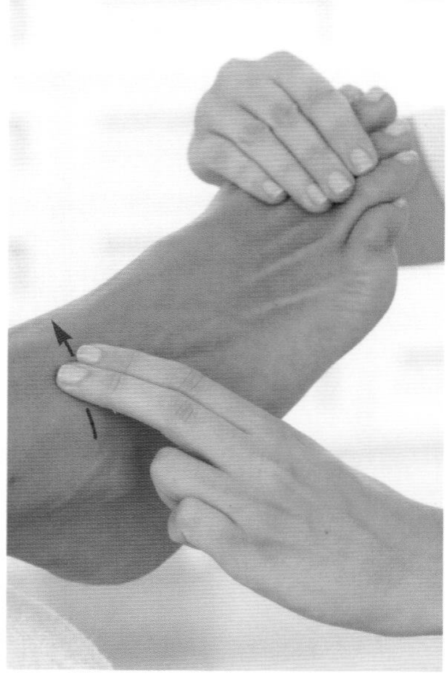

FALLOPIAN TUBE REFLEX AREA

You will find this reflex area across the top of the foot. Use your index and middle fingers to walk from the medial to the lateral aspect of the foot, connecting anklebone to anklebone, and back again. Continue in this manner 12 times.

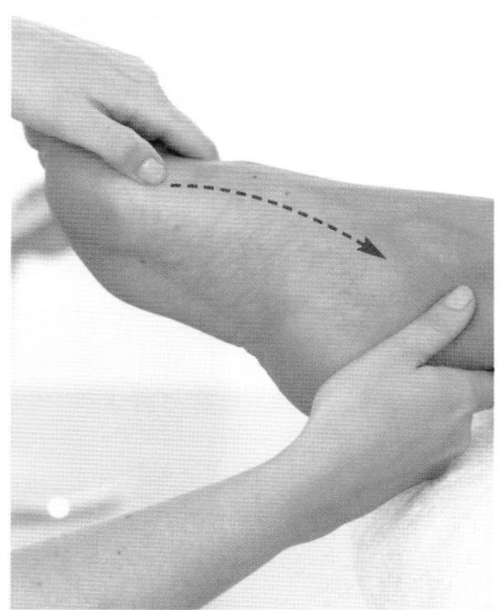

THORACIC AND LUMBAR VERTEBRAE REFLEX AREA

This lies on the medial aspect of the foot. Support the foot with one hand. Use your other thumb to take 12 gentle steps underneath the bone from the base of the joint of the big toe to work the thoracic vertebrae. You should end up on a bone called the navicular, which feels like a knuckle and is halfway between the bladder point and the ankle. Walk around the navicular bone, which represents lumbar one, taking five steps up to the dip in front of the ankle bone, which represents lumbar five. Repeat this movement four times.

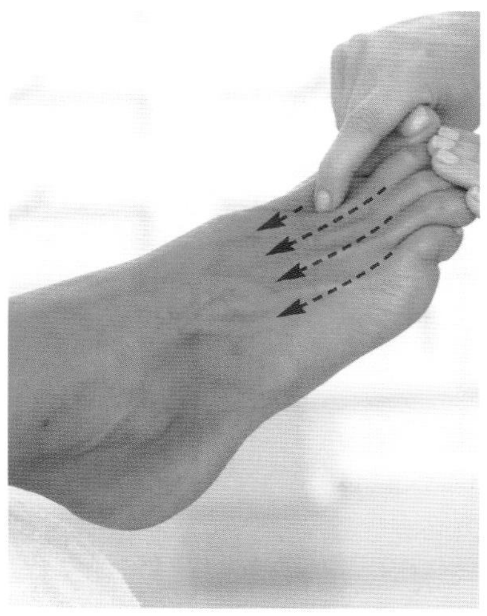

UPPER LYMPHATIC REFLEX AREA

Work on the dorsal aspect of the foot. Use your index finger and thumb to walk up from the base of the toes towards the ankle in between the metatarsals. Work with a medium pressure up as far as you can, then slide back to make circles lightly between the clefts of the toes. Repeat this movement six times.

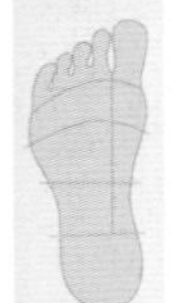

Pregnancy, weeks 14–36

Reflexology is able to facilitate a state of harmony and well-being. During pregnancy the body changes constantly according to the needs of the unborn baby, and reflexology can help relieve pregnancy-associated problems. Treatment should start at week 14 – this is because reflexology is rarely used in the first trimester (three months), so that the body can settle naturally. It is important to eat a well-balanced diet, avoiding junk food, highly seasoned or fried foods, in order to provide the growing baby with the correct vitamins and minerals. Limit tuna to once a week because of its mercury content.

REFLEX AREAS/POINTS TO WORK

- Pancreas
- Liver
- Ascending colon
- Descending colon
- Bladder
- Kidneys/adrenals
- Entire spine

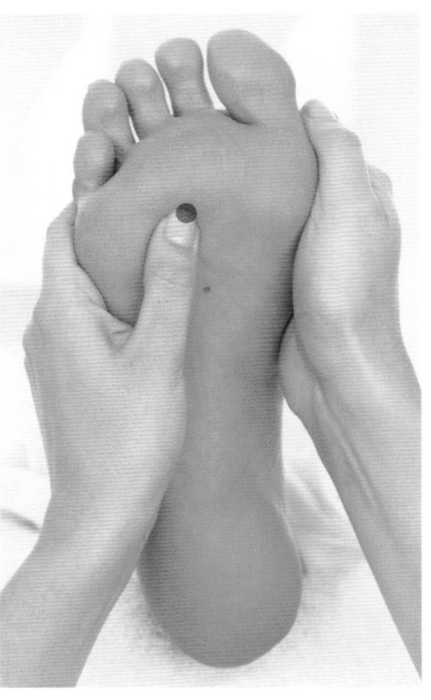

PANCREAS REFLEX POINT

This reflex point is only found on the right foot. Place your thumb on the third toe and trace a line down to below the diaphragm line. Push up into the joint and make small circles for six seconds.

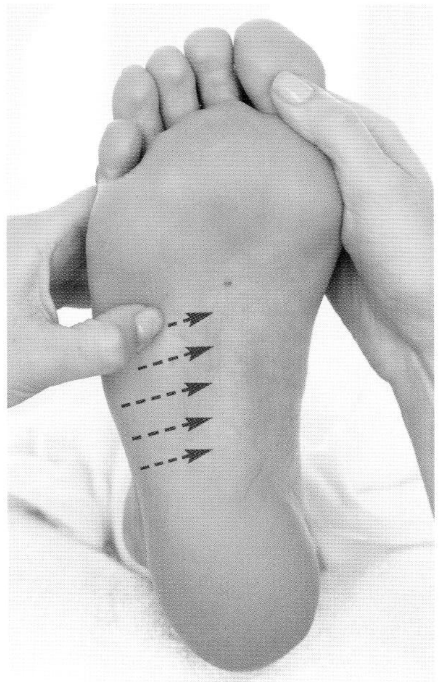

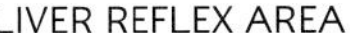

LIVER REFLEX AREA

This reflex area is only found on the right foot. Support the foot with your right hand, and place your left thumb just underneath the diaphragm line. Work slowly and precisely, horizontally across the foot, into zones five and four and just into zone three. Proceed in one direction. Continue in this manner until just above the redness of the heel. Complete the liver reflex movement six times.

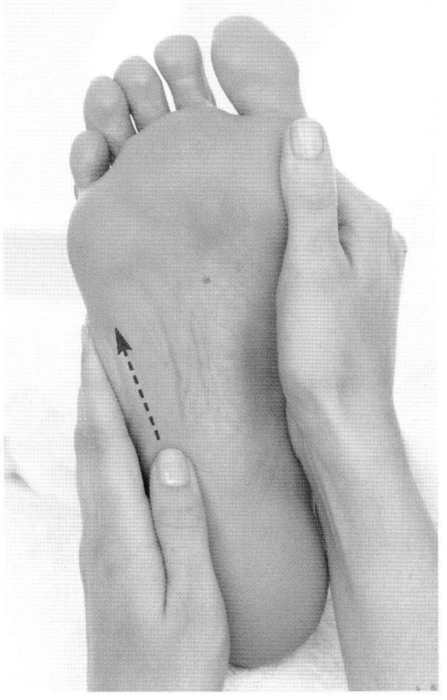

ASCENDING COLON REFLEX AREA

This reflex area is only found on the right foot. Use your left thumb to walk up zone four from the redness of the heel. Continue in this manner until you get halfway up the foot. Work the ascending colon reflex area four times in slow movements to help eliminate waste products and toxins.

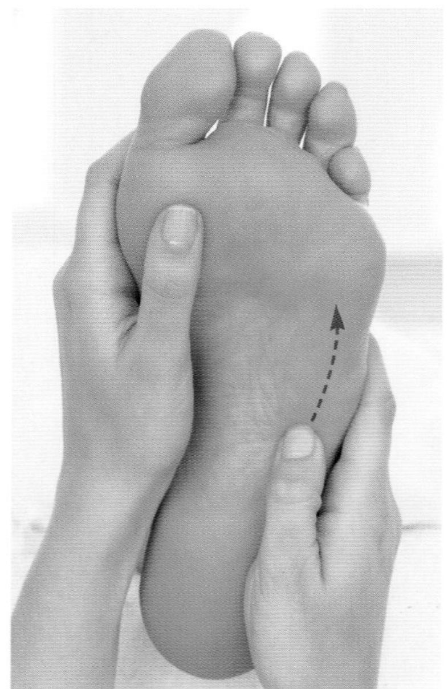

DESCENDING COLON REFLEX AREA

This reflex area is only found on the left foot. Use your right thumb to walk up zone four from the redness of the heel, to work this part of the colon. Continue in this manner until you arrive halfway up the foot. Work this reflex area six times and in slow movements to help stimulate the peristaltic muscular action of the colon.

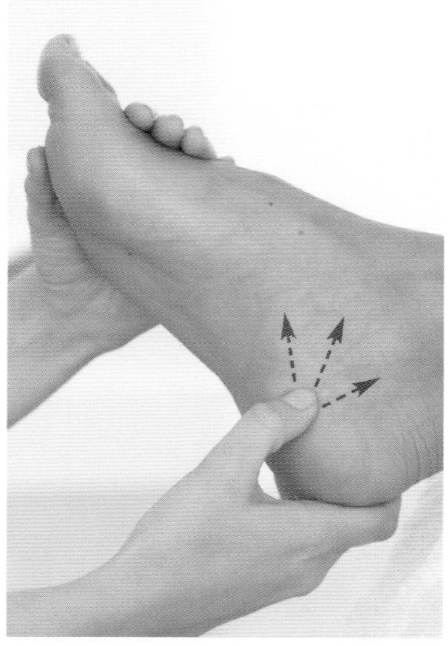

BLADDER REFLEX AREA

Work on the medial aspect of the foot. Place your thumb at the bladder point, which is at the edge of the soft area about one-third of the way from the back of the heel. Use your thumb to fan out over the area, like the spokes of a bicycle wheel, always returning to the bladder point. Work on this area six times.

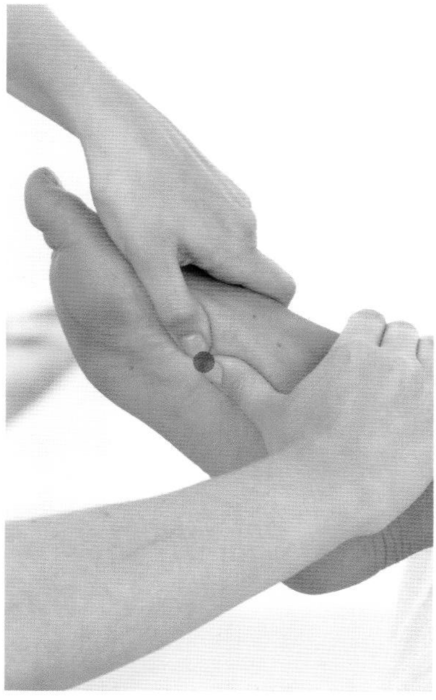

KIDNEY/ADRENAL REFLEX POINTS

You can find these reflexes in zone one, three steps down from the ball of the foot. Place your two thumbs together and gently push into the kidney/adrenal reflexes, making small circles. Work in this manner for 20 seconds.

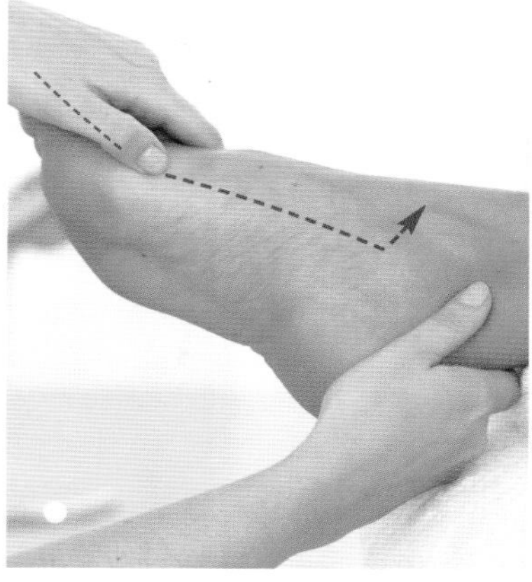

ENTIRE SPINE

Work on the medial aspect of the foot. Support the foot with one hand, and use your other thumb to walk gently seven steps in between the joints of the big toe, remembering that each step represents a specific vertebra. Walk towards the foot. Then take 12 gentle steps underneath the bone from the base of the joint of the big toe to work the thoracic vertebrae. You should end up on a bone called the navicular, which feels like a knuckle and is halfway between the bladder point and the ankle. Walk around the navicular bone, which represents lumbar one, taking five steps up to the dip in front of the ankle bone, which represents lumbar five. Repeat this movement gently three times.

Pregnancy, weeks 37–40

Use reflexology to prepare for birth – physically, psychologically and, most importantly, to balance the hormones. Insomnia is very common during the last few weeks of pregnancy, due to the anxiety of birth and difficulty in finding a comfortable sleeping position; it is also linked to low levels of the B vitamins. Arrange pillows to suit your needs, including beneath your abdomen to relieve breathlessness. Avoid bacon, cheese, sugar, tomatoes, chocolate, potatoes and wine close to bedtime, because these foods contain a brain stimulant. In the evening eat bananas, figs, yoghurt and wholegrain crackers because they contain sleep-promoting agents. Most women want to have a natural labour and, by working on the pituitary reflex, you can help promote the production of oxytocin, which causes the uterus to contract during labour. Synthetic oxytocin can be used to induce childbirth and can sometimes be used to expel the placenta after delivery. Drinking one or two cups of raspberry leaf tea a day can help in the final stages of pregnancy and can even be sipped throughout labour. However, it is only recommended during the last two months of pregnancy. The tea is believed to strengthen the walls of the uterus and shorten the second stage of labour.

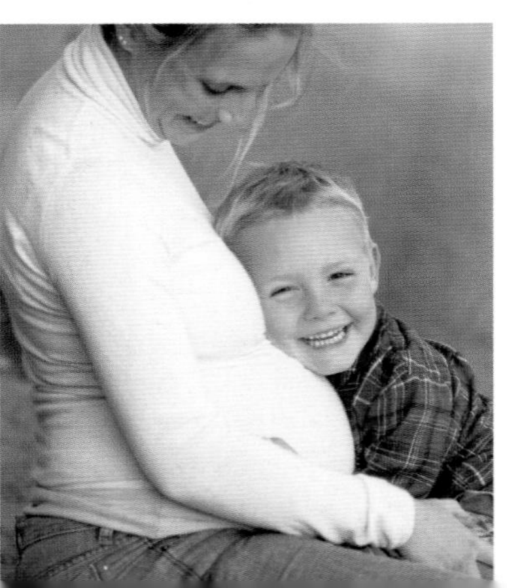

REFLEX AREAS/POINTS TO WORK

- Pituitary
- Thyroid
- Uterus
- Ovaries
- Kidneys/adrenals
- Entire spine

It is common for the baby to be active after you have had a reflexology treatment.

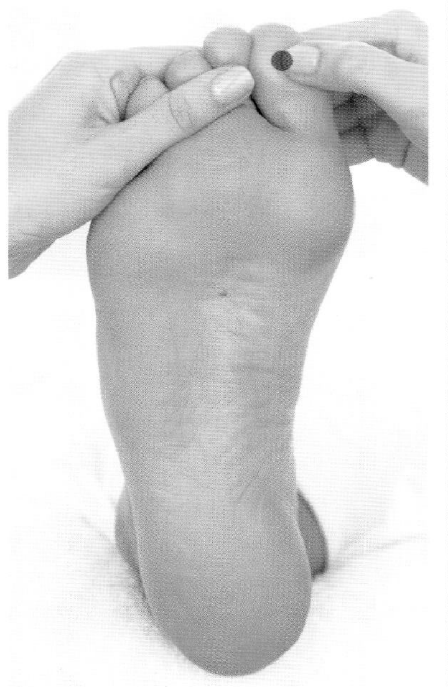

PITUITARY REFLEX POINT

Support the big toe with the fingers of one hand, and use your other thumb to make a cross to find the centre of the big toe. Place your thumb into the centre, push in and make circles for 25 seconds.

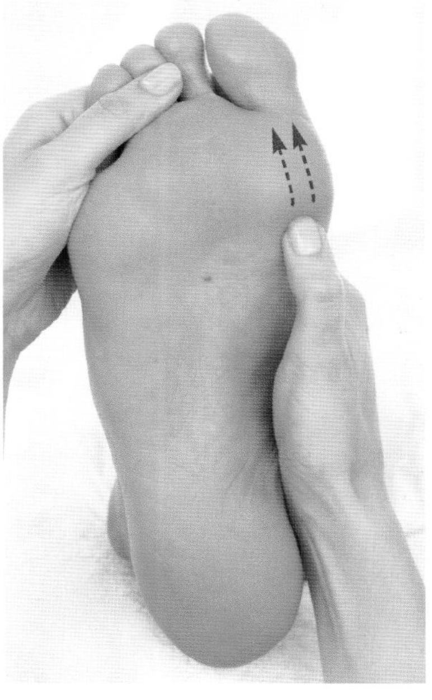

THYROID REFLEX AREA

Use your thumb to work the ball of the foot from the diaphragm line all the way up to the neckline. Repeat this movement slowly seven times over the area.

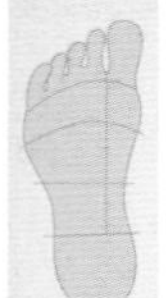

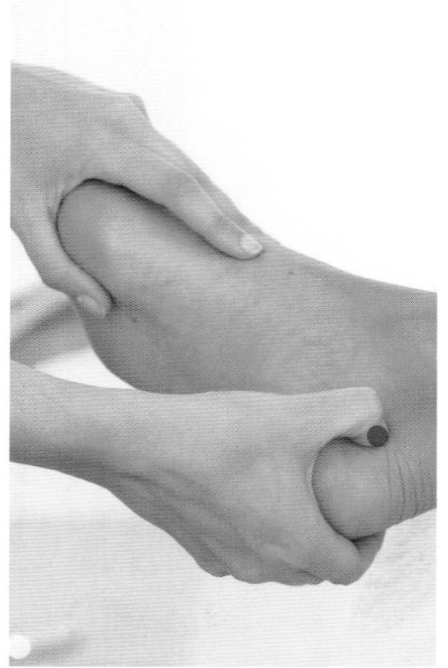

UTERUS REFLEX POINT

Work on the medial aspect of foot. Place your index finger approximately halfway between the back of the heel and the ankle bone. Push in gently and make circles for ten seconds.

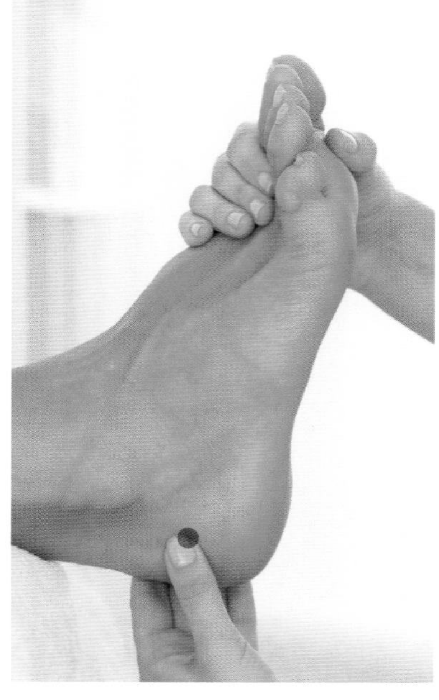

OVARY REFLEX POINT

Work on the lateral aspect of foot. Place your index finger approximately halfway between the back of the heel and the ankle bone. Push in gently and make circles for 15 seconds.

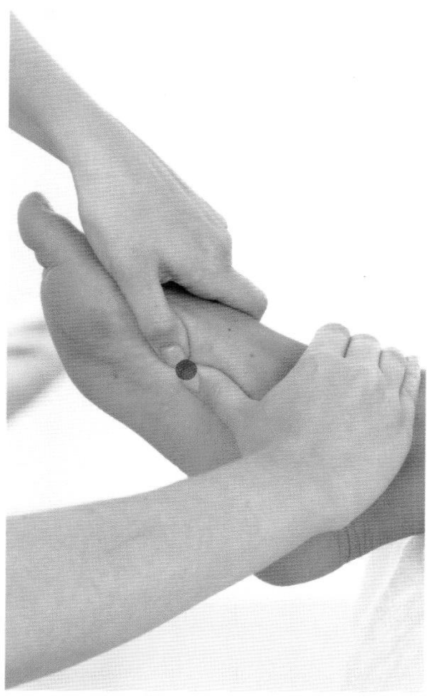

KIDNEY/ADRENAL REFLEX POINTS

You can find these reflexes in zone one, three steps down from the ball of the foot. Place your two thumbs together and gently push into these reflexes, making small circles. Work in this manner for 25 seconds to help relax the body.

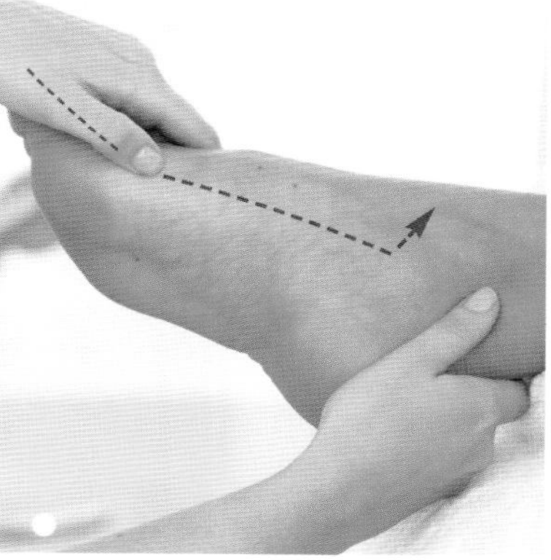

ENTIRE SPINE

Work on the medial aspect of the foot. Support the foot with one hand, and use your other thumb to walk gently seven steps in between the joints of the big toe, remembering that each step represents a specific vertebra. Walk towards the foot. Then take 12 gentle steps underneath the bone from the base of the joint of the big toe to work the thoracic vertebrae. You should end up on a bone called the navicular, which feels like a knuckle and is halfway between the bladder point and the ankle. Walk around the navicular bone, which represents lumbar one, taking five steps up to the dip in front of the ankle bone, which represents lumbar five. Repeat this movement gently five times.

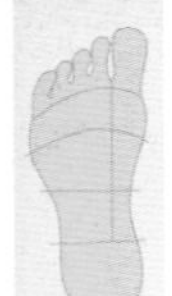

After the birth

During pregnancy the levels of oestrogen and progesterone rise, smoothing the muscles of the uterus, intestines and veins. After the birth they drop within minutes, and by the second day are very low. Reflexology can assist the return of tissues to a pre-pregnant state and can support emotional and mental well-being. Post-natal depression may be experienced as overwhelming and debilitating listlessness. Simple tasks surrounding the baby (or life in general) may be hard to cope with. This may not surface until weeks after the birth, and the true depths of post-natal depression may not occur until the baby is three to six months old.

REFLEX AREAS/POINTS TO WORK

- Pituitary
- Thyroid
- Liver
- Lungs
- Kidneys/adrenals
- Entire spine

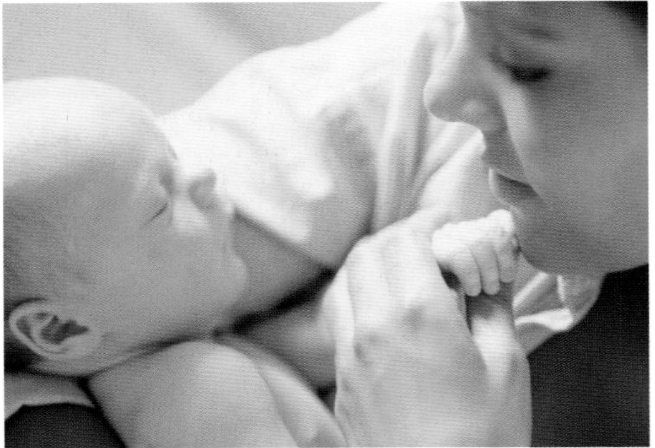

After the birth, reflexology can help re-balance the mother's hormone levels.

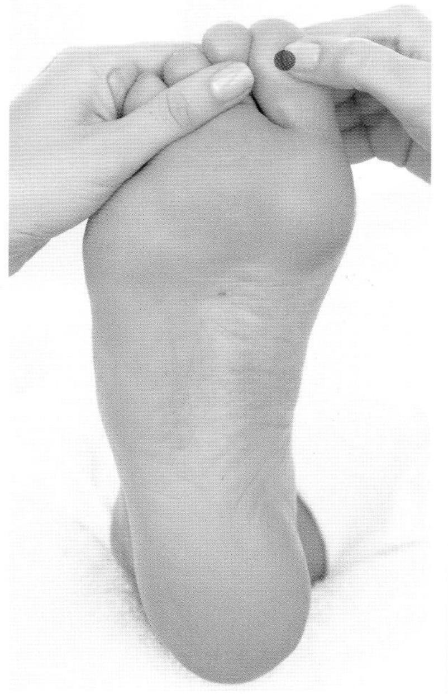

PITUITARY REFLEX POINT

Support the big toe with the fingers of one hand, and use your other thumb to make a cross to find the centre of the big toe. Place your thumb into the centre, push in and make circles for 25 seconds.

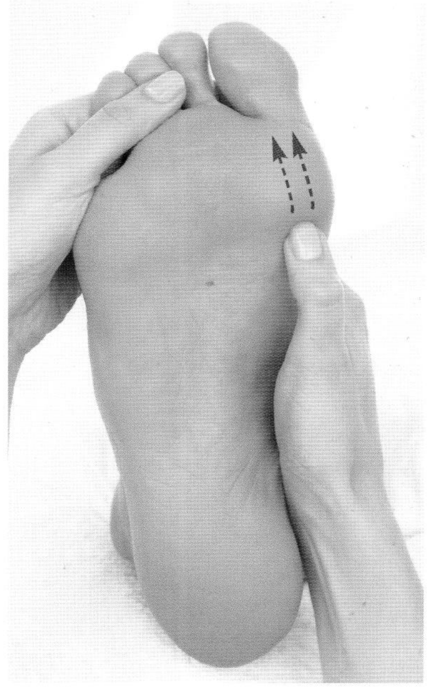

THYROID REFLEX AREA

Use your thumb to work the ball of the foot from the diaphragm line all the way up to the neckline. Repeat this movement slowly ten times over the area to help restore energy levels.

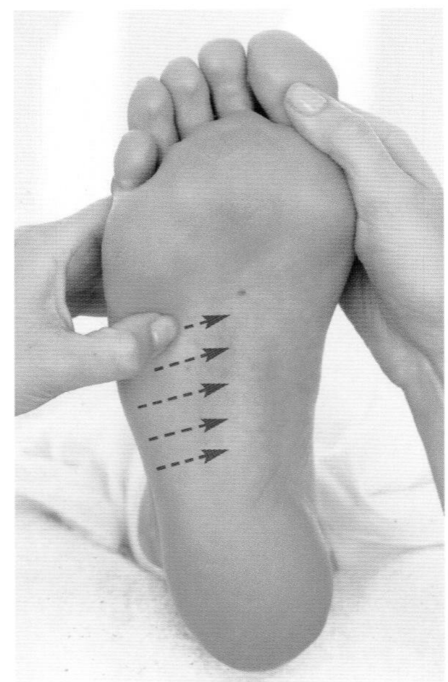

LIVER REFLEX AREA

This reflex area is only found on the right foot. Support the foot with your right hand, and place your left thumb just underneath the diaphragm line. Work slowly and precisely, horizontally across the foot, into zones five and four and just into zone three. Proceed in one direction. Continue in this manner until just above the redness of the heel. Complete the liver reflex movement six times.

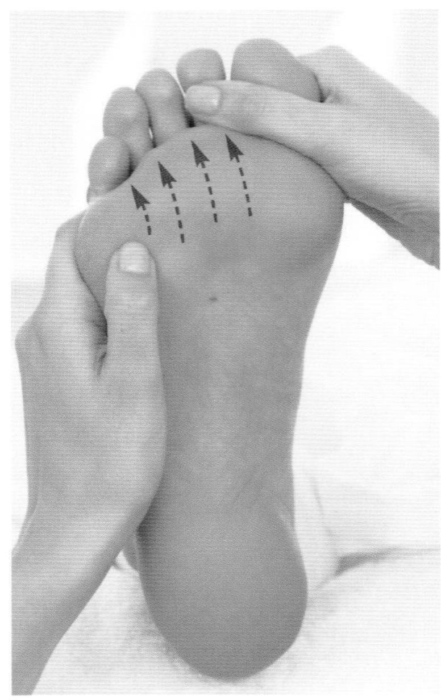

LUNG REFLEX AREA

Flex the foot back with one hand to create skin tension. Use the thumb of your other hand to work up from the diaphragm line to the eye/ear general area. You should be working in between the metatarsals. Repeat this process seven times, making sure you have worked in between all the metatarsals.

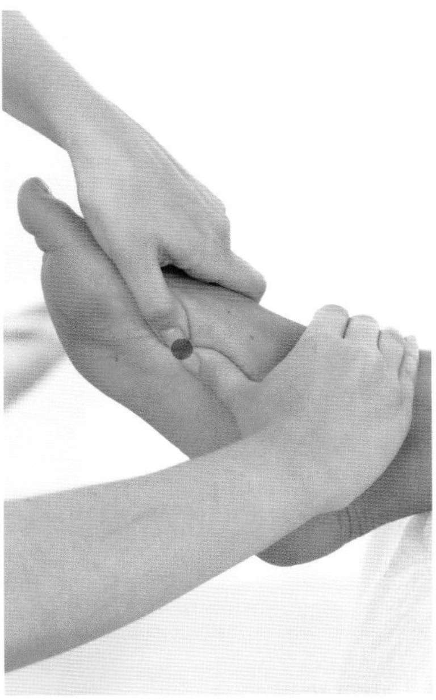

KIDNEY/ADRENAL REFLEX POINTS

You can find these reflexes in zone one, three steps down from the ball of the foot. Place your two thumbs together and gently push into the kidney/adrenal reflexes, making small circles. Work in this manner for 20 seconds.

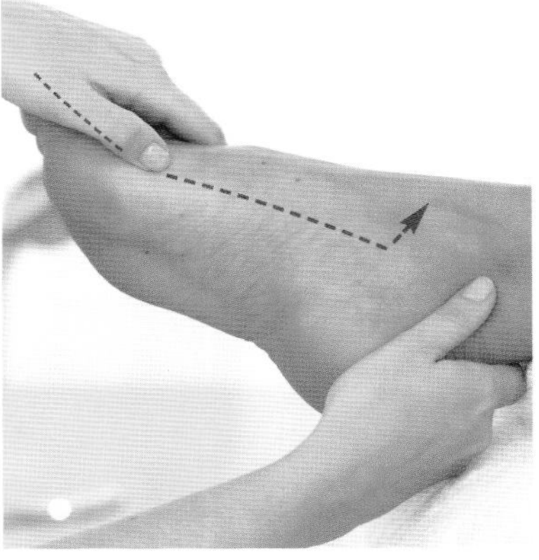

ENTIRE SPINE

Work on the medial aspect of the foot. Support the foot with one hand, and use your other thumb to walk gently seven steps in between the joints of the big toe, remembering that each step represents a specific vertebra. Walk towards the foot. Then take 12 gentle steps underneath the bone from the base of the joint of the big toe to work the thoracic vertebrae. You should end up on a bone called the navicular, which feels like a knuckle and is halfway between the bladder point and the ankle. Walk around the navicular bone, which represents lumbar one, taking five steps up to the dip in front of the ankle bone, which represents lumbar five. Repeat this movement gently three times.

TREATING YOUNG CHILDREN

Reflexology is beneficial to young children, and can help stimulate the healing processes as well as ensuring that the body's systems are functioning on all levels. Sometimes the anxiety of the mother or father can cause distress in the child, so it is always advisable that a parent receives reflexology as well, to help with issues affecting them. When both parent and child are receiving treatment, this can only reinforce the bond between them, and the relationship between child and

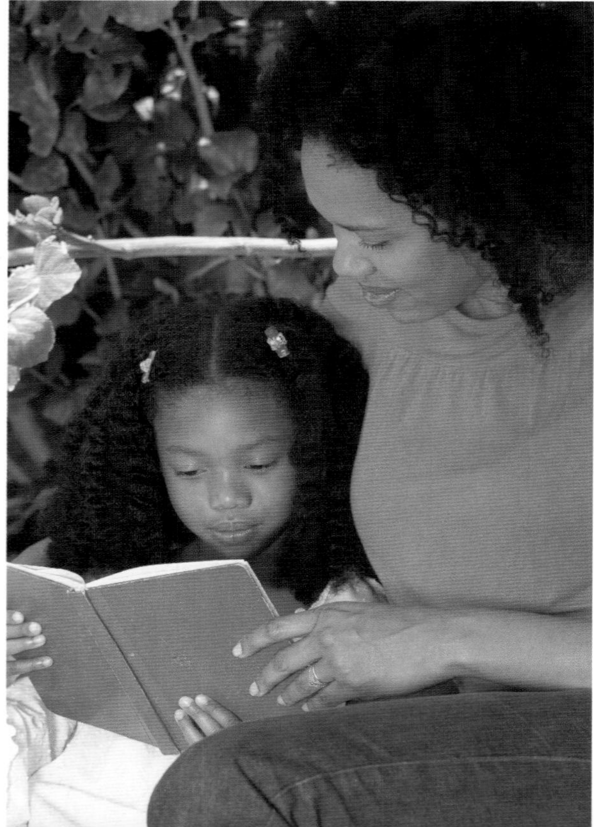

Reflexology can strengthen the bond between parent and child; if possible perform the sequence just before or after their bedtime story.

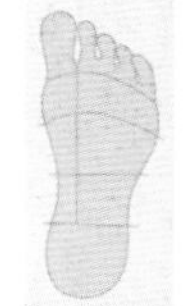

LIFESTYLE TIPS

Around one in every 200 children under 12 years old suffers from depression, attention-deficit hyperactivity disorder (ADHD, see page 332–335) and mild obsessions and compulsions. The most common cause is stress or a change in their circumstances either at home or at school. Other holistic factors include food allergies, additives, vitamin and nutrient deficiencies, blood-sugar imbalances, Lyme disease, an imbalance in the brain chemical serotonin, and occasionally a bacterial infection. Use the holistic approach to health by giving your child organic fruit and vegetables every two hours; include fish oils in their diet; and avoid sugar, processed foods, additives, caffeine and wheat. Carbohydrates raise serotonin levels in the brain, which has a calming effect, and fish oils are known to improve concentration and help with dyslexia. See a doctor to rule out Lyme disease or strep throat.

parent is an important aspect of the healing process. Applying gentle pressure to the reflexes causes physiological changes to take place in the body, because its own healing potential is stimulated. The sequence should be performed in a quiet room, with low lighting, no phones and tranquil music; ensure the child is comfortable and can fall asleep if necessary, and that if any toys or comforters are needed they are within reach. It is best for the parent to perform this sequence at night, either just before or after a bedtime story. Obviously, if a child has anything medically wrong with them, it is advisable to take them immediately to a doctor or the nearest hospital emergency department.

Poor appetite

This is not in itself a disorder, but is usually a symptom of some other problem that is affecting the child. Often emotional factors – such as stress, anxiety, depression, illness, trauma, worries at school, concerns about friendships, bullying or problems at home – may cause a child's appetite to diminish noticeably. An undetected underlying problem may also be the reason, and might include a food disorder or a junk-food diet, resulting in nutritional deficiencies. To stimulate a poor appetite, a healthy, interesting and fun diet is necessary, depending on the child's tolerances and tastes. Reflexology can help to stimulate the appetite, as well as reducing appetite-sapping anxiety in a child.

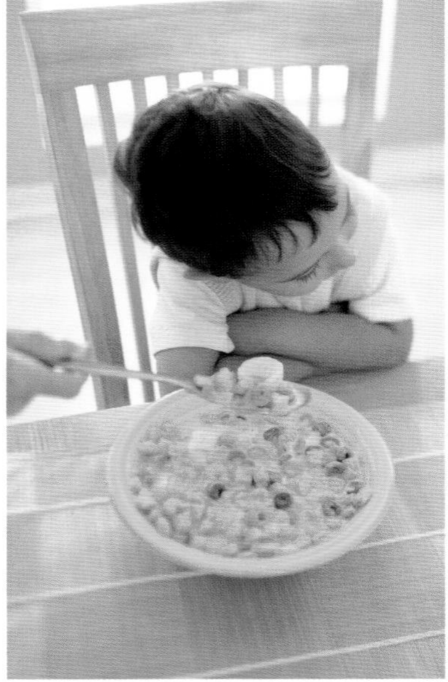

Several factors can contribute to a child's poor appetite, including stress and anxiety or problems at school or home.

REFLEX AREAS/POINTS TO WORK

- Hypothalamus/pituitary
- Diaphragm
- Stomach
- Ascending/transverse colon
- Adrenals
- Entire spine

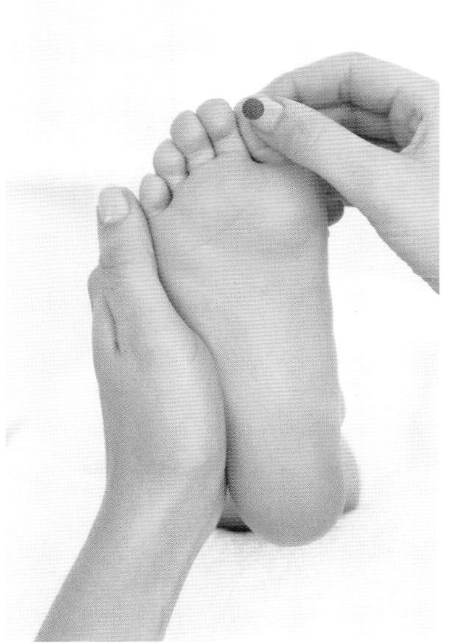

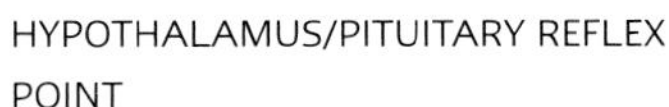

HYPOTHALAMUS/PITUITARY REFLEX POINT

Support the big toe with the fingers of one hand and find the centre of the big toe. Place one thumb on the centre of the big toe for the pituitary reflex. Then take one step up from the pituitary and one small step laterally. Make circular movements for 30 seconds.

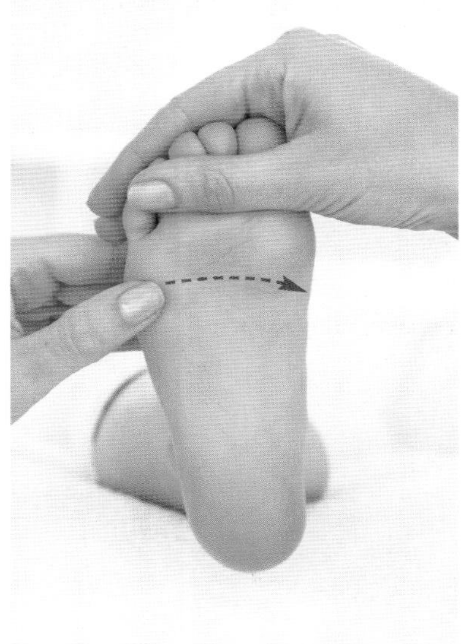

DIAPHRAGM REFLEX AREA

Flex the foot back with one hand to create skin tension. Use the thumb of your other hand to work under the metatarsal heads, across from the lateral to the medial aspect of the foot. Use slow steps and repeat this movement eight times.

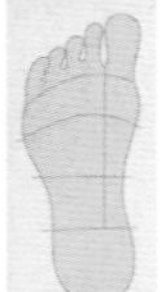

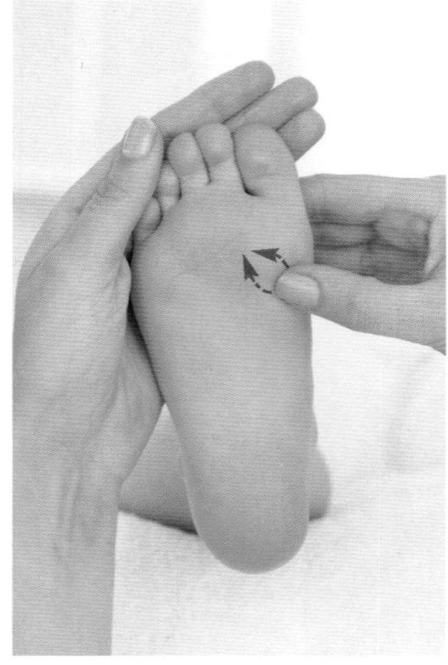

STOMACH REFLEX AREA

You will find this reflex area just under the ball of the foot. Support the foot with one hand, and place your other thumb just below the thyroid reflex area. Gently work up laterally to the solar plexus reflex, stopping there to stimulate it with circles for four seconds. Repeat this movement eight times.

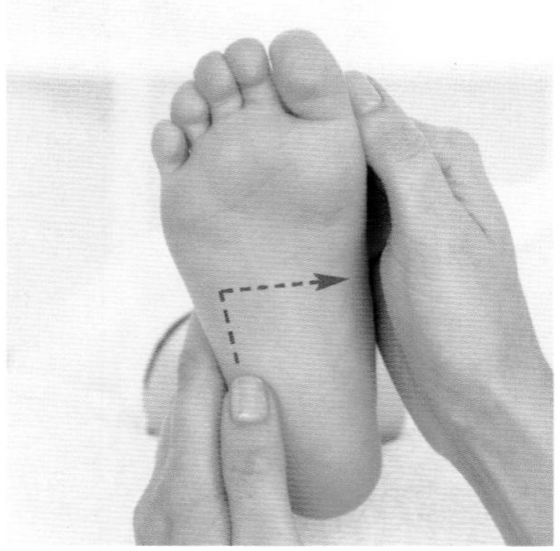

ASCENDING/TRANSVERSE COLON REFLEX

This reflex area is only found on the right foot. Use your left thumb to walk up zone four from the redness of the heel. Continue in this manner until you get halfway up the foot. Work the ascending colon reflex area four times in slow movements. Then walk across the transverse colon.

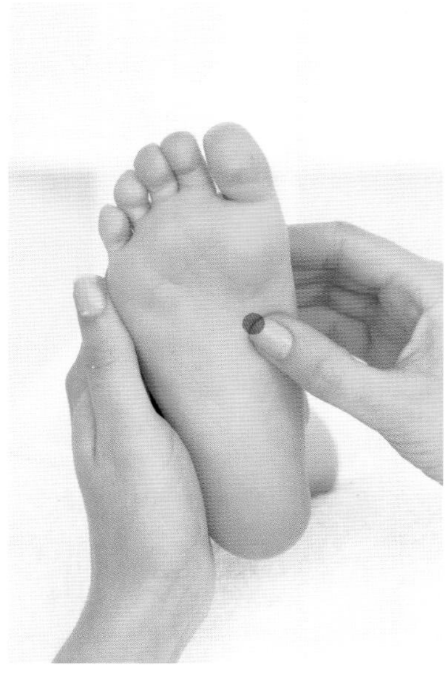

ADRENAL REFLEX POINT

You can find the adrenal reflexes in zone one, three steps down from the ball of the foot. Place your two thumbs together and gently push into the adrenal reflexes, making small circles. Work in this manner for 15 seconds.

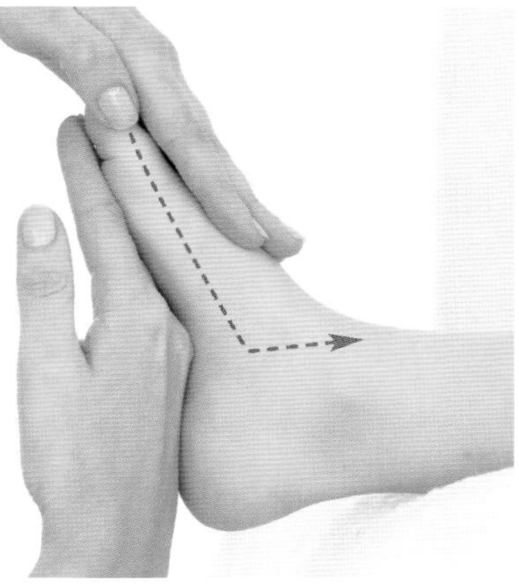

ENTIRE SPINE

Work on the medial aspect of the foot. Support the foot with one hand, and use your other thumb to walk gently seven steps in between the joints of the big toe, remembering that each step represents a specific vertebra. Walk towards the foot. Then take 12 gentle steps underneath the bone from the base of the joint of the big toe to work the thoracic vertebrae. You should end up on a bone called the navicular, which feels like a knuckle and is halfway between the bladder point and the ankle. Walk around the navicular bone, which represents lumbar one, taking five steps up to the dip in front of the ankle bone, which represents lumbar five. Repeat this movement gently three times.

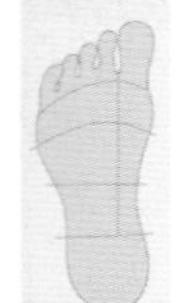

Croup

This is a respiratory infection that causes the throat to narrow, due to swelling. It can be very serious and needs to be treated properly by a medical practitioner if a child is having difficulty breathing. It commonly occurs in young children, whose airways are much narrower than those of adults. Most attacks occur at night, when mucus may increase and clog up the airways. The symptoms include spasms in the throat, difficulty in breathing, a wheezing noise, hoarseness, a feeling of suffocation, tightness in the lungs and a harsh, barking cough. Fits of coughing are another characteristic sign. Croup is usually preceded by an allergy attack, a cold, bronchitis or inhalation of a foreign body. To help thin the mucus it is a good idea to give a child plenty of fluids, including herbal teas and homemade soups. Warm ginger herb baths can help; then immediately wrap the child in a heavy towel and put him or her to bed to perspire, which can help loosen the mucus and rid the body of toxins. Reflexology can work on all the systems of the body to relieve the stress that the child is suffering and relax the airways.

Place a child with croup in a warm ginger herb bath then wrap in a heavy towel to perspire, which can help loosen the mucus.

REFLEX AREAS/POINTS TO WORK

- Oesophagus
- Diaphragm
- Lungs
- Adrenals
- Upper lymphatics
- Entire spine

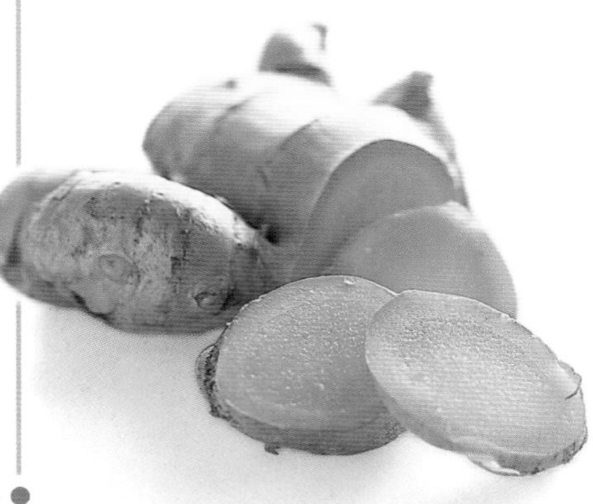

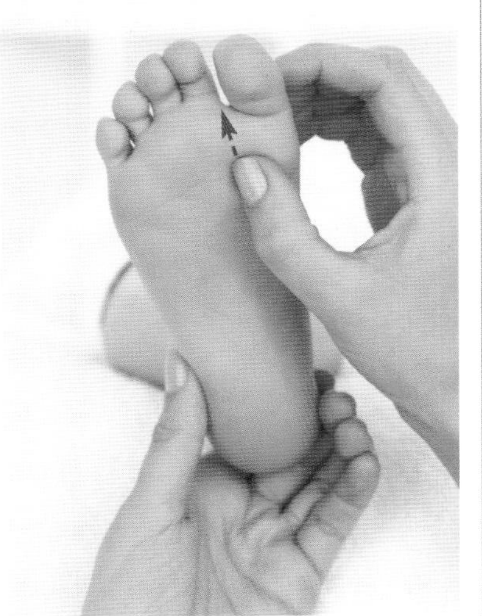

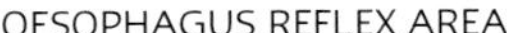

OESOPHAGUS REFLEX AREA

Flex the foot back with one hand to create skin tension. Place the thumb of your other hand at the diaphragm line in between zones one and two. Work up in between the metatarsals from the diaphragm line to the eye/ear general area. Continue in this manner six times. Working this area can help with disorders of the oesophagus, bad breath, trouble in swallowing and heartburn and strengthen the oesophagus.

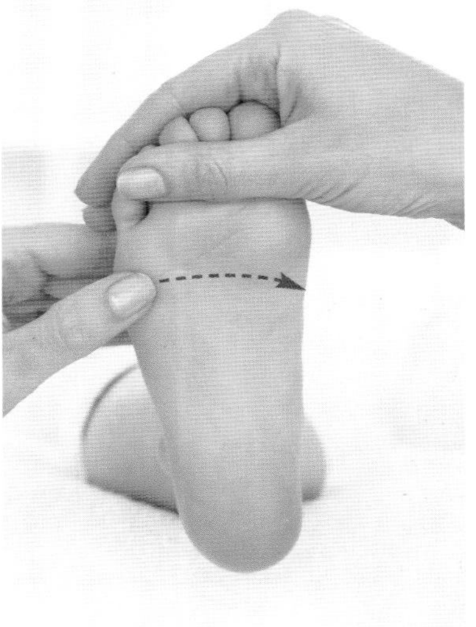

DIAPHRAGM REFLEX AREA

Flex the foot back with one hand to create skin tension. Use the thumb of your other hand to work under the metatarsal heads, across from the lateral to the medial aspect of the foot. Use slow steps and repeat this movement six times.

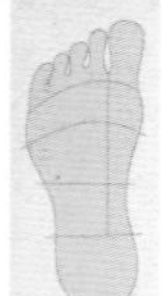

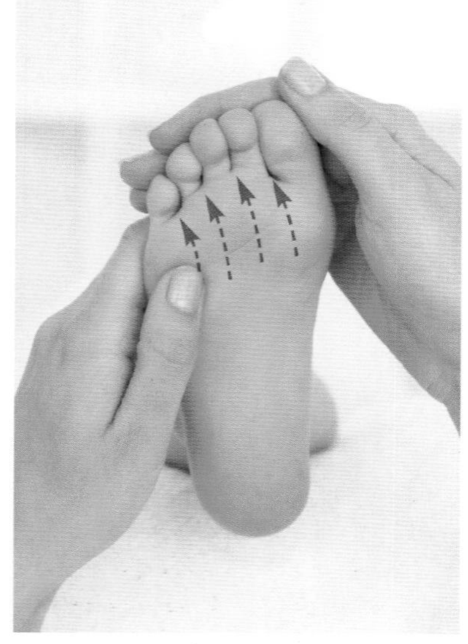

LUNG REFLEX AREA

Flex the foot back with one hand to create skin tension. Use the thumb of your other hand to work up from the diaphragm line to the eye/ear general area. You should be working in between the metatarsals. Repeat this process seven times, making sure you have worked in between all the metatarsals.

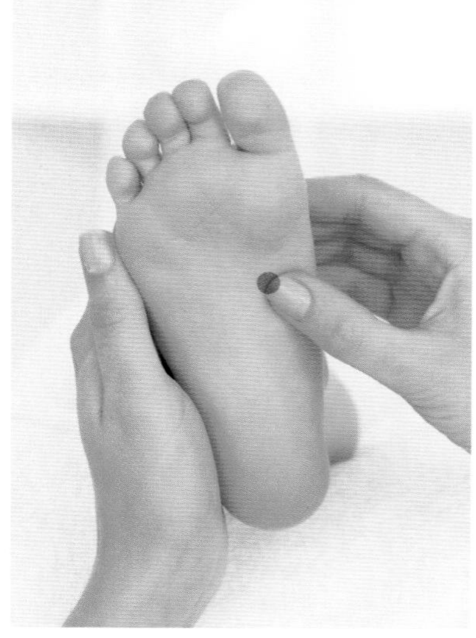

ADRENAL REFLEX POINT

You can find the adrenal reflex in zone one, three steps down from the ball of the foot. Place your thumb in the point and gently push into the adrenal reflexes, making small circles. Work in this manner for 15 seconds.

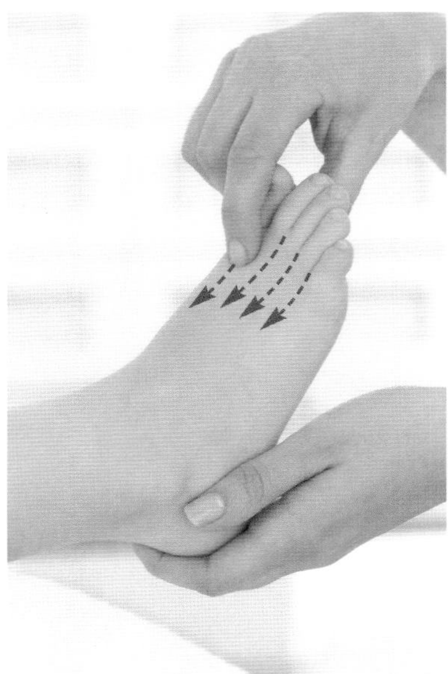

UPPER LYMPHATIC REFLEX AREA

Work on the dorsal aspect of the foot. Use your index finger and thumb to walk up from the base of the toes towards the ankle in between the metatarsals. Work with a medium pressure up as far as you can, then slide back to make circles lightly between the clefts of the toes. Repeat this movement six times to strengthen the body's immune system.

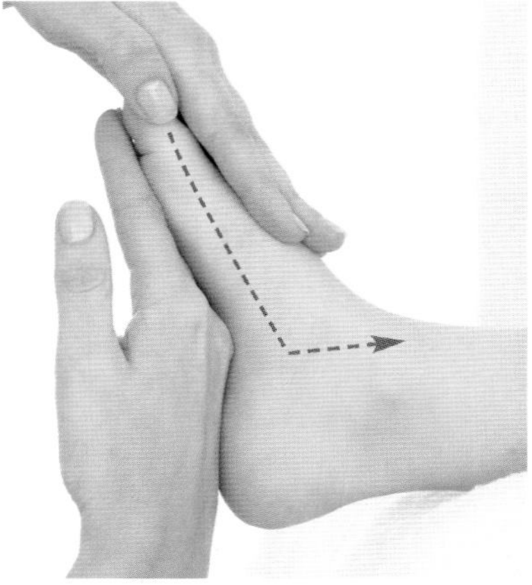

ENTIRE SPINE

Work on the medial aspect of the foot. Support the foot with one hand, and use your other thumb to walk gently seven steps in between the joints of the big toe, remembering that each step represents a specific vertebra. Walk towards the foot. Then take 12 gentle steps underneath the bone from the base of the joint of the big toe to work the thoracic vertebrae. You should end up on a bone called the navicular, which feels like a knuckle and is halfway between the bladder point and the ankle. Walk around the navicular bone, which represents lumbar one, taking five steps up to the dip in front of the ankle bone, which represents lumbar five. Repeat this movement gently three times.

Hyperactivity

Medically, this condition is termed attention-deficit hyperactivity disorder (ADHD). It causes a variety of learning and behavioural problems and mainly affects children. Hyperactivity may be characterized by a number of different behavioural problems, including an inability to finish tasks, head-knocking, self-destructive behaviour, temper tantrums, learning disabilities, low tolerance of stress and a lack of concentration. Factors linked to hyperactivity include heredity, smoking during pregnancy, oxygen deprivation at birth and food allergies. The consumption of sugar and additives in food has been strongly connected with hyperactive behaviour. It is therefore best to avoid the following: bacon, butter, carbonated drinks, mustard, confectionery, chocolate, soft drinks, coloured cheeses, hot dogs, ham, corn, milk, salt, salami, tea and wheat. If you think food allergies are contributing to your child's hyperactivity, see a qualified dietician who specializes in treating ADHD. Reflexology can work on the nervous and endocrine systems, to help encourage a state of calmness and balance, and on the digestive system, to help eliminate the allergens and other waste products.

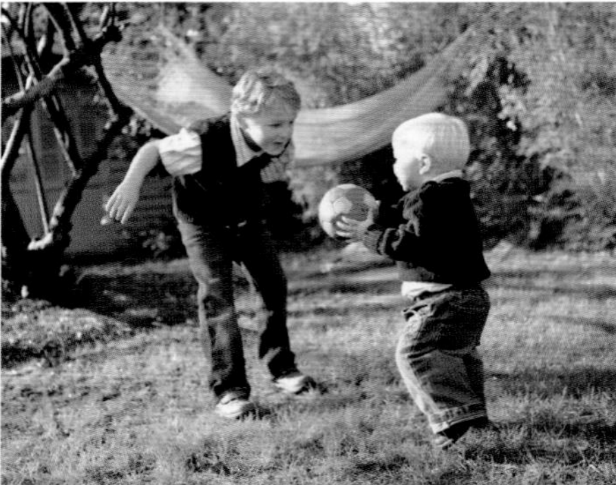

Research has shown that essential fatty acids may be of benefit when children have concentation problems.

REFLEX AREAS/POINTS TO WORK

- Pituitary
- Pancreas
- Adrenals
- Ascending/transverse colon
- Liver
- Entire spine

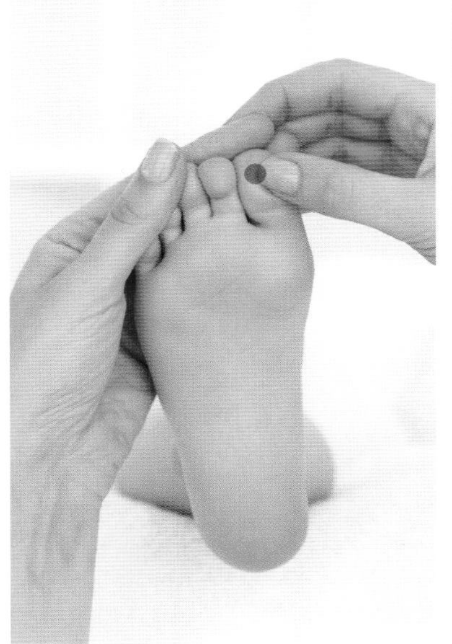

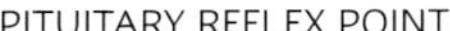

PITUITARY REFLEX POINT

Support the big toe with the fingers of one hand, and use your other thumb to make a cross to find the centre of the big toe. Place your thumb into the centre, push in and make circles for 15 seconds.

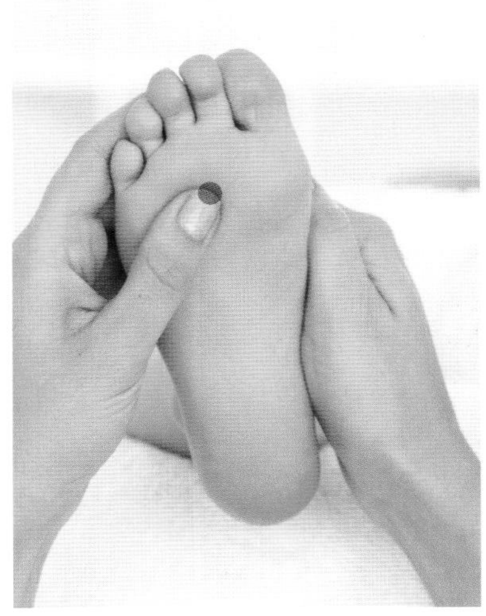

PANCREAS REFLEX POINT

This reflex point is only found on the right foot. Place your thumb on the third toe and trace a line down to below the diaphragm line. Push up into the joint and hook up for 12 seconds.

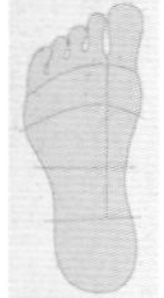

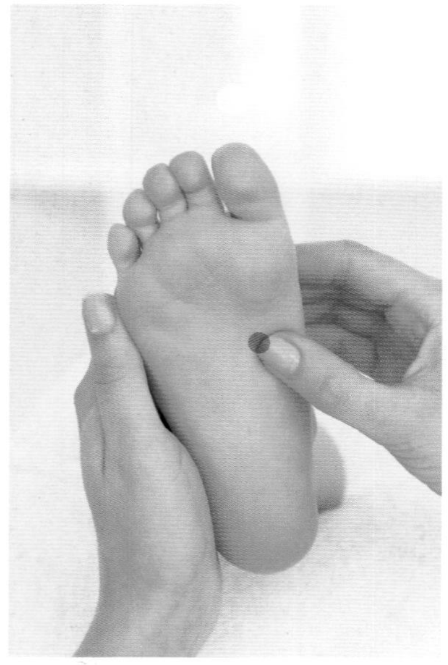

ADRENAL REFLEX POINT

You can find the adrenal reflexes in zone one, three steps down from the ball of the foot. Place your thumb in the point and gently push into the adrenal reflexes, making small circles. Work in this manner for 15 seconds.

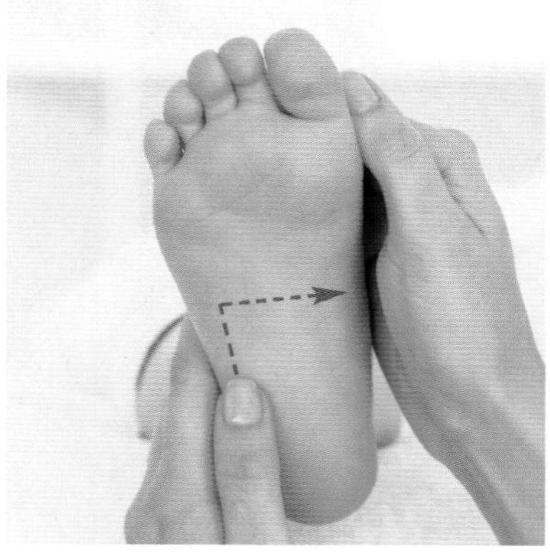

ASCENDING/TRANSVERSE COLON REFLEX

This reflex area is only found on the right foot. Use your left thumb to walk up zone four from the redness of the heel. Continue in this manner until you get halfway up the foot. Then turn your thumb to go right across the transverse colon. Repeat this four times in slow movements.

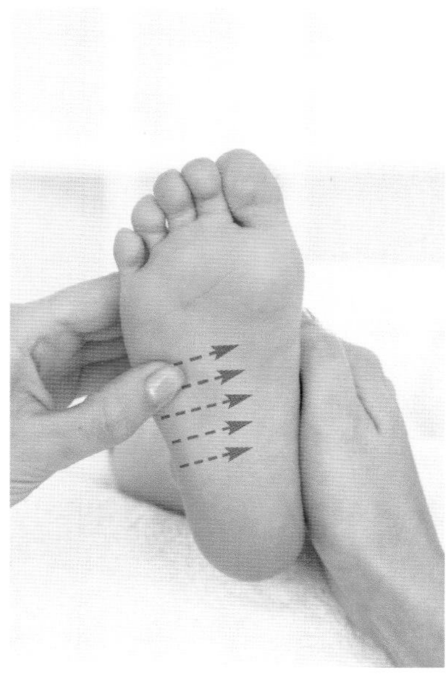

LIVER REFLEX AREA

This reflex area is only found on the right foot. Support the foot with your right hand, and place your left thumb just underneath the diaphragm line. Work slowly and precisely, horizontally across the foot, into zones five and four and just into zone three. Proceed in one direction. Continue in this manner until just above the redness of the heel, completing the liver reflex six times. Work with a light pressure.

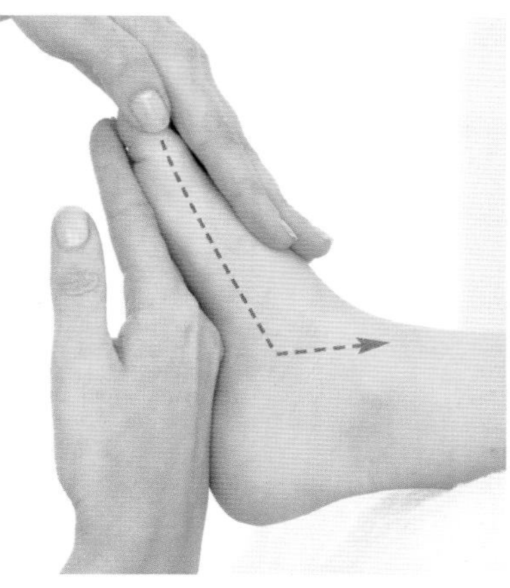

ENTIRE SPINE

Work on the medial aspect of the foot. Support the foot with one hand, and use your other thumb to walk gently seven steps in between the joints of the big toe, remembering that each step represents a specific vertebra. Walk towards the foot. Then take 12 gentle steps underneath the bone from the base of the joint of the big toe to work the thoracic vertebrae. You should end up on a bone called the navicular, which feels like a knuckle and is halfway between the bladder point and the ankle. Walk around the navicular bone, which represents lumbar one, taking five steps up to the dip in front of the ankle bone, which represents lumbar five. Repeat this movement gently three times.

THE GOLDEN YEARS

As we age, our immune system deteriorates and makes us more susceptible to disease. Most elderly people have at least three chronic illnesses, and they also lack vital energy and get tired very quickly. Ageing is a natural process and so is slowing down, because the body is becoming weaker – but this is not an indication that anything is wrong. We all feel tired after a hard day and our bodies slow down as a natural response; this is just part of the natural cycles and energies at different times in our lives. There are many factors that can sap an older person's enthusiasm for life, including a poor diet, insufficient money and loneliness, and this can create a sort of boredom and indifference to other family members, as well as to the world itself. A depressing self-fulfilling cycle can emerge whereby excessive worrying over minor aches and pains produces stress that further weakens the immune system, making someone even more susceptible to illness.

Reflexology is a very effective treatment for those in the golden years and can give them a sense of well-being, helping them to feel more balanced and better within themselves. It can also help with many aches and pains and can relieve the symptoms of chronic ailments. Always remember that on the most basic level reflexology can increase the circulation, which is very important for older people.

LIFESTYLE TIPS

Developing a healthy immune system is essential for the elderly. A good way to do this is by drinking chamomile tea during the day, because it increases levels of hippurate, which has been associated with increased antibacterial activity. This helps to explain why chamomile tea appears to boost the immune system and fight infections.

Gentle exercise is a wonderful way to boost the immune system and is key to promoting good health and longevity.

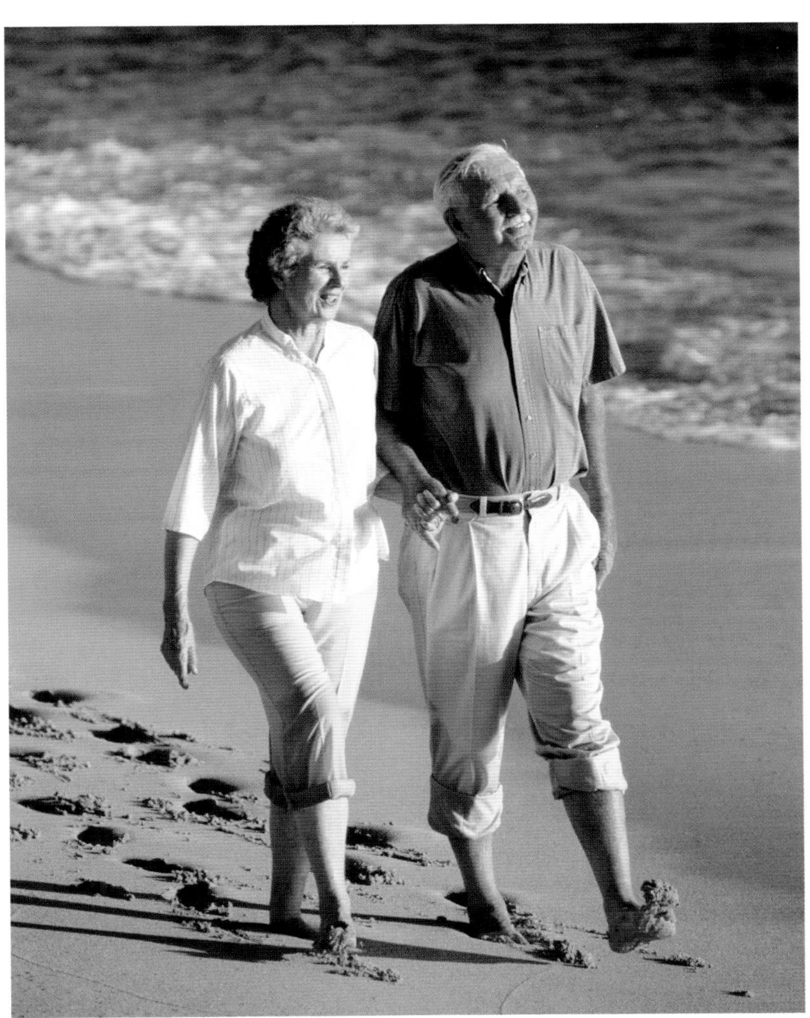

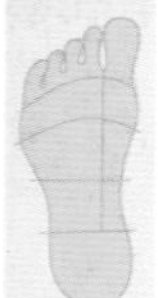

Alzheimer's disease

Alzheimer's disease is a type of dementia that commonly affects the elderly, although it can also strike people in their forties. Up to 50 per cent of Americans over 85 have Alzheimer's, which is characterized by a progressive mental degeneration that interferes with their ability to function at home or at work. Symptoms include memory loss, depression and severe mood swings, and death usually occurs within five to ten years. The precise cause is unknown, although research points to nutritional deficiencies, particularly of vitamins B12, A, E, boron, potassium and zinc. Autopsies of people who have died of Alzheimer's reveal excessive amounts of mercury and aluminium in the brain. It is useful to be aware that deep-water fish like tuna contain large amounts of mercury, as do fish liver oil supplements. But eating a well-balanced organic diet can help to increase the levels of vitamins and minerals in the body. Include lots of relaxation techniques to help your client feel they are in a safe place.

In 2006 a team at the University of Newcastle's Medicinal Plant Research Centre, led by Dr Ed Okello, found that both green and black tea inhibited the activity of enzymes connected with the development of Alzheimer's.

REFLEX AREAS/POINTS TO WORK

- Head
- Hypothalamus/pituitary
- Diaphragm
- Lungs
- Kidneys/adrenals
- Entire spine

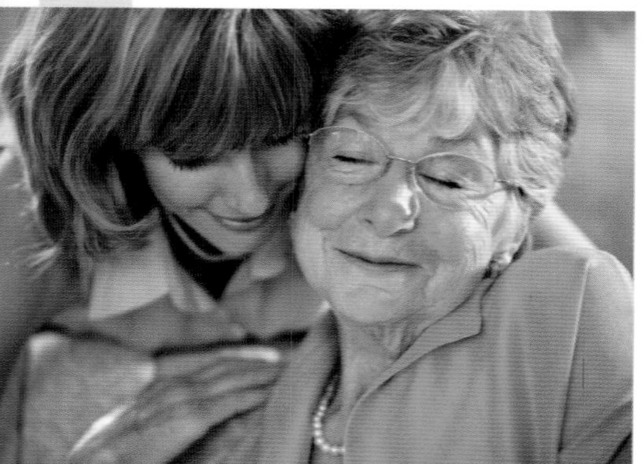

Reflexology is a calm and reassuring non-verbal method of communication.

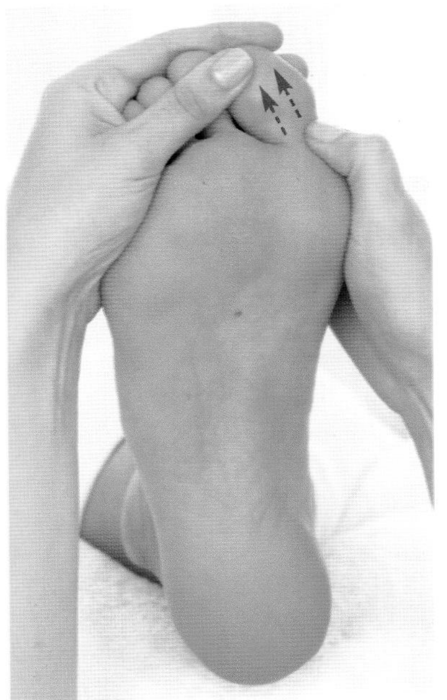

HEAD REFLEX AREA

Support the big toe with the fingers of one hand. Use your other thumb to walk up from the neckline to the top of the big toe. Repeat this several times in lines up the toe in a slow and gentle manner.

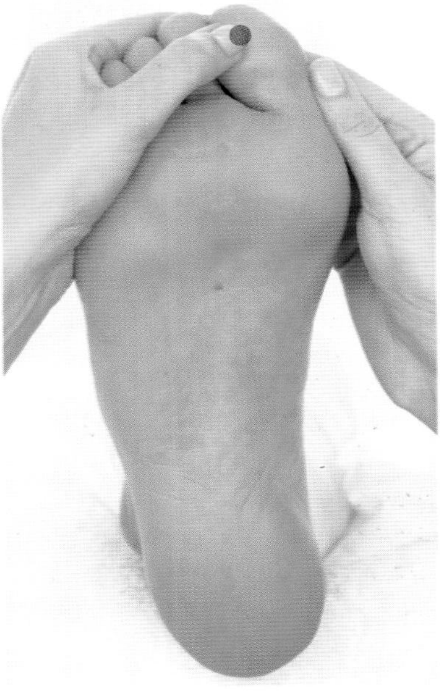

HYPOTHALAMUS/PITUITARY REFLEX POINT

Support the big toe with the fingers of one hand, then find the centre of the big toe. Place one thumb on the centre for the pituitary gland, and stimulate then take thumb one step up from the pituitary and one small step laterally and make circles for 30 seconds.

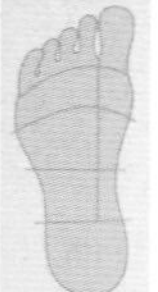

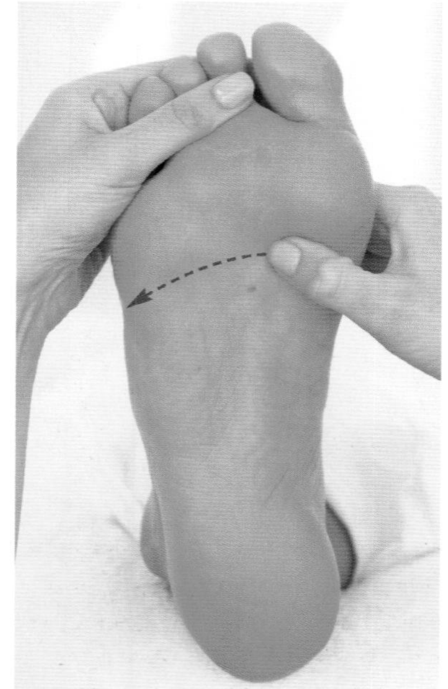

DIAPHRAGM REFLEX AREA

Flex the foot back with one hand to create skin tension. Use the thumb of your other hand to work under the metatarsal heads, across from the lateral to the medial aspect of the foot. Use slow steps and repeat this movement six times.

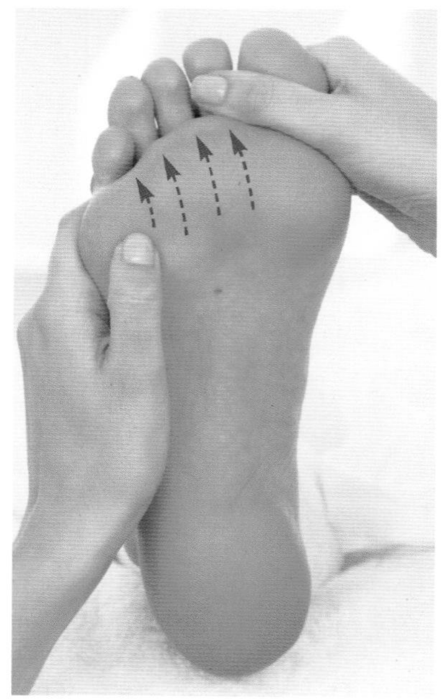

LUNG REFLEX AREA

Flex the foot back with your hand to create skin tension. Use the thumb of your other hand to work up from the diaphragm line to the eye/ear general area. You should be working in between the metatarsals. Repeat this process seven times, making sure you have worked in between all the metatarsals.

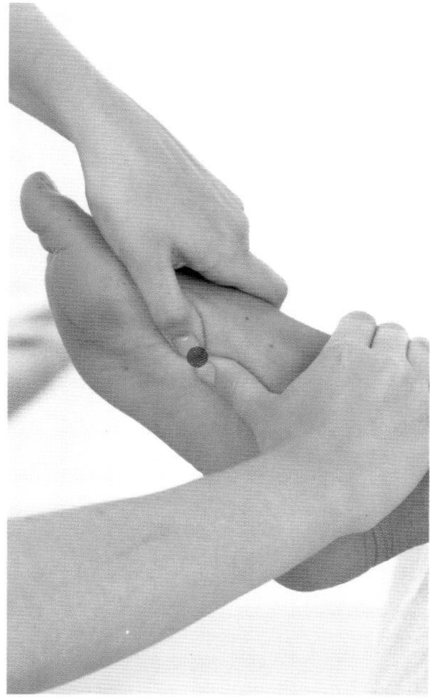

KIDNEY/ADRENAL REFLEX POINTS

You can find these reflexes in zone one, three steps down from the ball of the foot. Place your two thumbs together and gently push into the adrenal reflexes, making small circles. Work in this manner for 15 seconds.

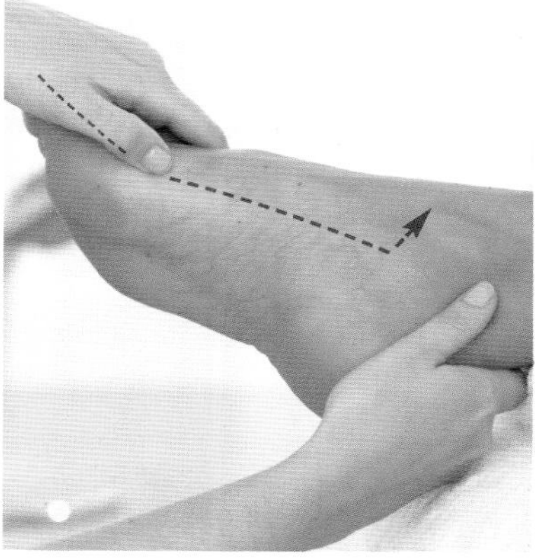

ENTIRE SPINE

Work on the medial aspect of the foot. Support the foot with one hand, and use your other thumb to walk gently seven steps in between the joints of the big toe, remembering that each step represents a specific vertebra. Walk towards the foot. Then take 12 gentle steps underneath the bone from the base of the joint of the big toe to work the thoracic vertebrae. You should end up on a bone called the navicular, which feels like a knuckle and is halfway between the bladder point and the ankle. Walk around the navicular bone, which represents lumbar one, taking five steps up to the dip in front of the ankle bone, which represents lumbar five. Repeat this movement gently three times.

Arthritis

This is one of the most common conditions in the elderly. Arthritis is the inflammation of one or many joints and is characterized by stiffness, pain and swelling. There is often a diminished range of motion, which can make it very difficult to do everyday activities. Arthritis is not a single disorder, but is the name for a joint problem with a number of causes. In most cases the sufferer will experience nearly constant pain. The overall pressure should be light, as older joints can be brittle and less flexible than younger ones, and should not cause any discomfort; if it does, reduce the pressure to a comfortable level.

REFLEX AREAS/POINTS TO WORK

- Pituitary
- Parathyroids
- Kidneys/adrenals
- Ascending colon
- Descending colon
- Entire spine
- Liver

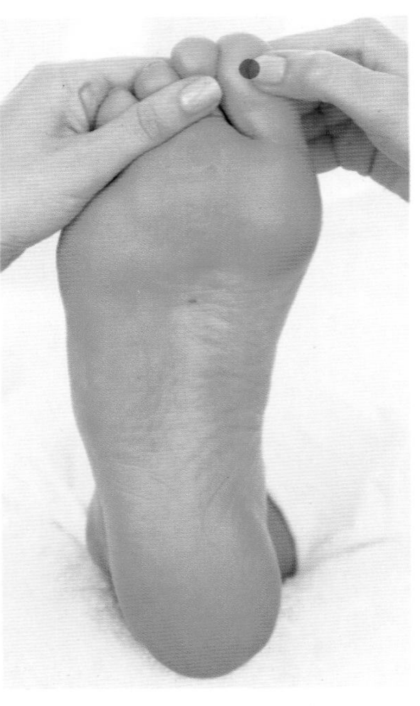

PITUITARY REFLEX POINT

Support the big toe with the fingers of one hand, and use your other thumb to make a cross to find the centre of the big toe. Place your thumb into the centre, push in and make circles for 15 seconds.

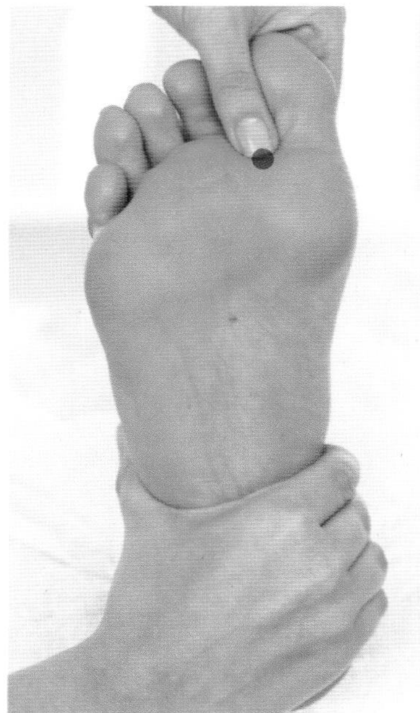

PARATHYROID REFLEX POINT

You can find this point in between the big toe and second toe. Use your index finger and thumb to pinch the section of skin between the first and second toes. Hold the pressure and gently make circles for six seconds.

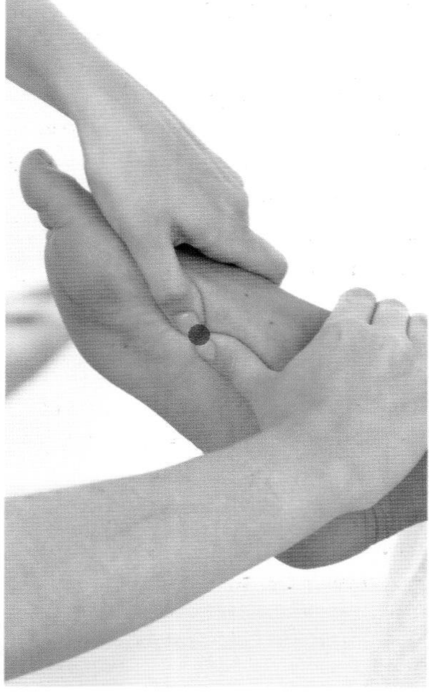

KIDNEY/ADRENAL REFLEX POINTS

You can find these reflexes in zone one, three steps down from the ball of the foot. Place your two thumbs together and gently push into the kidney/adrenal reflexes, making small circles. Work in this manner for 15 seconds.

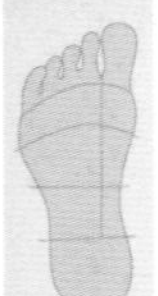

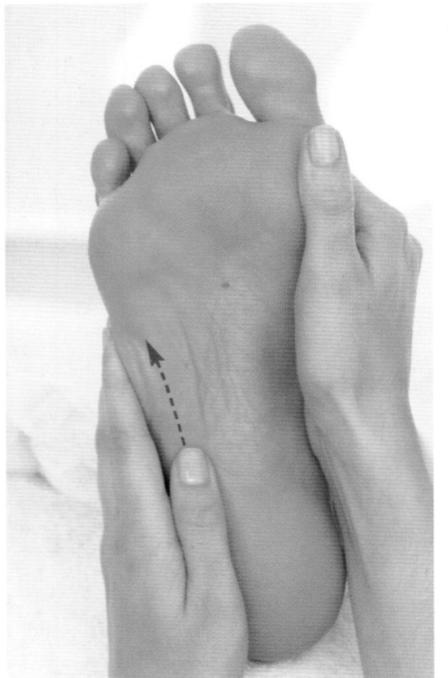

ASCENDING COLON REFLEX AREA

This reflex area is only found on the right foot. Use your left thumb to walk up zone four from the redness of the heel. Continue in this manner until you get halfway up the foot. Work the ascending colon reflex area four times in slow movements to help clean out the colon.

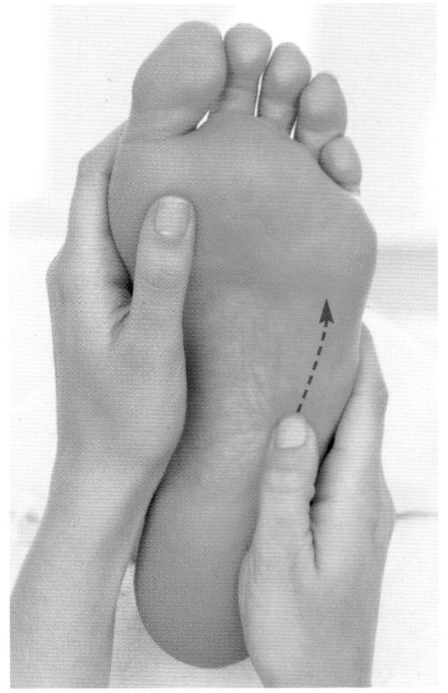

DESCENDING COLON REFLEX AREA

This reflex area is only found on the left foot. Use your right thumb to walk up zone four from the redness of the heel, to work this part of the colon. Continue in this manner until you arrive halfway up the foot. Work this reflex area six times and in slow movements to help stimulate the peristaltic muscular action of the colon.

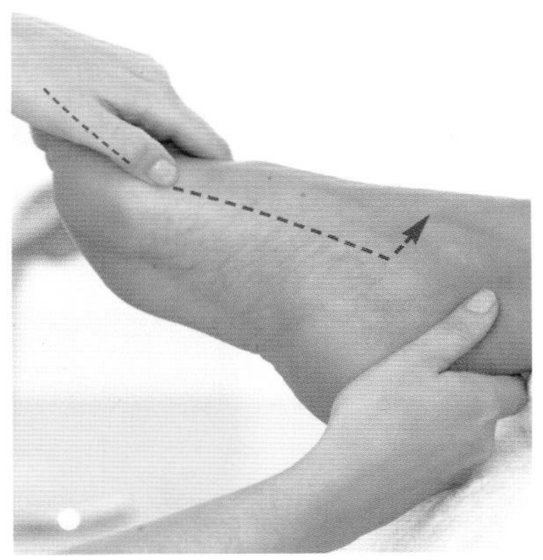

ENTIRE SPINE

Work on the medial aspect of the foot. Support the foot with one hand, and use your other thumb to walk gently seven steps in between the joints of the big toe, remembering that each step represents a specific vertebra. Walk towards the foot. Then take 12 gentle steps underneath the bone from the base of the joint of the big toe to work the thoracic vertebrae. You should end up on a bone called the navicular, which feels like a knuckle and is halfway between the bladder point and the ankle. Walk around the navicular bone, which represents lumbar one, taking five steps up to the dip in front of the ankle bone, which represents lumbar five. Repeat this movement gently three times.

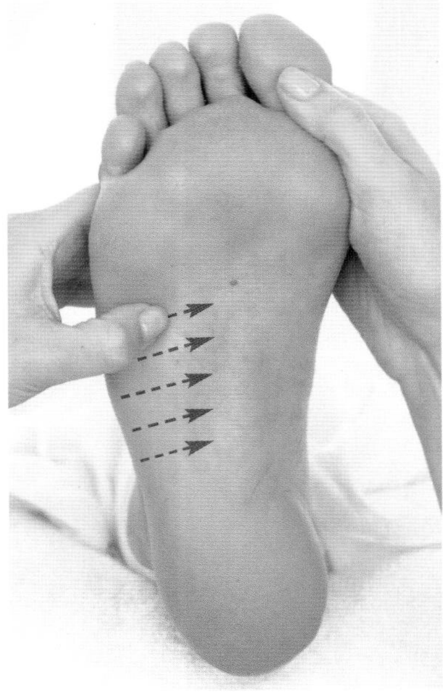

LIVER REFLEX AREA

This reflex area is only found on the right foot. Support the foot with your right hand, and place your left thumb just underneath the diaphragm line. Work slowly and precisely, horizontally across the foot, into zones five and four and just into zone three. Proceed in one direction. Continue in this manner until just above the redness of the heel. Complete the liver reflex movement six times.

REFLEXOLOGY FOR COUPLES

Touch is one of the best ways to improve intimate relationships. Being intimate with each other is important for your self-esteem and positive personal regard. It can open up the energy lines flowing through the body, helping you to relax and making it easier to express yourself both verbally and physically. Regular reflexology is a simple step towards regaining intimacy and can help to rejuvenate a positive relationship. Agree a time to give your loved one a reflexology session and to receive one. Once you have both enjoyed the treatments, sit opposite each other and use relaxation techniques playfully.

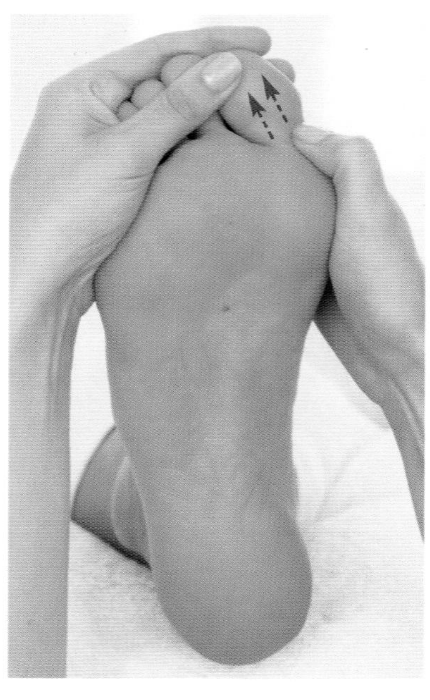

HEAD REFLEX AREA

Support the big toe with the fingers of one hand. Use your other thumb to walk up from the neckline to the top of the big toe. Repeat this several times in lines up the toe.

REFLEX AREAS/POINTS TO WORK

- Head
- Entire spine
- Diaphragm
- Thyroid
- Lungs
- Ascending colon
- Descending colon

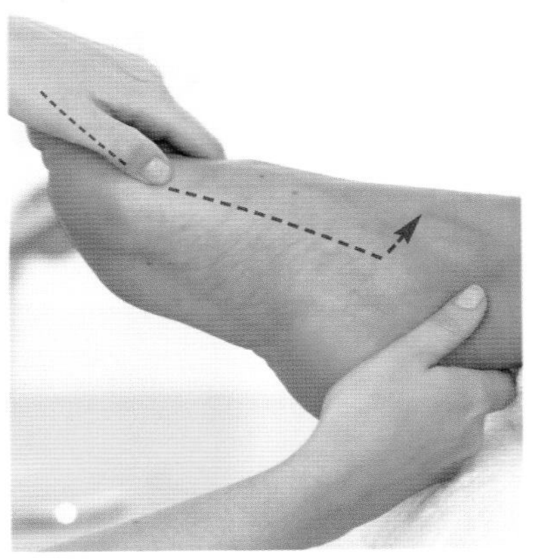

ENTIRE SPINE

Work on the medial aspect of the foot. Support the foot with one hand, and use your other thumb to walk gently seven steps in between the joints of the big toe, remembering that each step represents a specific vertebra. Walk towards the foot. Then take 12 gentle steps underneath the bone from the base of the joint of the big toe to work the thoracic vertebrae. You should end up on a bone called the navicular, which feels like a knuckle and is halfway between the bladder point and the ankle. Walk around the navicular bone, which represents lumbar one, taking five steps up to the dip in front of the ankle bone, which represents lumbar five. Repeat this movement gently three times.

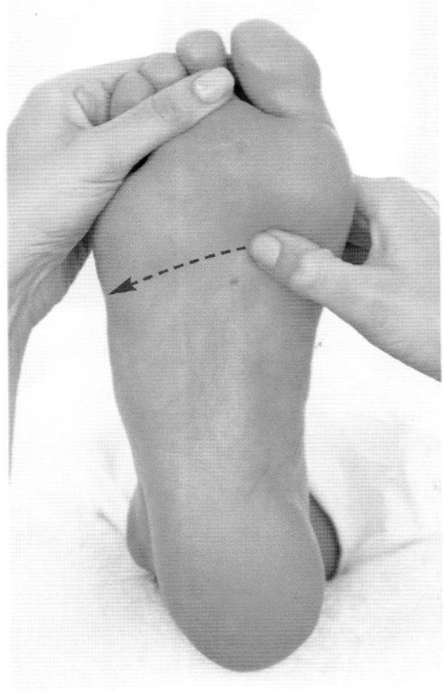

DIAPHRAGM REFLEX AREA

Flex the foot back with one hand to create skin tension. Use the thumb of your other hand to work under the metatarsal heads, across from the lateral to the medial aspect of the foot. Use slow steps and repeat this movement six times.

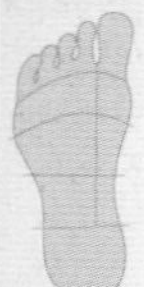

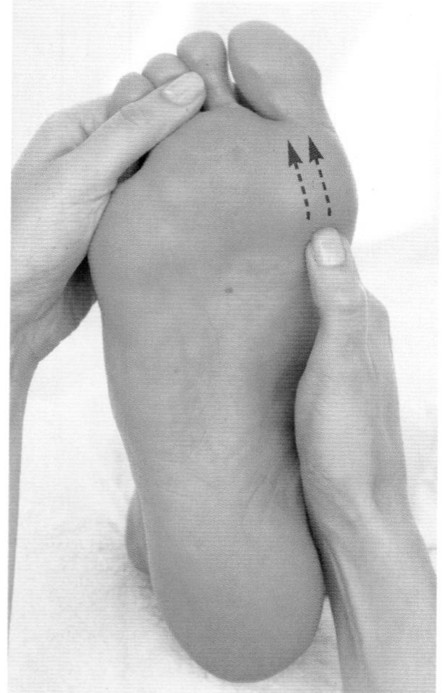

THYROID REFLEX AREA

Use one thumb to work the ball of the foot from the diaphragm line all the way up to the neckline. Repeat this movement slowly six times over the area to help boost energy levels.

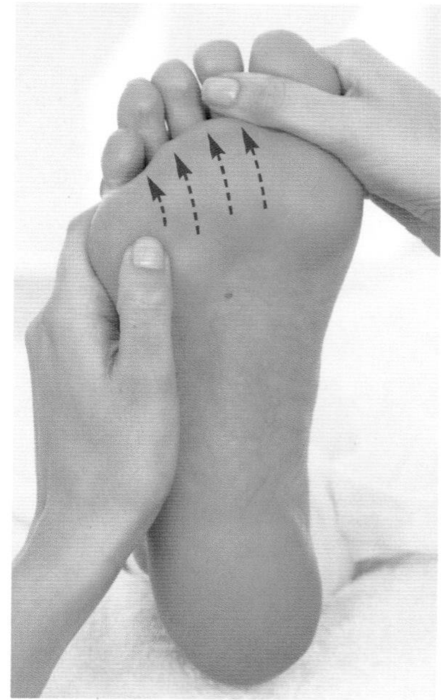

LUNG REFLEX AREA

Flex the foot back with one hand to create skin tension. Use the thumb of your other hand to work up from the diaphragm line to the eye/ear general area. You should be working in between the metatarsals. Repeat this process seven times, making sure you have worked in between all the metatarsals.

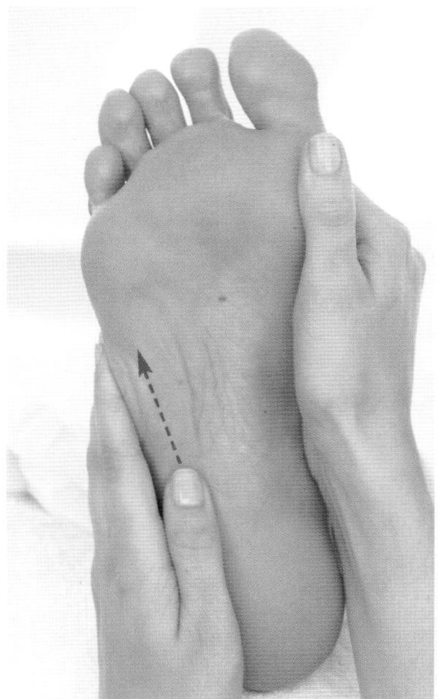

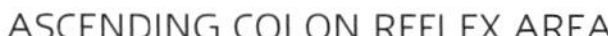

ASCENDING COLON REFLEX AREA

This reflex area is only found on the right foot. Use your left thumb to walk up zone four from the redness of the heel. Continue in this manner until you get halfway up the foot. Work the ascending colon reflex area four times in slow movements to help keep the colon clean.

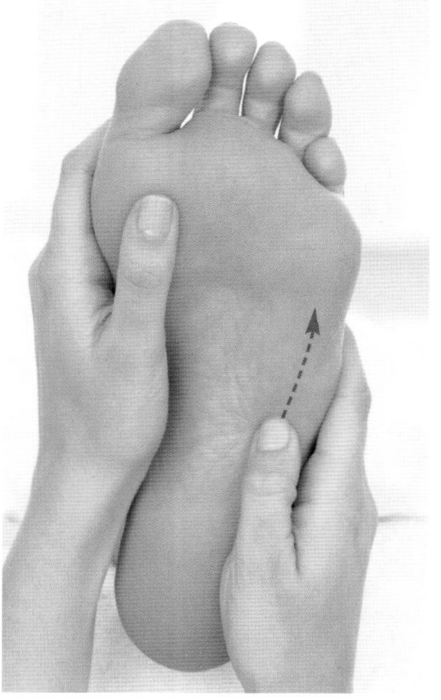

DESCENDING COLON REFLEX AREA

This reflex area is only found on the left foot. Use your right thumb to walk up zone four from the redness of the heel, to work this part of the colon. Continue in this manner until you arrive halfway up the foot. Work this reflex area six times and in slow movements to help stimulate the peristaltic muscular action of the colon.

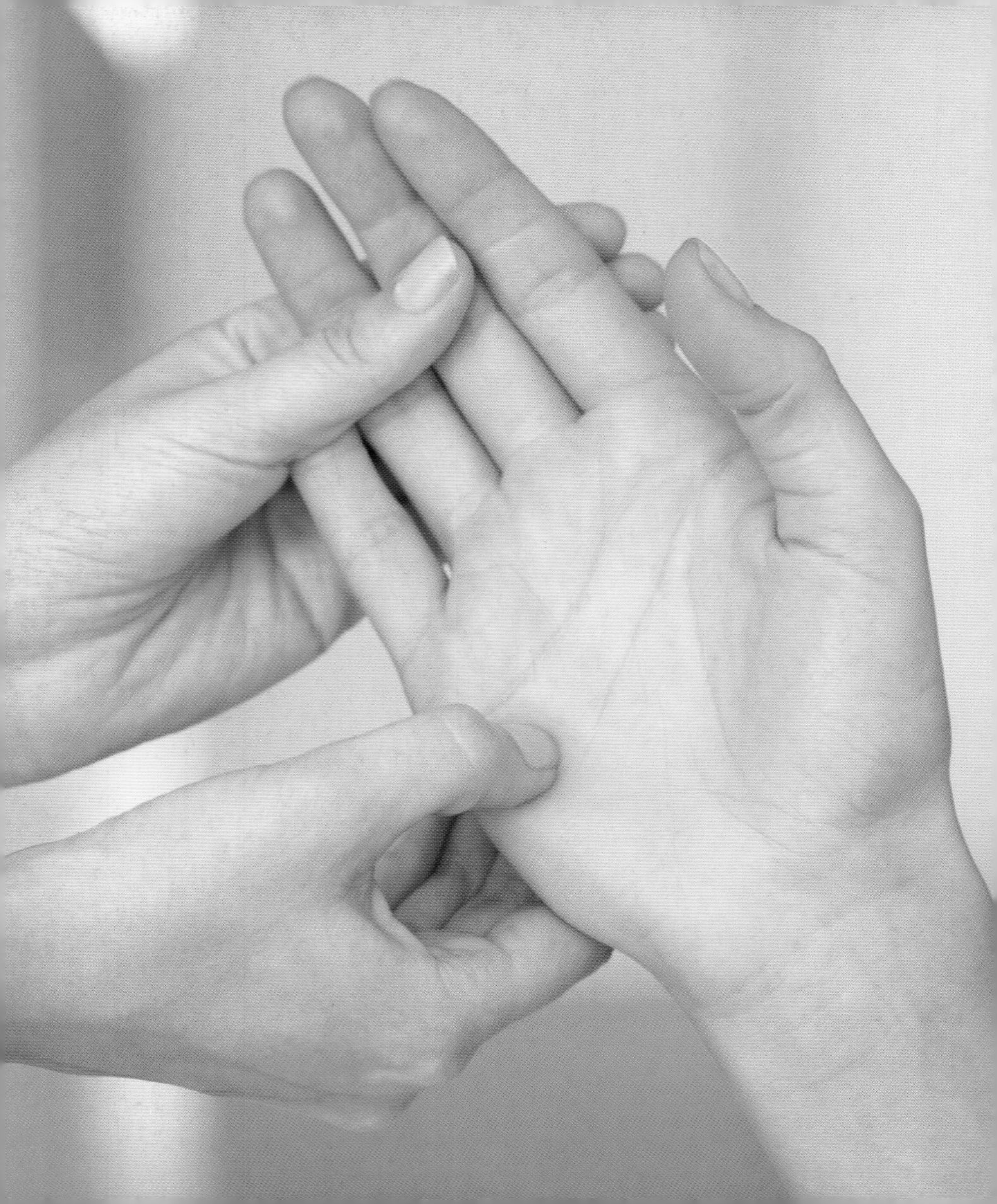

PART 7

Treating the hands

Working on the hands

Hand reflexology is an exceptionally relaxing treatment to receive and provides the recipient with the chance to unwind fully. The wonderful thing about giving a hand-reflexology treatment is that you can treat someone virtually anywhere, from an aeroplane, train or car to an office, shop or home. It is a safe, natural healing art that you can also use to treat yourself, wherever and whenever you wish.

Hand reflexology is empowering because, whether someone suffers from irritable bowel syndrome, sinusitis, headaches or needs relief from stress, it can help. It can be used as an alternative

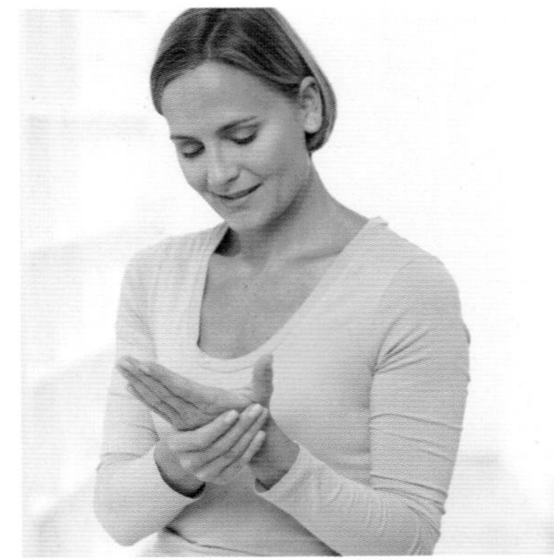

Working on your own hands, whenever you feel the need, can be self-empowering.

SITUATIONS WHERE HAND REFLEXOLOGY IS PREFERABLE

- The feet are badly infected with a fungal infection like athlete's foot
- The feet have many verrucae that cover large areas of the foot
- The feet have been injured recently by a sprain or strain
- A bone in the foot is broken
- The feet are in a plaster cast
- One foot (or both) has been amputated
- The client is embarrassed by their feet
- The feet are too ticklish for treatment
- The feet have extreme structural pain (perhaps from arthritis).

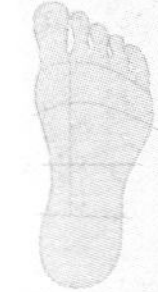

to foot reflexology; for example if someone has a foot injury, a leg and foot in a cast, ticklish feet, or if they don't want you to work on their feet for personal reasons. It also makes a good alternative for those suffering from infections such as athlete's foot and for amputees.

Self-treatment

There are very few body therapies that you can use effectively on yourself. Although foot reflexology is widely known, it is not easy to give yourself a treatment because on the whole it is uncomfortable to do so. With hand reflexology you can give yourself treatment and get amazing results. Treatments can focus on just two or three reflex points, so that you can work on them throughout the day to stimulate your body's own healing mechanisms.

Believing that you will be doing yourself good uses the power of the mind and, together with the positive action of hand reflexology, can help on many different levels. Just think of the power you can have over your own body. You can help to relieve common ailments such as constipation, frozen shoulder and anxiety attacks by working the relevant reflex point on your own hands.

Benefits of hand reflexology

Hand reflexology has many benefits, including the following:

- The hands are more accessible than the feet.
- If time is short, hand reflexology can be gentler and less disruptive.
- It is a treatment the elderly generally prefer as it is so relaxing.
- The hands are closer to the spine and the nerve roots, so treatments can really relax the central nervous system.
- Helps with any stress-related condition.
- Helps to relieve pain in the hands and arms associated with conditions such as multiple sclerosis, tenosynovitis, frozen shoulder, tennis elbow, whiplash, carpal tunnel syndrome, repetitive strain injury and rheumatoid arthritis.
- You can work on your own hands.
- Clients can work on their own hands between treatments.

Aspects of the hands

There are four different views or 'aspects' in hand reflexology, just as there are in foot reflexology. All the reflexology points and areas are located in very specific places, as in foot reflexology, and familiarizing yourself with the various aspects will help you locate these points and areas when you come to the basic hand-reflexology treatment (see pages 374–389). The aspects are as follows:

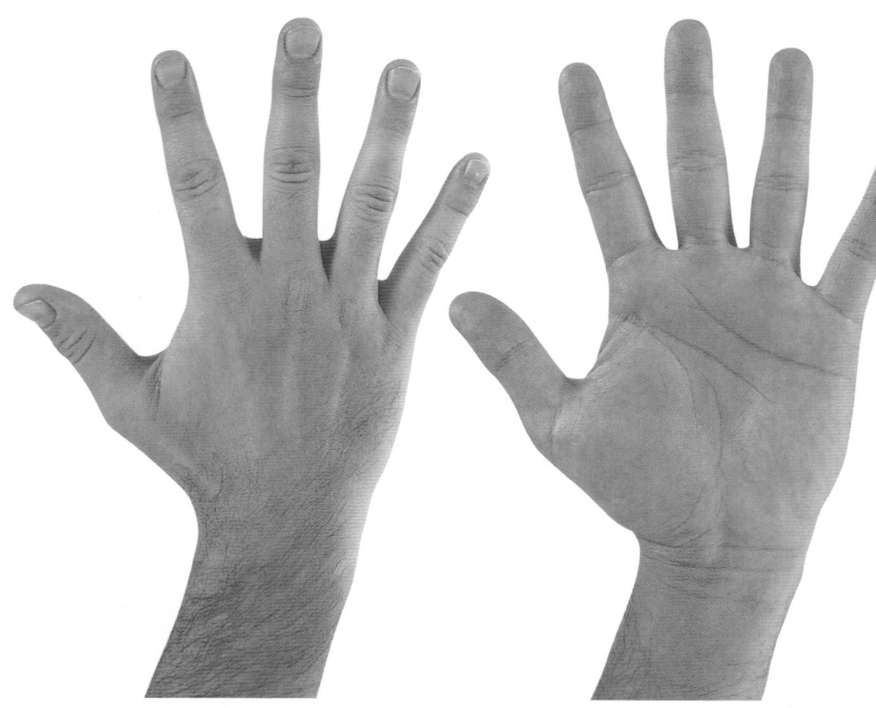

DORSAL ASPECT

PALMAR ASPECT

- **Dorsal aspect:** the view of the top of the hand as you look down at it.
- **Palmar aspect:** the view of the palm or underside of the hand.
- **Medial aspect:** the inside edge of the hand, running from the thumb to the wrist.
- **Lateral aspect:** the outside edge of the hand, running from the little finger to the wrist.

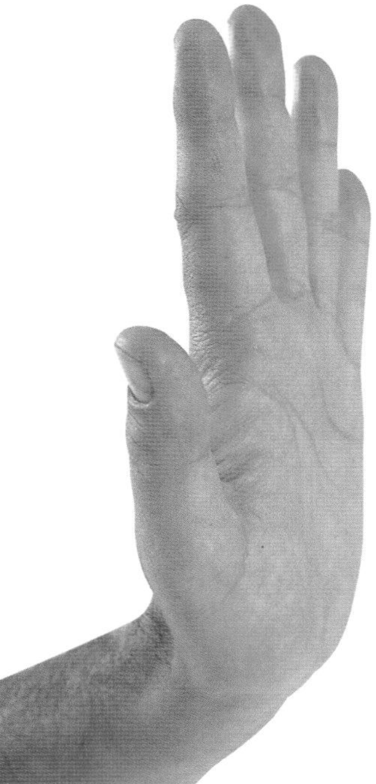

MEDIAL ASPECT

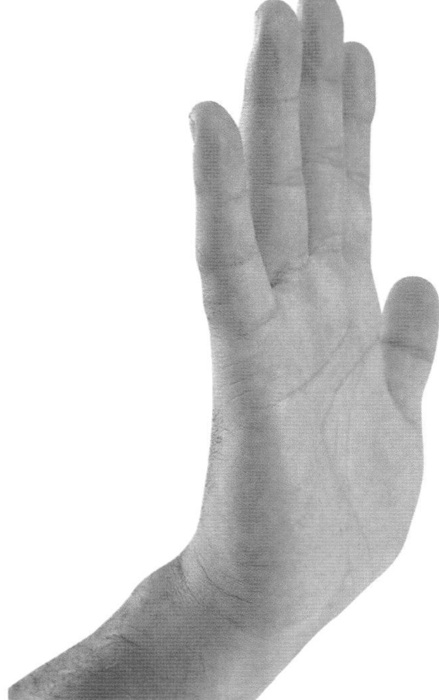

LATERAL ASPECT

Hand reflexology charts

The hand reflexology charts will help you identify where to find the reflexology points that correspond to different parts of the body. The more you look at these charts, the easier it will be when you give a treatment, because you will have familiarized yourself with the location of many of the reflex points.

HAND REFLEXOLOGY DORSAL ASPECT

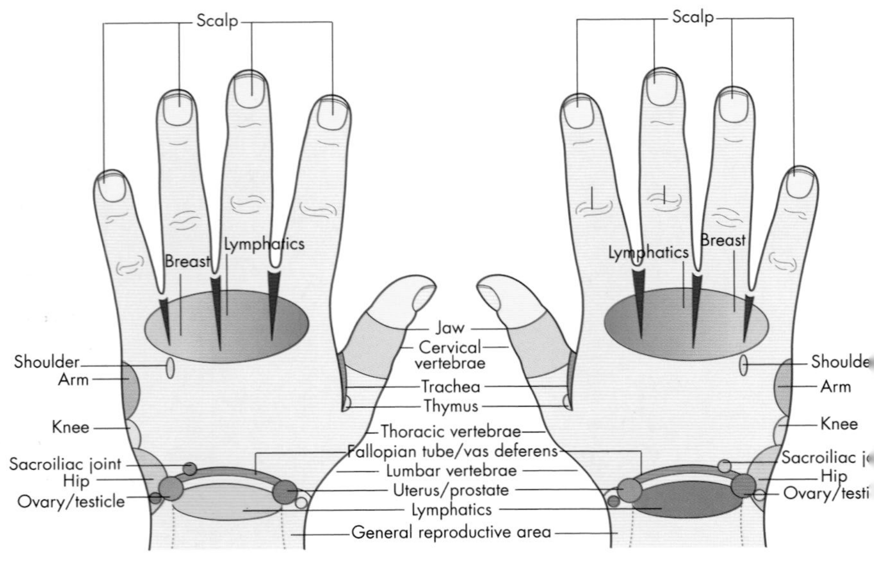

LEFT HAND

RIGHT HAND

HAND REFLEXOLOGY PALMAR ASPECT

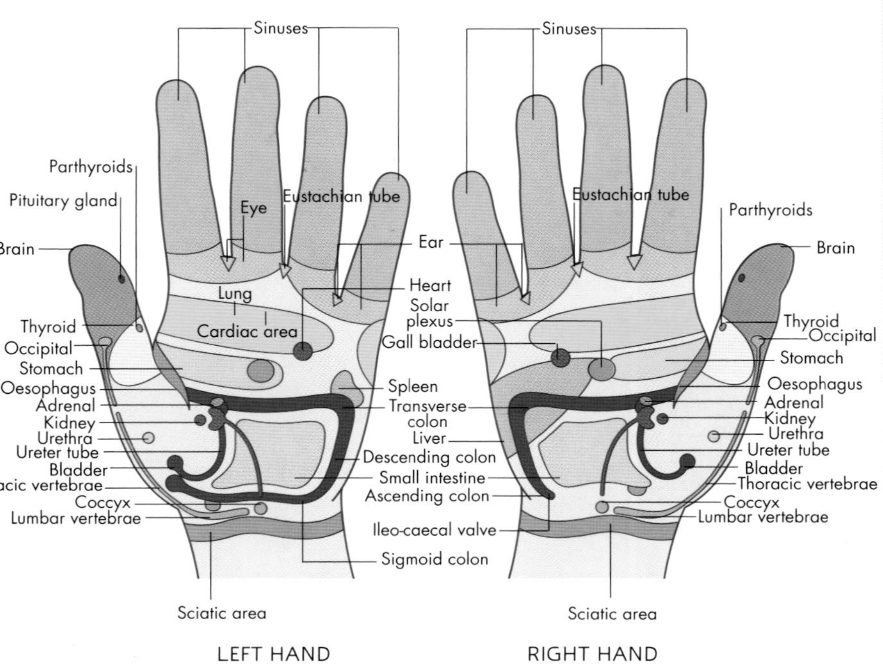

Preparing to treat

Treating someone with hand reflexology can simply involve taking their hand and working the reflex points. You can do this either standing up or sitting down, and it may take anything from 20 seconds to a couple of minutes. However, the basic hand reflexology treatment should take around 40 minutes. Here are some points to consider before giving a treatment:

- Try to look professional (see page 106), because it shows that you respect the treatment and the person you are treating; it is also the best way to ensure that your client will respect the treatment.
- Always have clean, short nails when giving reflexology treatments.
- Prepare a warm, comfortable environment.
- Cover a pillow with a towel before placing your client's hands on it; this keeps their hands well supported, and you can use the towel to keep warm the hand that you are not working on.
- Make sure that both you and your client are comfortable throughout the treatment.
- Establish eye contact with your client so that you can adjust the pressure to avoid any discomfort.
- Remove your own jewellery and ask your client to do the same.

Massage media

I like to use cornflour, with which I have created a signature scent and which is a safe alternative to talcum powder. If you use this, you are looking after your own hands, too. Alternatively you can also use a good base oil, such as grapeseed oil, which will feel relaxing for your client and will not dry out the skin on the hands. Older clients often prefer to have oil used on them, but it all depends on what you feel your client would like.

Before you start a treatment I suggest you rinse your hands under warm water: if your hands are cold the treatment will certainly not be as relaxing for your client! It is a good idea not to eat spicy foods or food containing garlic before a hand reflexology treatment because the client may smell it on your breath. You may even wish to use a mouthwash because you are so close to them during treatment.

Always remember to support the hands as best you can so your client can relax and be comfortable through the treatment.

It is essential to remove all jewellery before starting a treatment and wash your own hands to cleanse and warm them.

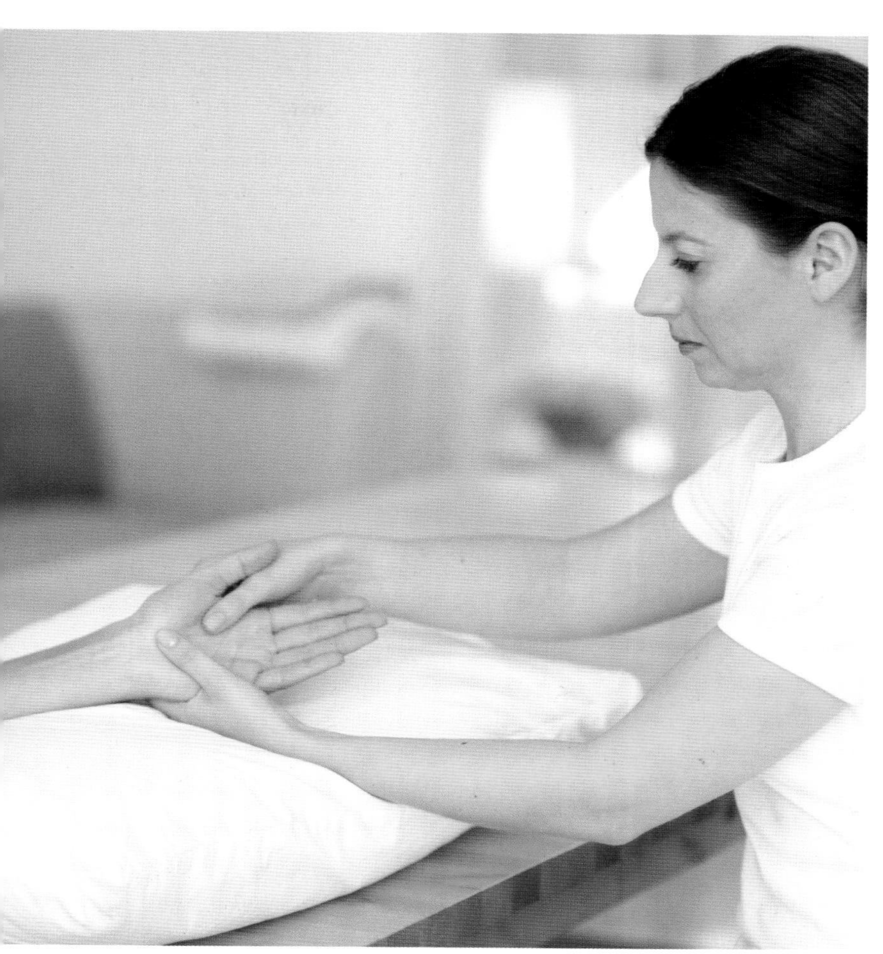

The healing space

You do not need any specific equipment to give a hand reflexology treatment. You can simply use whatever is available and adapt the environment to make both you and your client comfortable.

Treatment positions

There are six different positions in which you can give a hand reflexology treatment, depending on where you are. One great benefit of hand reflexology is that it is very versatile. The more comfortable you both are, the longer you can make your session last, resulting in a more fulfilling treatment.

1 Standing up

Stand up facing your client, who should also be standing and should be very close to you. If you take their hands in turn, you can access the reflex points. This is not the ideal position for giving a full treatment, but can be used successfully to work on certain reflexes.

2 Lying on a bed/sofa

Ask your client to lie down comfortably on the bed or sofa. Sit on a stool next to the client's right hand, which should ideally be placed on a pillow on your lap for support. Face your client so that you can observe any reactions to the treatment. Move yourself to the other side of the bed to begin treatment on the left hand.

3 Sitting opposite each other on the floor close enough to reach hands

Put two cushions on the floor so that you can sit comfortably opposite each other. Place your client's right hand on a cushion positioned on your lap. When you have finished treating it, work on the left hand. Try to keep your back straight throughout the session. This is a good position to use if you do not have any suitable furniture available.

4 Sitting opposite each other across a table on comfortable chairs

Find a small table, then place a pillow in the centre of the table and sit on a chair facing your client across the table. Your hands should be able to reach across the table while you are both sitting comfortably.

5 Sitting on chairs facing each other

Find two chairs and place them facing each other, but side by side (so that if the chairs had arms, they would be touching). Sit in the chairs facing each other. Place

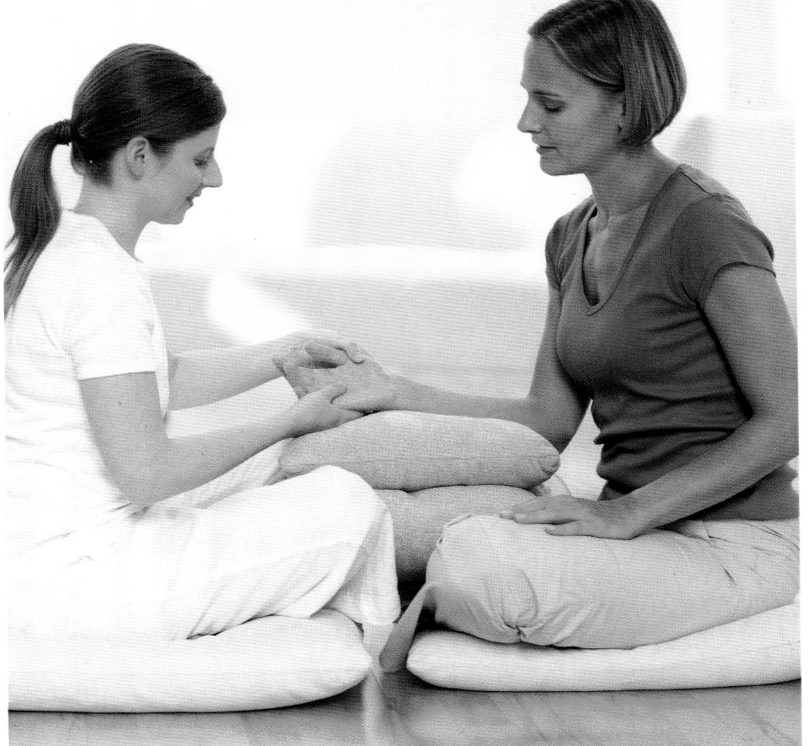

your client's right hand on a pillow on your lap and begin the session. Move to the other side of the client's chair to begin treatment on their left hand.

6 Sitting on a sofa

Ask your client to sit or lie down comfortably on a sofa. Make yourself comfortable on a chair, stool or the edge of the sofa next to their right hand. Place their hand on a pillow on your lap. Once you have finished treating it, ask your client to change direction so that you can easily reach their left hand.

If you choose the floor, sit on cushions for comfort and place the client's hand on further cushions at the right height.

Strengthening your hands

Keeping your hands strong is important in reflexology, because if you overuse them it could cause repetitive strain injury (RSI). So keep to a light to medium pressure and use both hands so that they share the work. On the whole you can use a much lighter pressure than you would for foot reflexology. Preventing many hand injuries revolves around one very important thing: warming up. Before you start, stretch out your hands and fingers and use the exercises shown here. Strengthening your hands can prevent damage and injuries from over use. Exercising the hands can strengthen grip, increase dexterity and improve mobility of the wrist. It promotes coordination, increases the range of motion and is also a neuromuscular and balance-training aid.

You don't necessarily need to spend more than a minute or two on these exercises, but please do warm up your hands for at least that long. Once you have done this, your hand and wrist muscles will be sufficiently warm to prevent major injuries.

Techniques

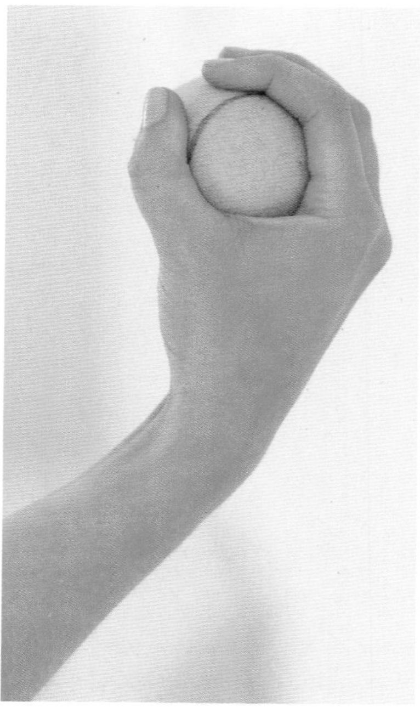

Place a tennis ball in the palm of your hand and squeeze it as hard as you can for two minutes, then swap hands. This will help to stimulate the blood supply throughout your hands and strengthen the muscles, nerves and joints.

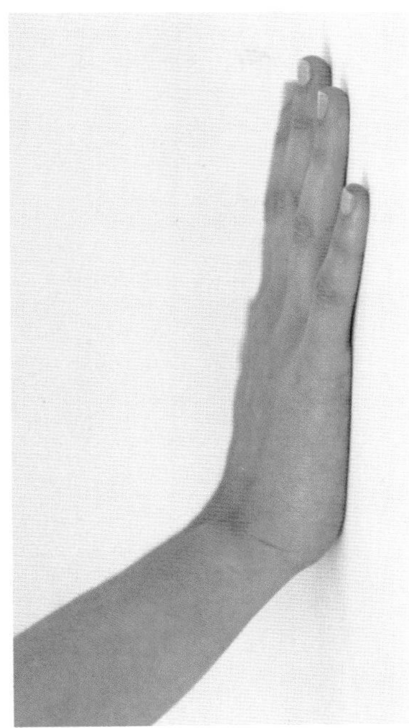

Place the palm of your hand on the surface of a flat wall. Push your hand against the wall, which will flex the hand and wrist. Hold this movement for ten seconds and then swap hands. Repeat this for two minutes each day.

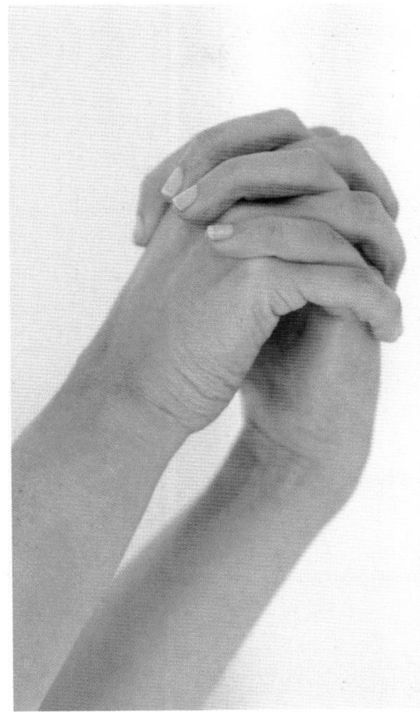

Interlock the fingers of one hand with the fingers of the other hand. Slowly rotate your hands in large clockwise circles for one minute. Then slowly rotate them in anticlockwise circles for one minute.

How to use the treatments

The basic hand reflexology sequence can be used on anybody, from the early years to the golden years of life. Your pressure should vary from light to medium, according to the person you are treating. Aim to create a smooth rhythm in the way your thumb or fingers flow throughout the therapy. You will always feel more crystals, and create a better flow of treatment, if you work in the direction of your thumb or fingernail. The techniques illustrated in this section include arrows showing the direction of movement, where applicable.

Flex your client's hand a lot during treatment, because this will enable you to feel more crystals, and your client will feel more fully the sensations from a reflex point. You also need to stay on a hand reflex point longer than in foot reflexology, because the hands are less sensitive to treatment. Keep in mind that an important objective is to meet the needs of your client and make it a relaxing, memorable treatment so they get the benefits.

If you are treating a baby, the techniques differ. You should still follow the directional arrows, but do not use the compression snake (see page 371), mole (see page 372) or crab-claw techniques (see page 373) with your thumb or finger. Instead, use the tip of your index finger and lightly stroke over the reflex areas as though you were the conductor of an orchestra. When you are working on babies with reflexology, they need far less pressure than adults.

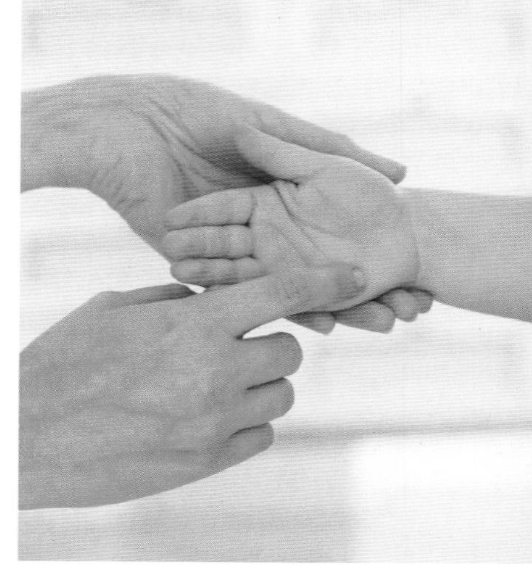

When performing a treatment on a baby or young child, the pressure you exert should be kept very light.

Reading reflexes in the hands

During treatment you are helping to restore energy throughout the body and to stimulate the body's natural healing abilities. You also want to 'read' the hands to try and identify weak areas with which your client needs help, by searching for crystals and looking for areas of pain or discomfort.

You can ask your client if they find any areas painful, or you may feel their fingers flinch when you work on a sensitive reflex area or point. There are fewer crystals to be felt in the hands than in the feet, but when you do find them, use the hand-reflexology techniques (see pages 370–373) to disperse them gently. Crystals or pain indicate an imbalance in the corresponding area of the body. For example, a crystal in the shoulder reflex may reflect a past, current or future problem in the shoulder.

The main difference from the feet is that we use our hands in many more ways. Our hands are also more exposed to pressure, which naturally breaks down a lot of the crystals that you would otherwise find. If someone tells you that an area is sensitive, reduce the pressure and continue to work very gently on that area for a further ten seconds.

Watch your client's face, holding eye contact if possible, so that you can relieve pressure if discomfort is evident.

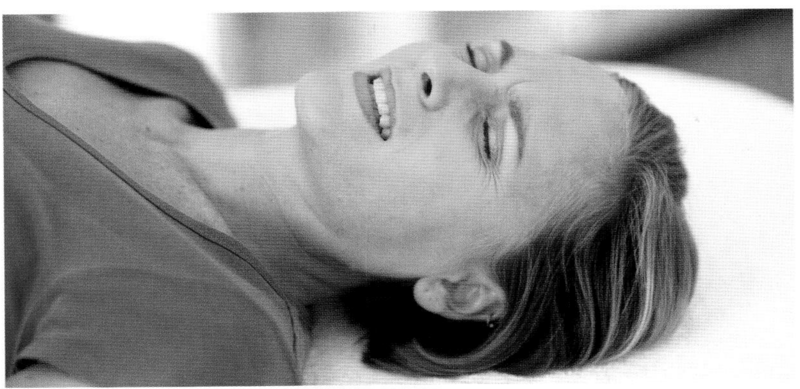

Relaxing the hands

The following relaxation movements are designed to convey your client to a state of calmness and balance and to a place of safety. As you work on their hands, watch your client's face relax and all their worries melt away. Their breathing will change to a deeper, slower rhythm. You will see their tension drop away from their shoulders down through their arms. The muscles in their hands will become easier to work on, as their body begins to explore its own self-healing capabilities.

Always start and end your treatment with these relaxation movements. They can last for as long or as short a time as you wish.

Having a hand reflexology treatment can be a wonderful way to relax and unwind.

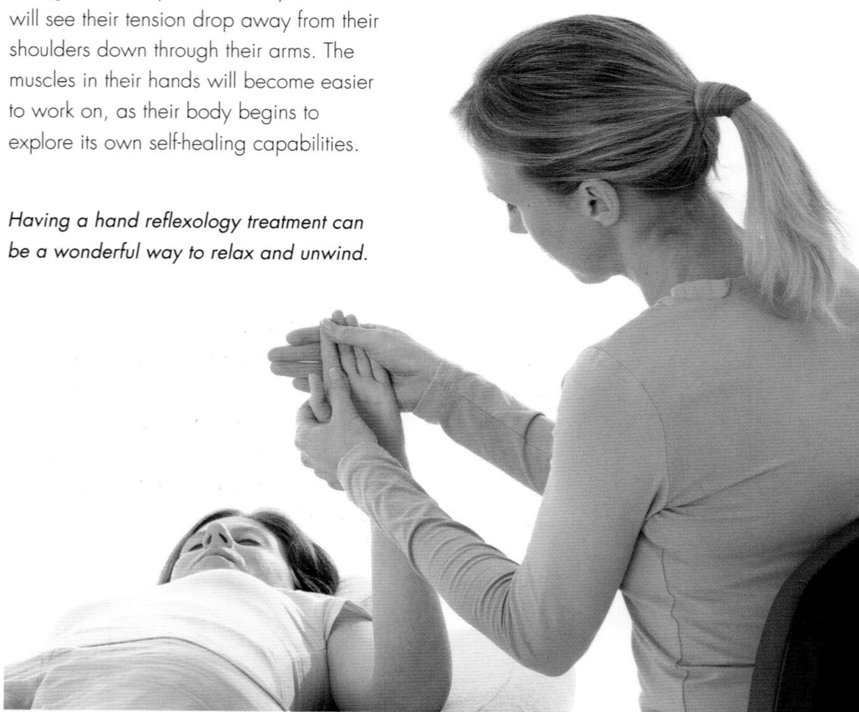

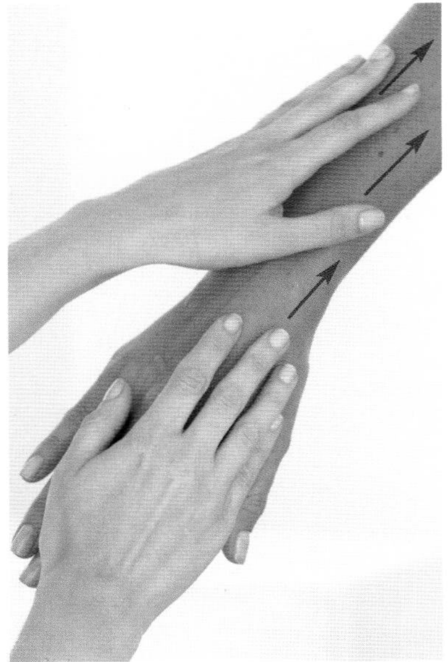

BUTTERFLY TOUCH

Place both of your palms on your client's right hand and gently move your hands up the arm and back down again. Both your hands should work together with a medium pressure. Now work on the left hand. Continue this movement for one minute on each hand.

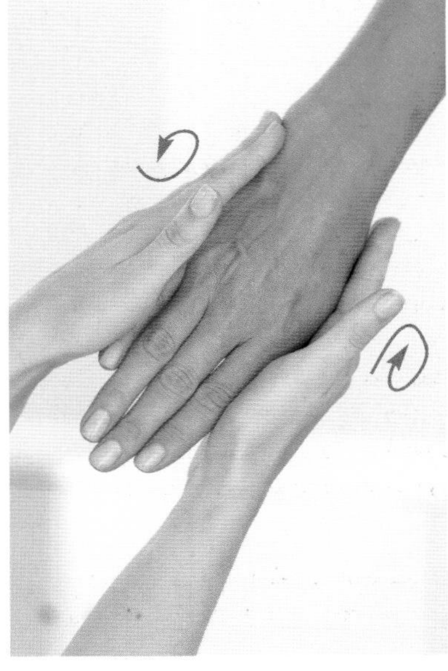

COMFORT CARESS

Place both of your palms on the edges of your client's right hand. Start rocking your hands towards and away from you, with a light pressure. Now work on the left hand. Continue this movement for 30 seconds on each hand.

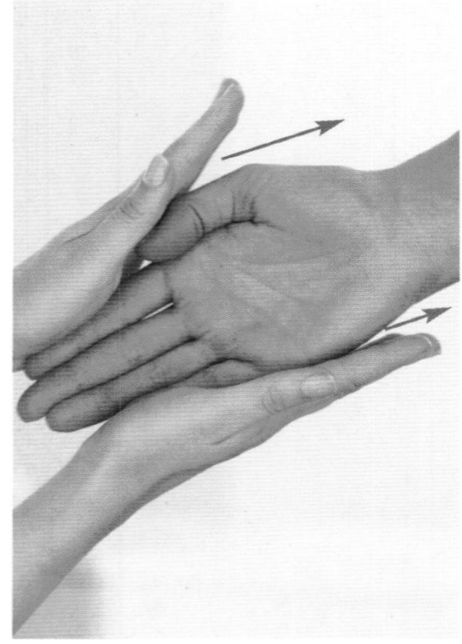

PHOENIX RISING

Place both of your palms on either side of the wrist on the client's right hand. Gently roll your hands all the way up from the base of the hand to the fingers. Hold the fingers softly for three seconds, then drop your hands back to either side of the wrist. Repeat this technique with a medium pressure five times and, as you do so, imagine healing energy building up in your hands ready for treatment. Now work on the left hand.

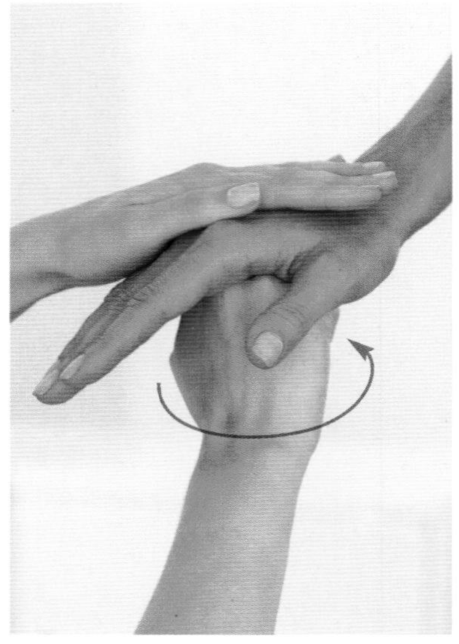

COYOTE CLASP

Place the fist of your hand on your client's right palm. Place your other hand palm down on the top of their hand. Slowly rotate your hands with a medium pressure while you amble through the landscape of their palm. Now work on the left hand. Continue this movement for 30 seconds on each hand.

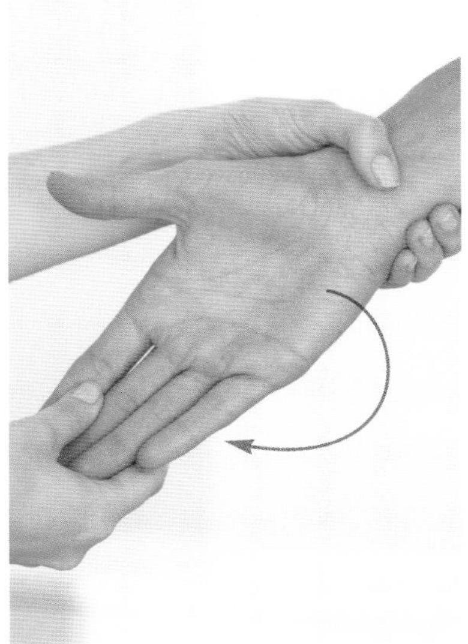

ANGEL'S WING

Support your client's right hand at the wrist with one hand, and use your other hand to gently rotate it, first clockwise and then anticlockwise, making big circles. Then gently flex the hand back and hold for five seconds. Now work on the left hand. Continue this movement for 30 seconds on each hand.

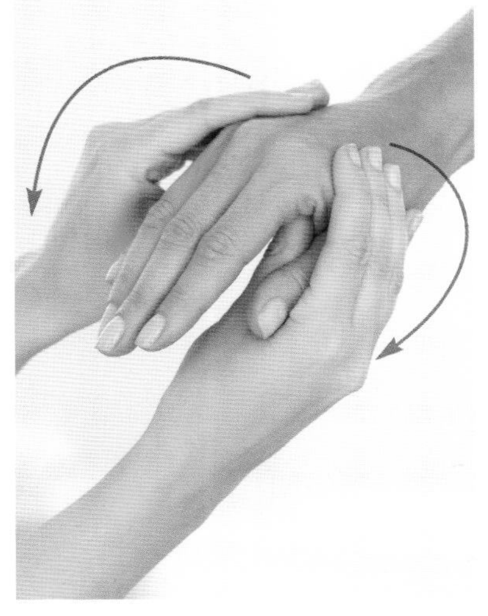

APOLLO'S BREATH

Put both your hands on your client's right hand, placing your fingers on the top of the hand and your thumbs on the palm. Your thumbs should be in the lung reflex area, 2.5 cm (1 in) apart. Gently pull your fingers towards you, while putting a little more pressure on your thumbs. Ask your client to visualize as they breathe in that their breath is healing the area of the body that needs help. Complete this movement five times. Now work on the left hand. Continue this movement for 30 seconds on each hand.

Basic techniques

On the following pages there are three simple hand-reflexology techniques that are easy to remember and use, as well as being very relaxing to experience. You should use these techniques throughout your treatment, so start building up your confidence in the use of them now. As you read the descriptions, practise the techniques on your own hand, focusing on the pressure you are using as well as the speed of treatment. Generally the slower you go, the greater chance you have of finding and dispersing crystals, and the more relaxing it will feel for your client.

These techniques will help you to give a professional treatment and to activate the body's own healing processes. Take deep breaths as you practise to help you relax.

If you are pregnant you can work your own pituitary reflex to stimulate the hormone oxytocin to help bring about a natural birth.

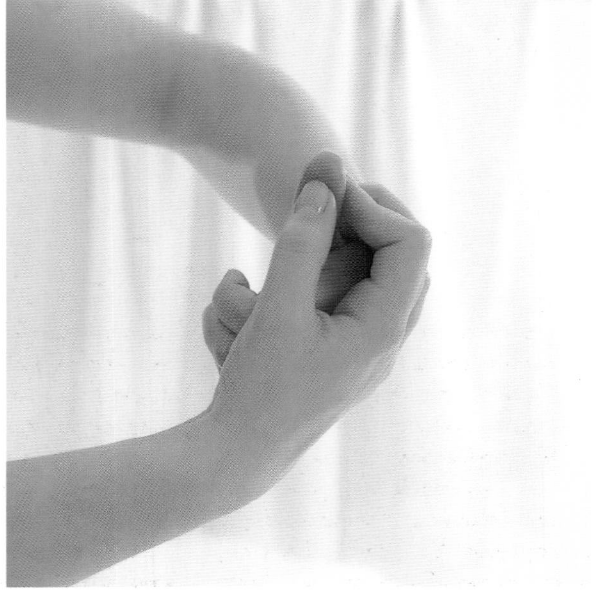

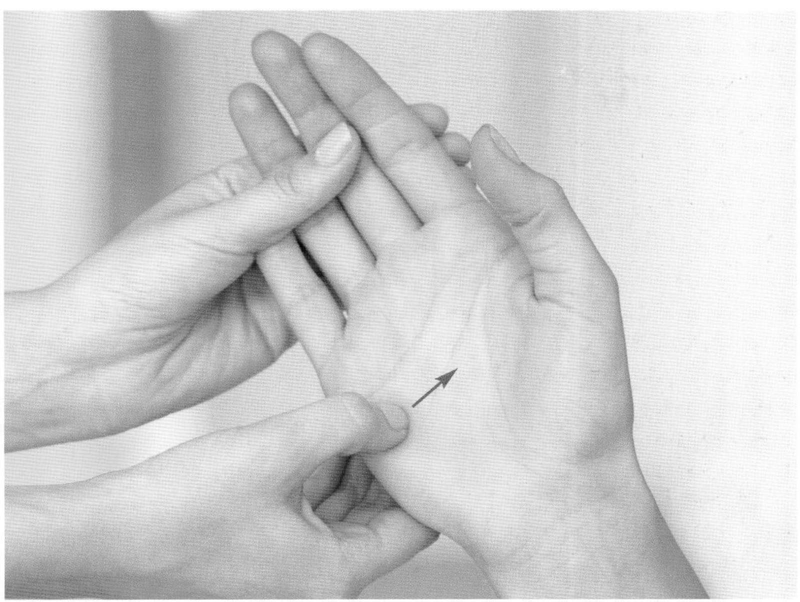

SNAKE

This is the most commonly used compression technique and you can use either your thumb or your index finger. To use the snake, unlock and relock your working thumb or finger as you move forward in tiny steps. Use the print of your thumb or finger, rather than the tip, for your own and your client's comfort. This is an alternating pressure technique, and your thumb or finger will apply pressure when pressed down and will release pressure as it slides forward a tiny step. As you press down you may be aware of crystals either popping under the skin or feeling like sugar granules. First practise this technique on the palm of your own hand to create a rhythm that you are happy working with. Keep the same slow pace throughout.

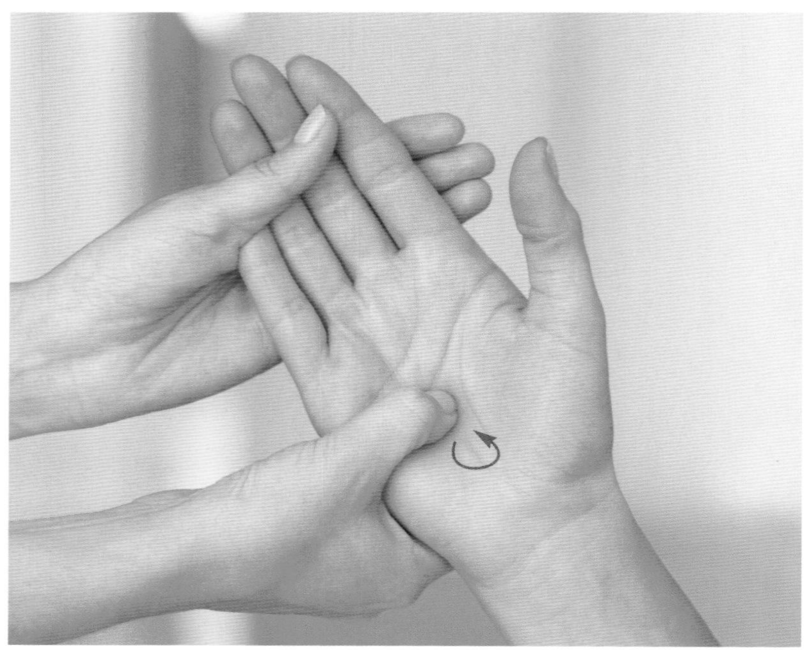

MOLE

Use the mole technique to burrow into a reflex point or within a reflex area to disperse crystals with a circular movement. You can use either your thumb or finger for this technique. Rotate it in a clockwise or anticlockwise direction to break down any crystals. Always use the print of your thumb or finger, rather than the tip, because however short your nails are, there is a good chance they will cause discomfort for your client. Try this movement on the centre of the palm of your own hand, keeping your fingers relaxed. You will notice that the longer you spend here, the more sensations your receiving hand will feel. This technique is effective even if a practitioner does not have very much strength in their hands, but wants to give a good therapeutic treatment.

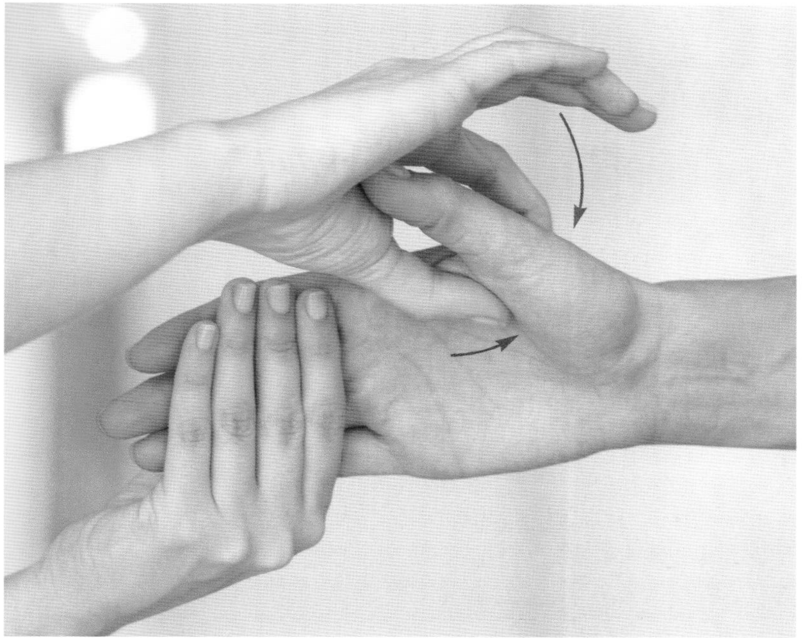

CRAB CLAW

Use the crab claw technique to access a reflex point effectively, working with ease to produce anything from a very light to hard pressure. Place your index finger on the top of the hand and your thumb on the palm of the hand. Always use the print of your thumb or finger, rather than the tip. You can walk up to a reflex point with this technique and access it by applying a little pressure, then rocking back and forth as though you were rocking a swing. You will find that your thumb and finger will start gently to tear the area they are on, and this skin movement will stimulate the reflex point. Always make eye contact with your client when using this powerful technique, so that you can adjust the pressure to avoid any discomfort.

General hand treatment

The best way to start and end your treatment is with the relaxation techniques described on pages 366–369. Then you should apply the following sequence, first on the right hand and then on the left hand, using slow, confident movements. Once you have completed work on the right hand, cover it with a towel to keep it warm and comfortable while you treat the left hand.

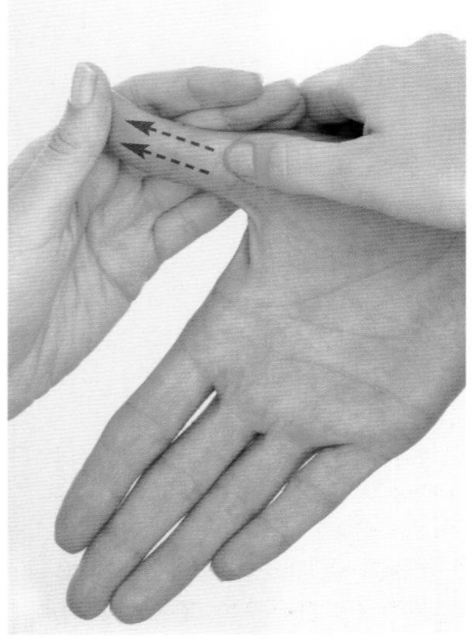

HEAD REFLEX AREA

Support the client's hand, and use your working thumb to snake up from the base to the tip of the thumb. Continue in this manner for 20 seconds, using a medium pressure, until you have covered the area.

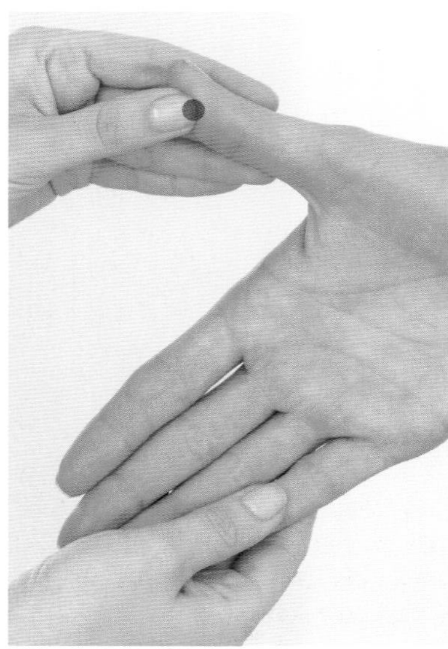

PITUITARY REFLEX POINT

Use your thumb to push into the centre of the client's thumb, using the mole technique to apply pressure and burrow into the pituitary point. Continue this for ten seconds with a medium pressure.

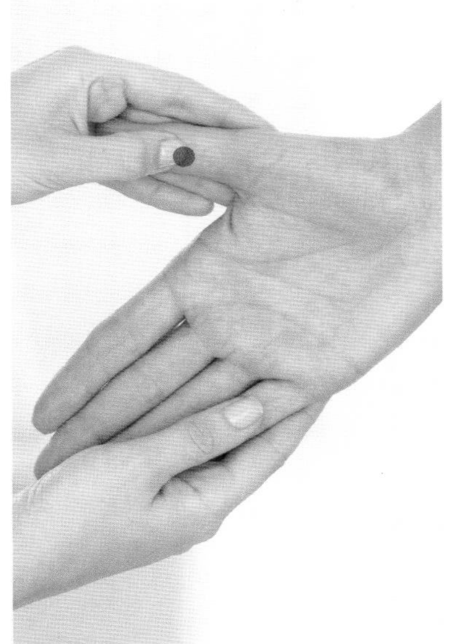

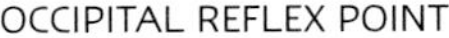

OCCIPITAL REFLEX POINT

Place your thumb on the occipital point on your client's hand, which is found at the base of the distal phalanx where it meets the proximal phalanx. Push up to the joint and use the mole technique to burrow in to the occipital with a medium pressure for ten seconds.

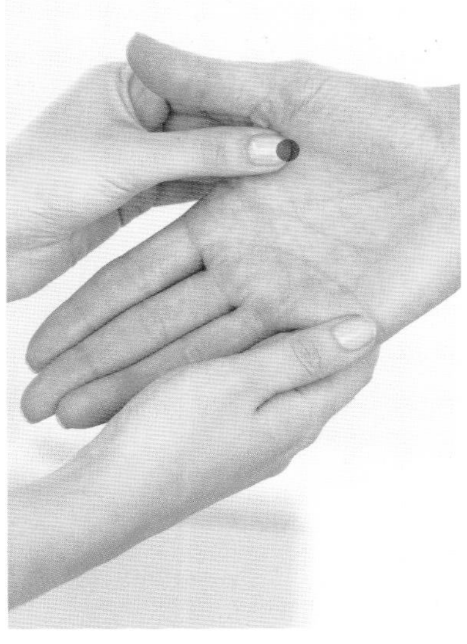

OESOPHAGUS REFLEX AREA

Use your thumb and index finger to pinch the webbing between the client's thumb and index finger, using the crab claw technique to make large circles. Apply a light pressure for ten seconds.

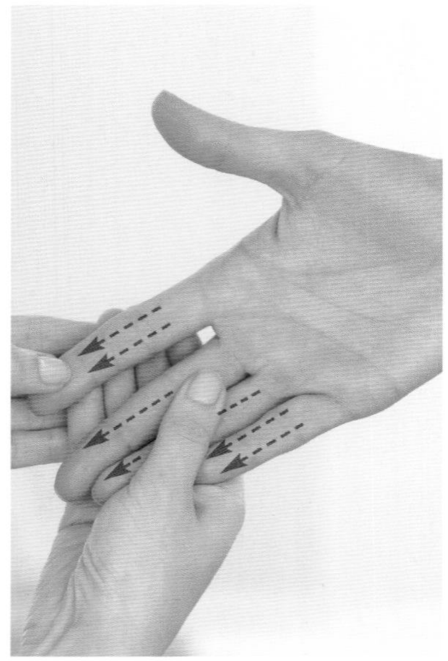

SINUS REFLEX AREA

Use your finger or thumb to snake up from the base to the tip of the client's fingers for the sinuses. Use slow movements with a medium pressure to help drain or strengthen the sinuses. Continue with a medium pressure for one minute.

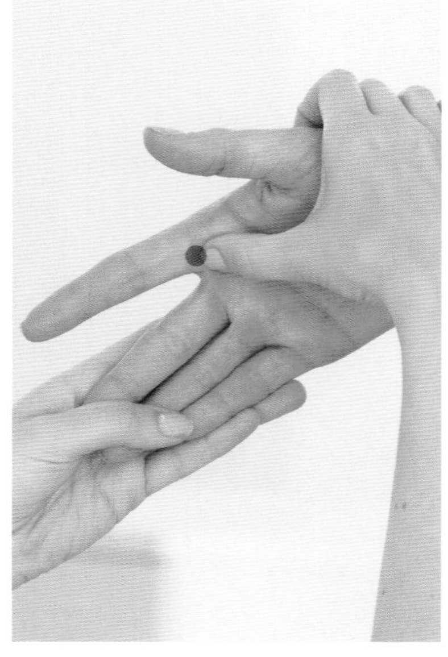

EYE REFLEX POINT

Place your thumb in between the client's index finger and second finger. Use the mole technique to burrow into the eye point for five seconds with a medium pressure making large circles.

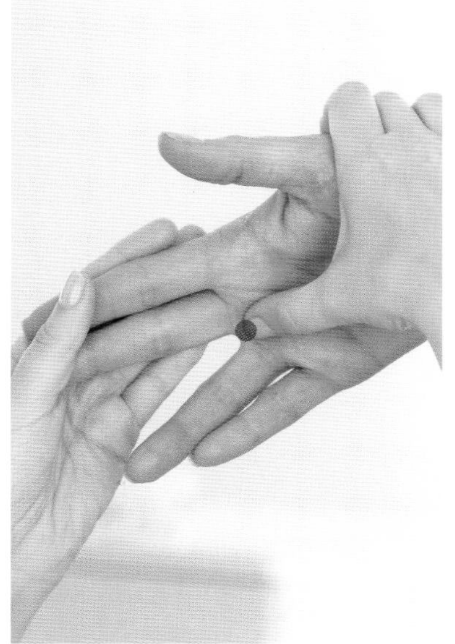

EUSTACHIAN TUBE REFLEX POINT

Place your thumb in between the client's second finger and third finger. Use the mole technique to burrow into the Eustachian point for five seconds with a medium pressure.

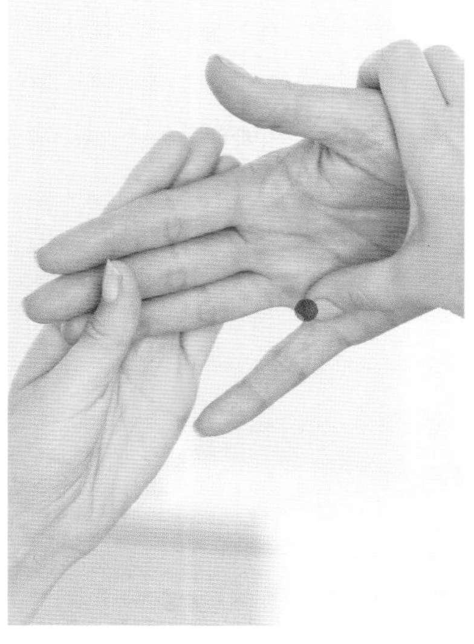

EAR REFLEX POINT

Place your thumb in between the client's fourth finger and fifth finger. Use the mole technique to burrow into the ear point for five seconds with a medium pressure.

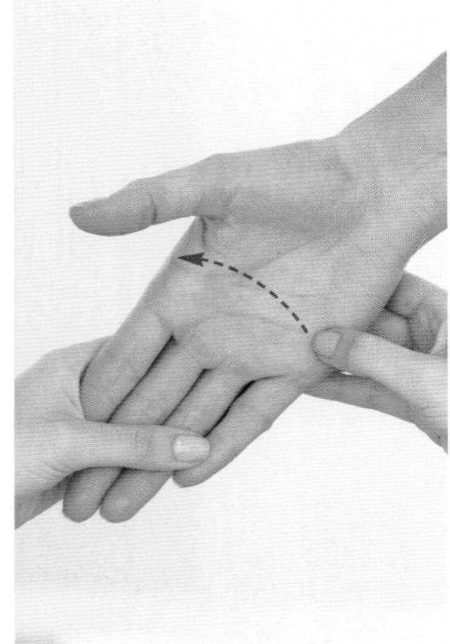

DIAPHRAGM REFLEX AREA

Support the client's hand and flex it back to create skin tension. Place your working thumb halfway down the palm of the client's hand. Slowly use the snake technique to walk across the hand from one side to the other. Continue this movement with a medium pressure for ten seconds, dispersing any crystals.

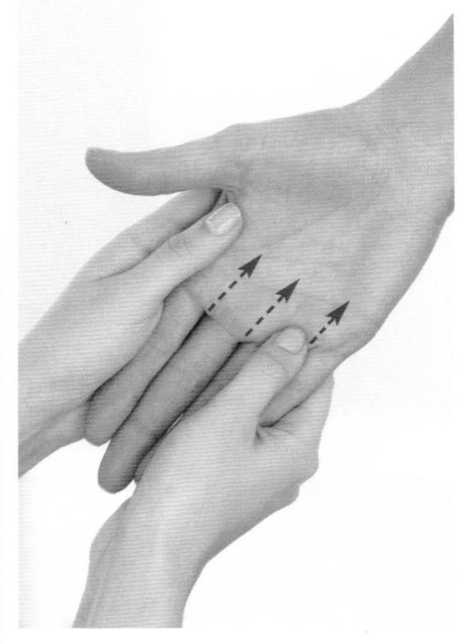

LUNG REFLEX AREA

Place your thumb in between the base of the fourth and fifth fingers. Use the snake technique to work up to the diaphragm line, working in between the bones. Continue in this manner for 20 seconds in between zones two and three, three and four, and four and five. Work this area with a medium pressure for 15 seconds.

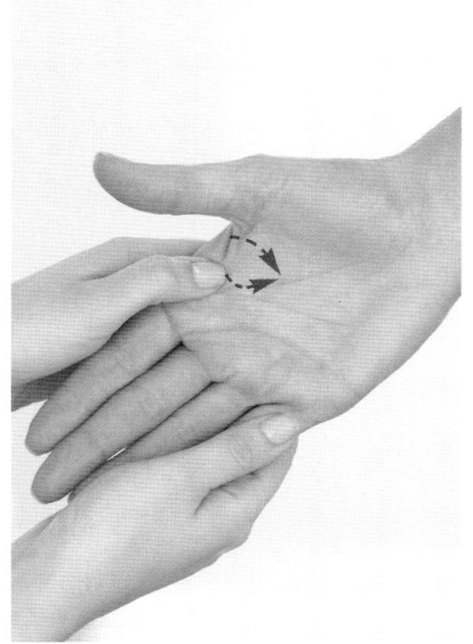

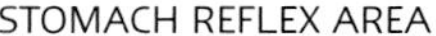

STOMACH REFLEX AREA

Flex the client's hand to create skin tension. Place your working thumb on the webbing in between the client's index finger and thumb. Slowly use the snake technique to walk from the edge of the hand, then slide back to your starting point. Continue in this manner with a light pressure for ten seconds until you have covered the area.

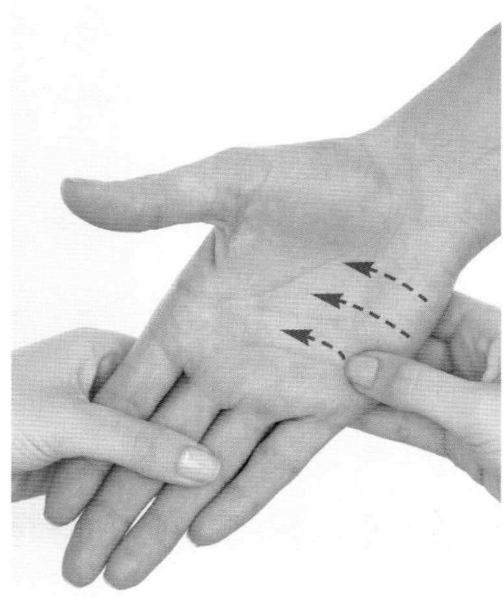

LIVER REFLEX AREA

This reflex area is only found on the right hand. Place your working thumb on the edge of the client's hand and just underneath the diaphragm line. Use the snake technique and work from the edge of the hand in a straight line to zone three. Slide back and take a step down towards the wrist, then repeat this technique in lines until you finish just above the wrist. Continue in this manner for ten seconds with a medium pressure.

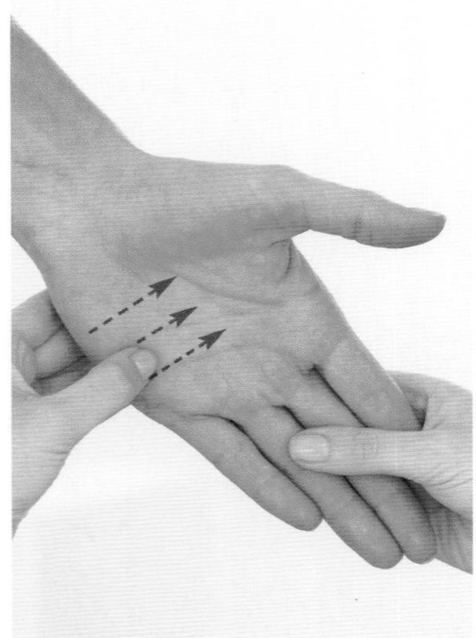

SPLEEN REFLEX AREA

This reflex area is only found on the left hand. Place your working thumb on the edge of the client's hand and just underneath the diaphragm line. Use the snake technique and work from the edge of the hand in a straight line to zone three. Slide back and take a step down towards the wrist, then repeat this technique for three lines. Continue in this manner for ten seconds with a medium pressure.

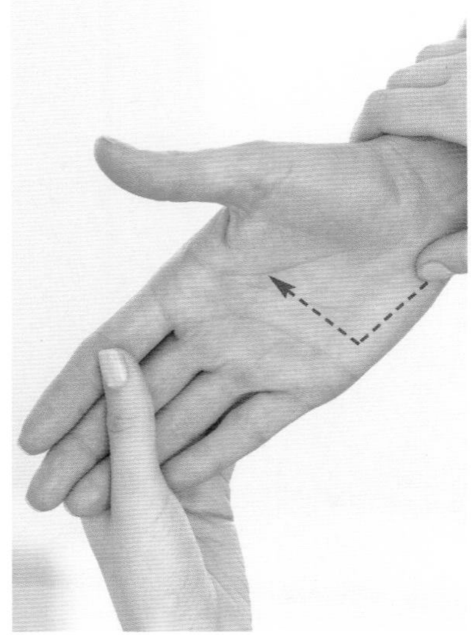

ASCENDING COLON/TRANSVERSE COLON REFLEX AREA

This reflex area is only found on the right hand. Place your working thumb at the base of the client's hand in zone four. Use the snake technique to work slowly up the ascending colon. Halfway up the hand, stop and use the mole technique for three seconds. Then turn your thumb and use the snake technique to work across the hand, ending up at the webbing between the index finger and thumb. Continue in this manner with a medium pressure for 30 seconds dispersing crystals as necessary.

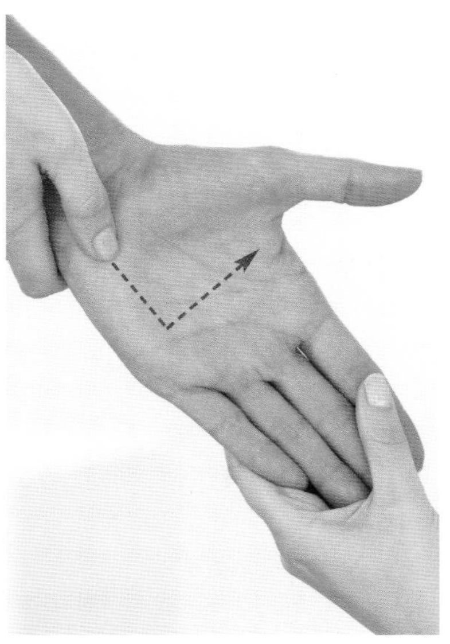

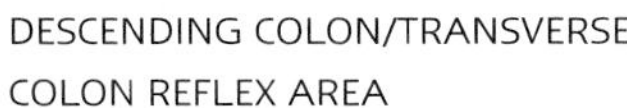

DESCENDING COLON/TRANSVERSE COLON REFLEX AREA

This reflex area is only found on the left hand. Place your working thumb at the base of the client's hand in zone four. Use the snake technique to work slowly up the descending colon. Halfway up the hand, stop and use the mole technique for three seconds. Then turn your thumb and use the snake technique to work across the hand, ending up at the webbing between the index finger and thumb. Continue in this manner with a medium pressure for 30 seconds to help clean the colon.

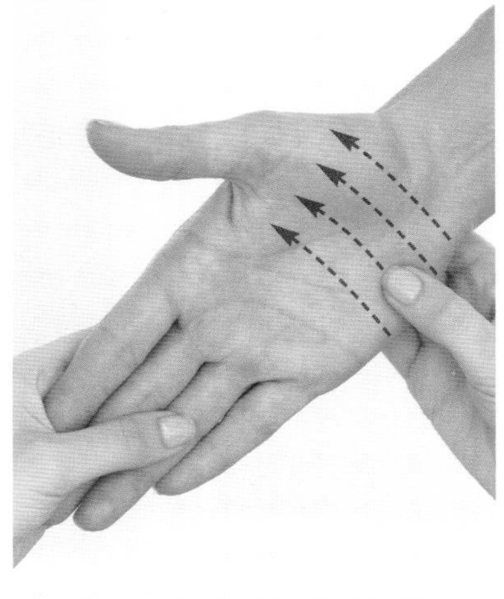

SMALL INTESTINE REFLEX AREA

Place your working thumb at the edge of the client's hand and just below the diaphragm line. Use the snake technique to walk across the palm in a straight line. Slide your thumb back and take a step down, then walk across the hand. Continue in this manner until you have reached the wrist. Work the small intestine area with a light pressure for ten seconds to help with proper absorption.

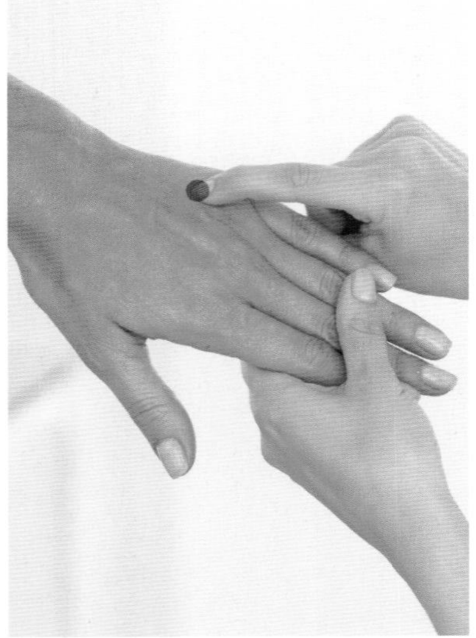

SHOULDER REFLEX POINT

Place your thumb and index finger at the base of the client's fourth and fifth fingers. Use the crab claw technique to walk down towards the wrist for three steps. Apply pressure and rock back and forth with a medium pressure for ten seconds.

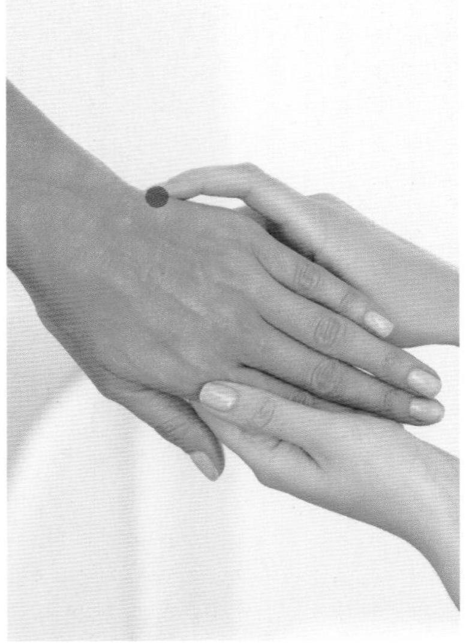

KNEE REFLEX POINT

Place your index finger halfway down the client's hand from the fifth finger. Apply pressure and use the mole technique to burrow into the knee reflex, making circles for ten seconds.

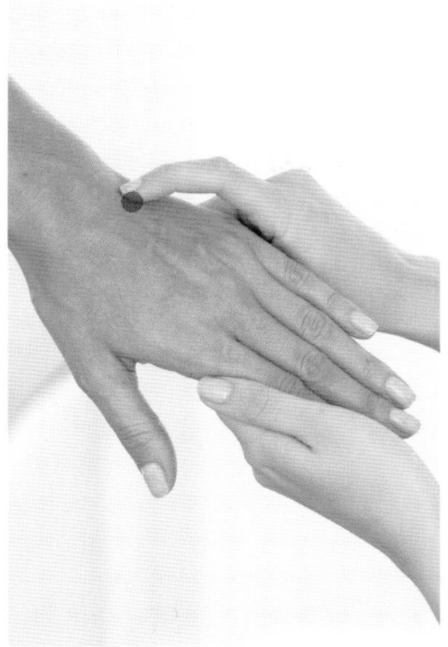
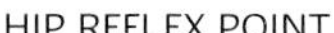

HIP REFLEX POINT

Place your left index finger on the hip point, which is at the base of the client's fourth metacarpal, and use the mole technique to work the hip point with a medium pressure for six seconds.

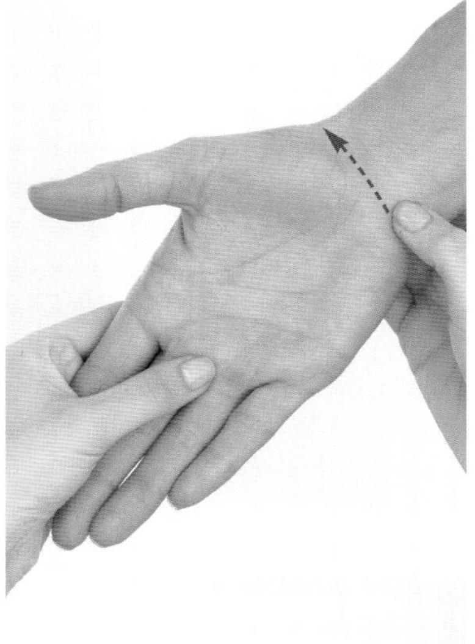

SCIATIC REFLEX AREA

Use the snake technique to walk across the base of the client's hand and just above the wrist with your thumb, from the lateral to the medial aspect, six times with a firm pressure.

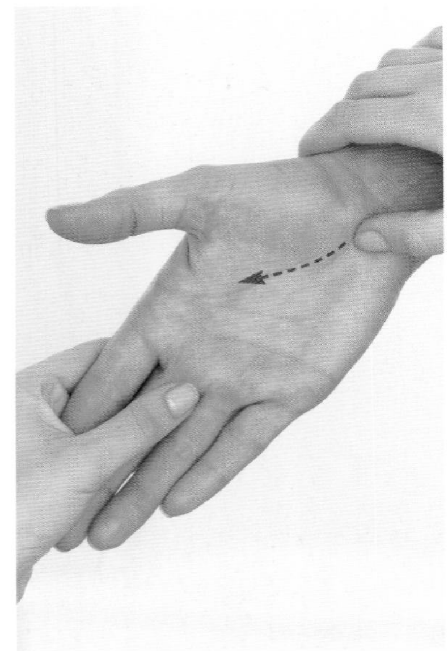

URETER TUBE REFLEX AREA

Find the base of the client's lifeline, which starts at the centre of the palm and just above the wrist. With your thumb use the snake technique to walk up from the base of the client's hand, finishing when you come to the webbing. Repeat this movement slowly three to five times with a medium pressure.

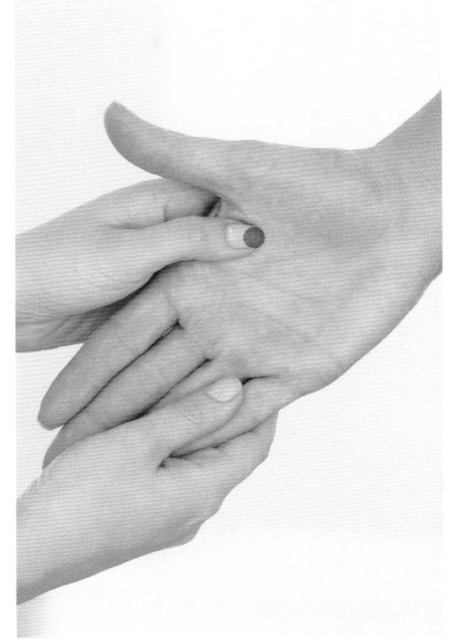

KIDNEY/ADRENAL REFLEX POINT

You will find the kidney/adrenal point at the top of the ureter tube. Support the client's hand and place your thumb in the webbing between their thumb and index finger. Your thumb should be halfway up the hand. Use the mole technique to burrow into the kidneys/adrenals with a light pressure for 15 seconds.

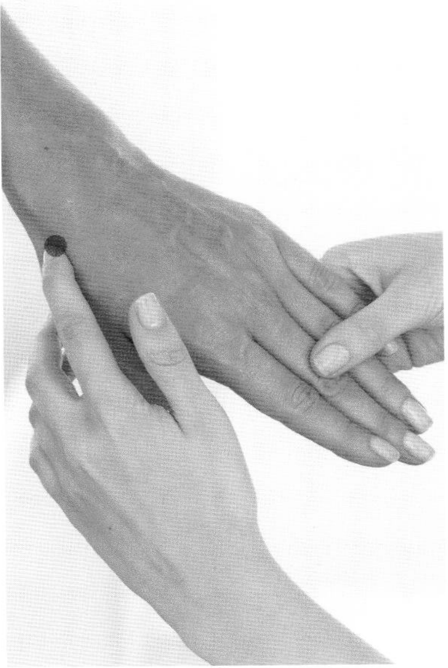

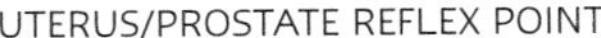

UTERUS/PROSTATE REFLEX POINT

Place your index finger on the client's thumb and slide it down to the base of the thumb, just above the wrist. Here you will find a small indentation, which is the uterus/prostate reflex point. Use the mole technique with a medium pressure for ten seconds making big circles.

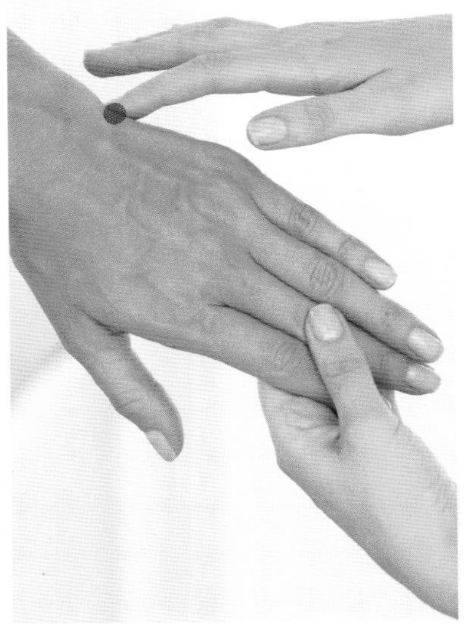

OVARIES/TESTES REFLEX POINT

Place your working finger on the client's fifth finger and slide it down to the base of the index finger, just above the wrist. Here you will find a small indentation, which is the ovary/testes reflex point. Use the mole technique with a medium pressure for ten seconds making big circles.

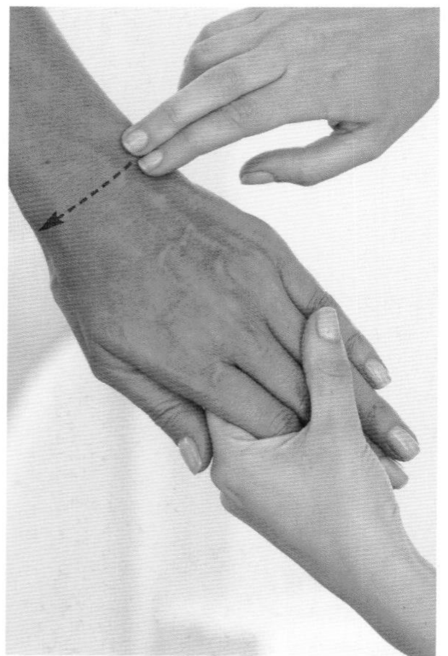

FALLOPIAN TUBE/VAS DEFERENS REFLEX AREA

Use the snake technique with your index and third fingers to walk across the top of the client's wrist, from the medial to the lateral aspect. Repeat this movement six times with a medium pressure.

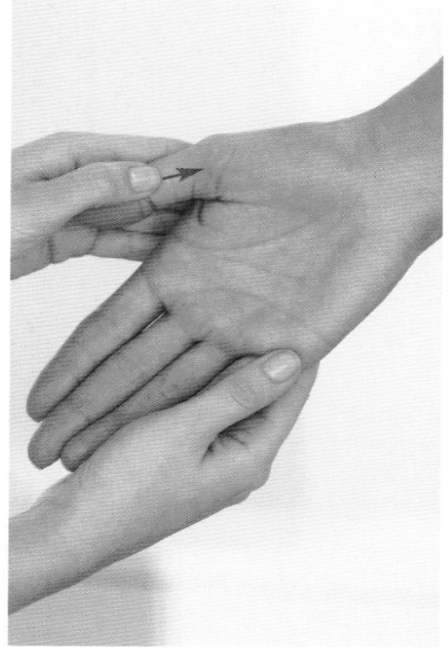

CERVICAL VERTEBRAE REFLEX AREA

Use the snake technique along the bone of the client's thumb from the first to the second joint. Make seven tiny steps along the bone, representing the seven cervical vertebrae of the neck. Use a firm pressure and, whenever you find a sensitive reflex, reduce this pressure.

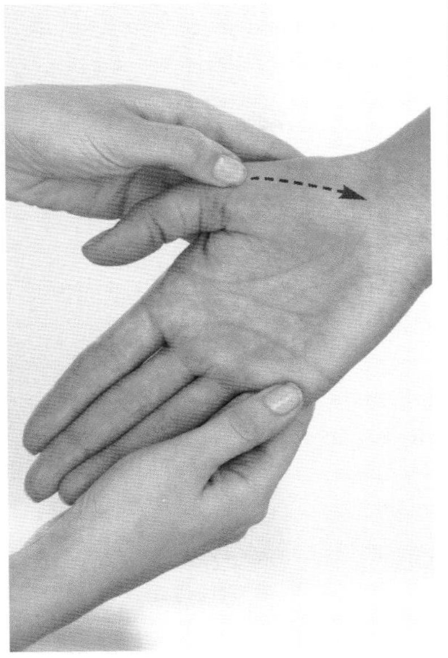

THORACIC VERTEBRAE REFLEX AREA

Place your thumb at the base of the client's hand and just above the wrist. Use the snake movement to walk up to the base of the thumb taking 12 steps, representing the 12 thoracic vertebrae. Use a firm pressure and repeat this movement six times to help the spine.

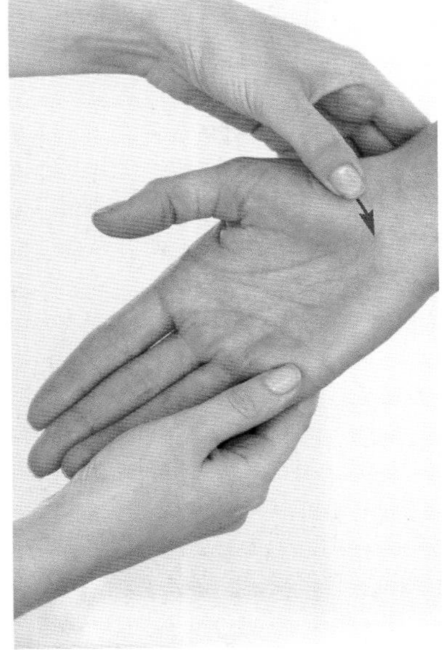

LUMBAR VERTEBRAE REFLEX AREA

Place your thumb just above the base of the client's thumb. Use the snake technique to walk along the bone for five very small steps to the middle of the palm of the hand, representing the five lumbar vertebrae. Use a firm pressure and repeat this movement six times.

Closing the treatment

End this powerful hand-reflexology sequence with all or some of the relaxation techniques described earlier (see pages 366–369).

Aftercare

Now that your treatment is complete, cover the client's hands with a towel and go and wash your hands. Give your client a glass of water, to flush away any toxins that have been released during the reflexology session. Ask them how they feel, and talk about any reflexes that you felt were out of balance, finding out from your client why these areas might be sensitive. Remember that it is important to refer them to a doctor or other complementary therapist if necessary, and to give no unqualified advice concerning their condition.

Closing the treatment is about giving good practical holistic lifestyle suggestions that will not get in the way of nature. The therapy of reflexology has a powerful effect on the body and the client's physical and emotional states. I always believe that the treatment gives a person what they most need for their body at that time. By increasing the blood and lymphatic ciruclation of the body through the feet and hands, you can help with the transportation of nutrients around the body. I sometimes give a client a healthy vegeatble or fruit juice which can provide them with an instant supply of these essential vitamins and minerals. Ending the treatment with something special to drink or eat can be what makes your treatment a personal and caring extension of your intention to heal.

Once a treatment is finished, wash your hands thoroughly before having a final chat to your client about the session.

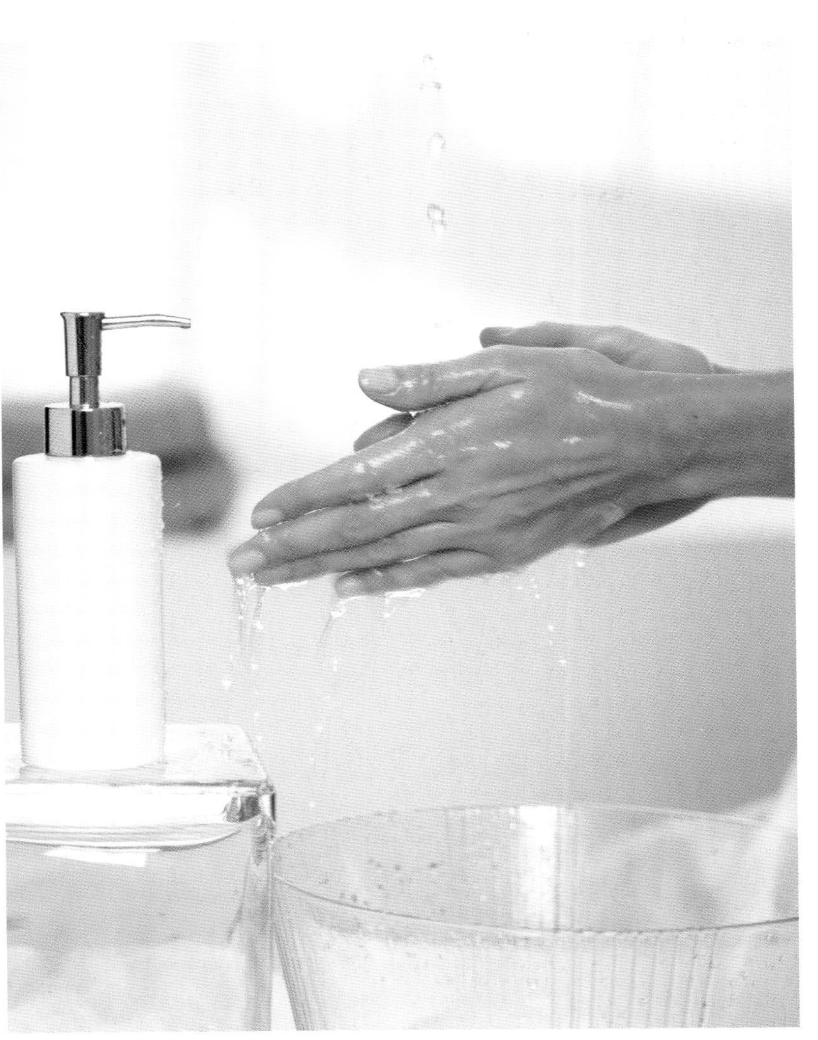

Index

Figures in *italics* indicate captions. Main references to reflex areas/points are indicated in **bold** type.

Acknowledgements

About the author

Louise Keet is Principal of the London School of Reflexology, which is London's largest reflexology school. www.learnreflexology.com

The Keet reflexology techniques used in this book have been developed to provide the most effective outcomes to the treatments. This powerful method was devised by Louise and Michael Keet and is practiced around the world. The Keet method is used by graduates of their respective schools; London School of Reflexology and Central London College of Reflexology and can be learnt on their vocational level 3 diplomas in Reflexology.

Author's acknowledgements

This book is dedicated to Ziggie and Phoenix Bergman, the epicentre of my life.

Thank you to Irene Lemos for the special closeness we have shared over the years, St John Wright for his love and patience, Deborah Dor and M.J. Low for their love, understanding and support, Beatrice McClennan for her wonderful friendship and the times we have spent together, Fanny Aubertin for her friendship and putting a smile on my face when I needed it most and Mr and Mrs Charles Longbottom for their kindness. Thank you to Sue Rickards a gifted teacher in Gabrielle Roth's 5Rhythms® and to all those who shared the space and helped me heal through dance.

Special thanks to Jessica Cowie and Jane McIntosh who gave me the opportunity to write this book, Camilla Davis, Mandy Greenfield, Kerenza Swift and Leigh Jones for their trust, expertise and guidance. Thank you to the Association of Reflexologists for all the excellent work they put into making reflexology the recognised and trusted complementary therapy that it is.

A special thought to all my graduates and students of the London School of Reflexology who are making a difference to so many people's lives.

Executive Editor: Jessica Cowie
Editors: Camilla Davis; Kerenza Swift
Executive Art Editor: Leigh Jones
Designer: Julie Francis
Photographer: Ruth Jenkinson
Production Manager: Simone Nauerth
Models: Samantha Whyman at ModelPlan, Poppy Gillioz, and Beatrice Sims
Special photography: Octopus Publishing Group Ltd/Ruth Jenkinson
Other photography: Corbis UK Ltd Allen Bell 204; Alessandra Schellnegger/zefa 14; Brooke Fasani 232; David Raymer 192; Flint 264; Image Source 252; Image100 228; Imagemore Co. Ltd. 188; Leslie Richard Jacobs 300; Martin Harvey 200; Norbert Schaefer 224; Pinnacle Pictures 116; Pixland 212; Tim Pannell 324; Timothy Tadder 58; **Getty Images** 3D4Medical.com 38; Altrendo Images 32; Ariel Skelley 282; STOCK4B 184; Kent Mathews 268; **istockphoto.com** George Peters 105; Jovan Nikolic 99; Sheryl Griffin 220; Will Johnson 196; **Octopus Publishing Group Limited** Clive Streeter 292; Peter Myers 244; Peter Pugh-Cook 26, 354, 370; Russell Sadur 90, 254, 332; Ruth Jenkinson 288, 336; William Reavell 28, 270, 328; **Royalty-Free Images** 304, 318; PhotoDisc 287; **Science Photo Library** Aj Photo 278; BSIP Laurent 180; Ian Hootan 172; **Shutterstock** Graham S. Klotz 98, Rene Jansa 30.